Curriculum Development and Evaluation in Nursing

Sarah B. Keating, EdD, MPH, RN, C-PNP, FAAN, served as endowed professor, Orvis School of Nursing, University of Nevada, Reno, where she coordinated and taught in the nurse educator track and coordinated the collaborative University of Nevada doctor of nursing practice (DNP) program for the Reno campus. She graduated with a BSN from the University of Maryland, and earned an MPH from the University of North Carolina, Chapel Hill. She has an EdD from SUNY–Albany and a certificate in primary care from the University of Rochester, and is a certified pediatric nurse practitioner. Dr. Keating taught community health nursing, nursing fundamentals, health assessment, health care policy, and nursing leadership in undergraduate and graduate programs. She served as graduate coordinator for the School of Nursing at Russell Sage College, director of nursing for San Francisco State University, and dean of the Saint Mary's–Samuel Merritt Colleges Intercollegiate Nursing Program. She served as chair of the board of directors for Hospice by the Bay in San Francisco and was chair of the California Strategic Planning Committee for Nursing for 10 years. Dr. Keating is the recipient of many awards and recognitions and has been published in a variety of journals, in addition to serving as editor for the *Journal of Home Health Care Nursing*. She received funding for over 15 research and program grants and led the development of numerous educational programs, including nurse practitioner, advanced community health nursing, clinical nurse leader, case management, entry-level master's programs, nurse educator tracks, and the DNP and MSN/MPH programs. In addition, she recently served as a curriculum development and evaluation consultant and reviewer for the Western Association of Senior Schools and Colleges (WASC) accreditation agency.

Curriculum Development and Evaluation in Nursing

Third Edition

Sarah B. Keating, EdD, MPH, RN, C-PNP, FAAN

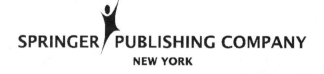

SPRINGER PUBLISHING COMPANY

NEW YORK

Springer Publishing Company, LLC
11 West 42nd Street
New York, NY 10036
www.springerpub.com

Acquisitions Editor: Margaret Zuccarini
Composition: diacriTech

ISBN: 978-0-8261-3027-3
e-book ISBN: 978-0-8261-3028-0
Instructor's PowerPoints: 978-0-8261-2223-0
Instructor's Manual: 978-0-8261-2284-1

Instructor's Materials: Qualified instructors may request supplements by emailing textbook@springerpub.com

14 15 16 17 / 5 4 3 2 1

The author and the publisher of this Work have made every effort to use sources believed to be reliable to provide information that is accurate and compatible with the standards generally accepted at the time of publication. The author and publisher shall not be liable for any special, consequential, or exemplary damages resulting, in whole or in part, from the readers' use of, or reliance on, the information contained in this book. The publisher has no responsibility for the persistence or accuracy of URLs for external or third-party Internet websites referred to in this publication and does not guarantee that any content on such websites is, or will remain, accurate or appropriate.

Library of Congress Cataloging-in-Publication Data

Keating, Sarah B., editor.
    Curriculum development and evaluation in nursing / Sarah B. Keating. — Third edition.
        p. ; cm.
    Preceded by Curriculum development and evaluation in nursing / [edited by] Sarah B. Keating. 2nd ed. c2011.
    Includes bibliographical references and index.
    ISBN 978-0-8261-3027-3 — ISBN 978-0-8261-3028-0 (e-book) — ISBN 978-0-8261-2223-0 (instructor's powerpoints) — ISBN 978-0-8261-2284-1 (instructor's manual)
    I. Title.
    [DNLM: 1. Education, Nursing. 2. Curriculum. 3. Evaluation Studies as Topic. 4. Evidence-Based Nursing. WY 18]
    RT71
    610.73071'1—dc23
                                    2014020375

Printed in the United States of America by McNaughton & Gunn.

To past and present contributors. Thank you for sharing your expertise with our colleagues and students in nursing education.

Contents

Contributors

Lori Candela, RN, EdD, FNP-BC, CNE   Associate Professor, School of Nursing, University of Nevada, Las Vegas, Nevada

Susan M. Ervin, MS, RN, CNE   Assistant Professor, Orvis School of Nursing, University of Nevada, Reno, Nevada

Karen E. Fontaine, MSN, RN, CNE   Instructor, Carrington College, Sacramento, California

Peggy Guin, PhD, ARNP, CNS-BC, CNRN, SCRN   Neuroscience Clinical Nurse Specialist, Nursing and Patient Services, University of Florida Health Shands Hospital, Gainesville, Florida

Abby Heydman, PhD, RN   Professor and Academic Vice President Emeritus, Samuel Merritt University, Palm Desert, California

Betty Jax, MSN, ARNP, RN-BC   Administrative Director, Nursing Education, University of Florida Health Shands Hospital, Gainesville, Florida

Melissa Jones, RN, MN   Assistant Professor, Good Samaritan School of Nursing, Linfield College, Sherwood, Oregon

Sarah B. Keating, EdD, MPH, RN, C-PNP, FAAN   Adjunct Professor, Orvis School of Nursing, University of Nevada, Reno, Nevada

Patsy L. Ruchala, DNS, RN   Director and Professor, Orvis School of Nursing, University of Nevada, Reno, Nevada

Arlene Sargent, EdD, RN   Associate Dean, School of Nursing, Samuel Merritt University, Lafayette, California

Coleen Saylor, PhD, RN   Professor Emeritus, School of Nursing, San Jose State University, El Dorado Hills, California

Nancy A. Stotts, RN, EdD, FAAN   Professor Emeritus, School of Nursing, University of California, San Francisco, San Francisco, California

Pamela Wheeler, PhD, MSN, RN   Associate Professor, Good Samaritan School of Nursing, Linfield College, Sherwood, California

Peggy Wros, PhD, RN   Senior Associate Dean for Student Affairs and Diversity, Oregon Health and Science University, West Linn, Oregon

Preface

In the short time since the publication of the first and second editions of this text, many changes have occurred that will directly affect nursing curricula now and in the near future. In my view, there are several major changes that will influence nursing curricula in these early decades of the 21st century. The most influential are the recommendations from the Institute of Medicine (IOM) for the need for higher education for nurses to meet health care demands, and the recommendation of the American Association of Colleges of Nursing (AACN) for the doctor of nursing practice (DNP) degree to be the level of entry for advanced practice by 2015. These recommendations resulted in increasing numbers of associate degree in nursing (ADN)-prepared nurses returning to school for their baccalaureates, and improved articulation between associate degree and baccalaureate programs, as well as the explosion of DNP programs across the nation. Other significant trends are the continuing growth and application of technology and informatics to the delivery of educational programs and instructional strategies, and the influence of the Affordable Care Act, which changed the way care is delivered, with nursing playing a major role in affecting this change. Although it is difficult to predict how these changes will play out over the next 5 to 10 years, they will surely force nursing programs to continually assess, evaluate, and revise their curricula.

This third edition continues to serve graduate students and nurse educators in schools of nursing and in the practice arena as a practical guide for developing, revising, and evaluating nursing curricula and educational programs. Overviews of the history of nursing education, changing educational environments, the role of faculty, learning theories, and educational taxonomies describe underlying concepts that help guide curriculum development and evaluation. The text goes into detail about conducting a needs assessment to determine the extent of revision or development needed to produce an up-to-date and vibrant curriculum. It is followed by a detailed description of the essential components of the curriculum and the various levels of nursing education from the ADN to doctorate. Educational evaluation and accreditation and the impact of technology and informatics on the curriculum are discussed. New chapters added to this edition include budget considerations related to curriculum development and research focused on nursing education. **Supplementary PowerPoint slides and an Instructor's Manual are available for nurse educators by contacting textbook@springerpub.com.**

Contributors to the text are experts in their field and provide up-to-date information on learning theories, educational taxonomies, and curriculum development and evaluation. Chapter 15 applies the concepts of curriculum development and evaluation to the practice setting for staff development purposes. The author and contributors review the current literature and add their expertise to assist readers in the application of these concepts in their educator roles. The final chapter of the text raises current issues facing nursing educators as changes in education and the health care system occur. The critical need for translational science, research, and evidence-based practice in education is reviewed along with ideas for investigation and application to practice. The continuing career and entry-level issues related to nursing are discussed, with a proposed unified nursing curriculum to use as a launching pad for debate.

Although the DNP is acknowledged as the final degree for advanced practice and the PhD/DNS (doctor of nursing science) for research, will nursing ever see an entry-level doctorate much like other professions? Will collaborative scholarly endeavors between the professional doctorate and the research doctorate take place? What effects will interprofessional collaboration have on practice, the health care system, and education? As technology and informatics become integral parts of nursing education and practice, how will the profession and education be affected and what permutations will they take in the curriculum? These are the issues to ponder and debate for the future.

On a personal note, this is the last edition for which I will serve as author/editor. As I read the history of nursing education, I identified with many of the high points, from graduating from one of the first 4-year BSN programs in the 1950s, to earning a master's in public health nursing through one of the universities in the Southern Council on Collegiate Education for Nursing, to earning a doctorate in education when PhDs, or practice doctorates, were few if nonexistent in the early 1980s, to participating in a fellowship to prepare nurse practitioners for the development of nurse practitioner programs in the mid-1970s. It is delightful to reflect on these times in nursing and to see how far nursing has come, and be able to see its bright future. I have great confidence in nursing's future for I have witnessed its transformation as a profession, the development of nursing science, the movement toward higher education, its advocacy for nursing's role in health care, and its contributions to the discipline of education and technology.

It is with pleasure that I introduce Stephanie DeBoor, PhD, RN, CCRN, assistant professor and associate director of the graduate program at Orvis School of Nursing, University of Nevada, Reno (UNR), who will assume the editorship of the next edition of this text. Dr. DeBoor is a certified critical care, clinical specialist and served as a nurse administrator in a large regional hospital prior to coming to UNR as a faculty member for the Orvis School of Nursing. She earned her PhD in nursing education and research and serves as the associate director for the graduate programs, which include the master of science in nursing and the University of Nevada Collaborative Doctor of Nursing Practice. In addition to her role as associate director, she teaches in both the undergraduate and graduate programs. She led the faculty in the development of an acute care nurse practitioner program and the BSN to DNP program, and is currently working with faculty on a clinical specialty program in psychiatric/mental health nursing. Her love of teaching, enthusiasm for student learning, commitment to quality education, philosophy about nursing education, and visions for the future of nursing will contribute to the continuation of this text as a resource for nursing educators. I wish the very best to Stephanie and my colleagues and look forward to observing the continued evolution of nursing education.

Sarah B. Keating

Overview of Nursing Education: History, Curriculum Development Processes, and the Role of Faculty

Sarah B. Keating

OVERVIEW

The third edition of this text devotes itself to the processes of curriculum development and evaluation that are critical responsibilities of nurse educators in schools of nursing and staff development in health care agencies. A curriculum provides the goals for an educational program and guidelines for how they will be delivered and ultimately, evaluated for effectiveness. This text focuses on curriculum development and evaluation and *not* instructional design and strategies that are used to deliver the program. Some major theories and concepts that relate to both curriculum development and instructional strategies are discussed but only in light of their contributions to the mission and philosophy of the educational program, for example, learning theories, educational taxonomies, and critical thinking.

To initiate the discourse on curriculum development, a definition is in order. For the purposes of the textbook, the definition is: *A curriculum is the formal plan of study that provides the philosophical underpinnings, goals, and guidelines for delivery of a specific educational program.* The text uses this definition throughout for the *formal* curriculum, while recognizing the existence of the *informal* curriculum. The informal curriculum consists of activities that students, faculty, administrators, staff, and consumers experience outside of the formal planned curriculum. Examples of the informal curriculum include interpersonal relationships, athletic/recreational activities, study groups, organizational activities, special events, academic and personal counseling, and so forth. Although the text focuses on the formal curriculum, nurse educators should keep the informal curriculum in mind for its influence and use to reinforce learning activities that arise from the planned curriculum.

To place curriculum development and evaluation in perspective, it is wise to examine the history of nursing education in the United States and the lessons it provides for current and future curriculum developers. Section I sets the stage through an examination of nursing's place in the history of higher education and the role of faculty and administrators in developing and evaluating curricula.

Nursing curricula are currently undergoing transformation. Today's emphases on the learner and measurement of learning outcomes, integration into the curriculum of quality and safety concepts, evidence-based practice, translational science and research, and the application of technology to the delivery of the program provide exciting challenges and opportunities for nurse educators. Nursing faculty and educators must consider all of these factors when examining the curriculum and considering change. Today and tomorrow's curricula call for an integration of processes that are learner- and consumer-based and, at the same time, ensure excellence by building in outcome measures to determine the quality of the program. In addition, there is a need for research on curriculum development and evaluation to provide the underpinnings for evidence-based practice in nursing education.

HISTORY OF NURSING EDUCATION IN THE UNITED STATES

Chapter 1 traces the history of American nursing education from the time of the first Nightingale schools of nursing to the present. The trends in professional education and society's needs impacted nursing programs that started from apprentice-type schools to a majority of the programs now in institutions of higher learning. Lest the profession forgets, liberal arts and the sciences in institutions of higher learning play a major role in nursing education and set the foundation for the development of critical thinking and clinical decision making so necessary to the nursing process.

Chapter 1 reviews major historical events in society and the world that influenced nursing practice and education as well as changes in the health care system. World War I and World War II increased the demand for nurses and a nursing education system that prepared a workforce ready to meet that demand. The emergence of nursing education that took place in community colleges in the mid-20th century initiated continuing debate about entry into practice. The explosive growth of doctor of nursing practice (DNP) programs in recent times and their place in advanced practice, nursing leadership, and education brings the past century happenings into focus as the profession responds to the changes in the health care system and health care needs of the population.

CURRICULUM DEVELOPMENT AND APPROVAL PROCESSES IN CHANGING EDUCATIONAL ENVIRONMENTS

Chapter 2 discusses the processes for programs undergoing change or creating new curricula. Curriculum committees in schools of nursing receive recommendations from faculty for curriculum changes and periodically review the curriculum for its currency, authenticity, and diligence in realizing the mission, philosophy, and goals. The chapter describes the classic hierarchy of curriculum approval processes in institutions of higher learning and the importance of nursing faculty's participation within the governance of the institution. The governance of colleges and universities usually includes curriculum committees or their equivalent composed of elected faculty members. These committees are at the program, college-wide, and/or university-wide levels and provide the academic rigor for assuring quality in educational programs.

Faculty and administrators continually assess curricula and program outcomes and based on the results of the assessment, refine existing curricula through major or minor revisions. An issue of contention during the assessment and development phase is what to take out of the curriculum when new content is indicated. The challenge faculty faces is to preserve critical content and, at the same time, bring current and future information into the curriculum. This means that faculty must be willing to compromise and give up outdated (but dear) content to make way for newer knowledge. In some instances, new programs are needed with the same processes of assessment used to produce the justification for the new programs.

It is a cardinal rule in academe that the curriculum "belongs to the faculty." In higher education, faculty members are deemed the experts in their specific discipline; or in the case of nursing, clinical specialties or functional areas such as administration, health care policy, case management, and so forth. They are the people who determine the content that must be transferred to and assimilated by the learner. At the same time, they should be expert teachers in the delivery of information, that is, pedagogy or in the case of adult learners, andragogy. Curriculum planning and the art of teaching are learned skills and nursing faculty members have a responsibility to include them in their repertoire of expertise as well as being content specialists.

Nursing faculty must periodically review a program to maintain a vibrant curriculum that responds to changes in society, health care needs of the population, the health care delivery system, and the learners' needs. It is important to measure the program's success in preparing nurses for the current environment and for the future. Currency of practice as well as that of the future must be built into the curriculum, because it will be several years before entering cohorts graduate. In nursing, there is an inherent requirement to produce caring, competent, and confident practitioners or clinicians. At the same time, the curriculum must meet professional and accreditation standards. Although it is unpopular to think that curricula are built upon accreditation criteria, in truth, integrating them into the curriculum helps administrators and faculty to prepare for program approval or review and accreditation by assuring that the program meets essential quality standards.

Administrators provide the leadership for organizing and carrying out the evaluation activities. To bring the curriculum into reality and out of the "Ivory Tower," faculty and administrators must include students, alumni, employers, and the people whom their graduates serve into curriculum building and evaluation processes. Outcomes from the total program are measured through summative evaluation methods such as follow-up surveys of graduates and NCLEX and certification exam results. Chapter 2 introduces the role of accreditation in curriculum development and evaluation. Section V continues the discussion on the processes that relate to accreditation and its related activities of program evaluation, review, and approval.

THE ROLE OF FACULTY IN CURRICULUM DEVELOPMENT AND EVALUATION

Both new and experienced faculty members have major roles in curriculum development, implementation, and program evaluation. Although there is a tendency to see only the part of the curriculum in which the individual educator is involved, it is essential that instructors have a strong sense of the program as a whole. In that way, the curriculum remains true to its goals, learning objectives (student learning outcomes), and the content necessary for reaching the goals. Following the curriculum plan results in an intact curriculum and, at the same time, provides the opportunity for faculty and students to identify gaps in the program or the need for updates and revisions. Such needs are brought to the attention of other instructors and the coordinators of the courses or levels in the program for assessment and follow-up.

Chapter 3 examines the overall responsibilities of faculty in curriculum development and evaluation. It describes how everyday teaching and clinical supervision activities implement the program and, in the process, lead to the identification of the need for revision or introducing new material in the curriculum. It is the responsibility of core faculty to ensure that the curriculum plan is followed by clinical instructors or adjunct professors who may not be as familiar with the total curriculum plan and its intended outcomes. At the same time, adjunct faculty and clinical instructors can provide valuable information for refining the curriculum and bringing it into focus to meet current health care demands. The chapter discusses how experienced faculty members should orient and mentor new nurse educators into this aspect of the nurse educator role, that is, curriculum development and evaluation. The roles of faculty participation and leadership on curriculum, program evaluation, and accreditation committees within the school and institution are elaborated upon. Trends, issues, and research needs related to curriculum development and evaluation are reviewed.

CHAPTER 1

History of Nursing Education in the United States

Susan M. Ervin

OBJECTIVES

Upon completion of Chapter 1, the reader will be able to:

1. Discuss the historical roots of formal nursing education
2. Compare important curricular events in the 19th century with those in the 20th and 21st centuries
3. Cite the impact that two world wars had on the development of nursing education
4. Differentiate among the different curricula that prepare entry-level nurses
5. Cite important milestones in the development of graduate education in nursing
6. Evaluate the decade most pivotal to the development of one type of nursing program, that is, diploma, associate degree, baccalaureate, master's, or doctoral degree
7. Evaluate the impact of the history of nursing education on current and future curriculum development and evaluation activities

OVERVIEW

The adventure that is labeled nursing education began at the close of the U.S. Civil War when it was recognized that nursing care was crucial to soldiers' survival and that nurses must have some formal education. Using Florence Nightingale's model of nursing education, hospital-based nursing programs flourished throughout the 19th and well into the 20th century. With few exceptions, however, Nightingale's model was abandoned and hospital schools trained students with an emphasis on service to the hospital rather than education of a nurse.

Early nurse reformers such as Isabel Hampton Robb, Lavinia Dock, and Annie W. Goodrich laid the foundation for nursing education built on natural and social sciences and, by the 1920s, nursing programs were visible in university settings. World War I and World War II underscored the importance of well-educated nurses and the Army School of Nursing and the Cadet Army Corps significantly contributed to the movement of nursing education into university settings.

Associate degree programs developed in the 1950s as a result of community college interest in nursing education, while Mildred Montag's dissertation related to the preparation of a different type of nurse. The situation of nursing in community colleges, along with the American Nurses Association (ANA) proposal that nursing education be located within university settings, sparked a civil war in nursing that has yet to be resolved.

By the latter half of the 20th century, graduate education in nursing was established with master's and doctoral programs growing across the country. Graduate education continues to strengthen the discipline as it moves into the 21st century.

IN THE BEGINNING

American nursing programs changed dramatically over the past 150 years in response to milestones such as world wars, the Great Depression, and changing U.S. demographics. The initial milestone that catalyzed the founding of formal education for nurses was the Civil War. Prior to the Civil War, most women only provided nursing care in the home to their family. Every woman expected to nurse family members. Older women, who had extensive family experience and needed to earn a living, would care for neighbors or contacts that were referred by word of mouth (Reverby, 1987). As women began to care for the soldiers during the war, they transferred their skills and knowledge from home to the battlefield. The value of nursing care in the soldiers' recovery and the need for formal education for nurses were both recognized as the Civil War came to a close.

The New England Hospital for Women and Children, located in Boston, was the first American school to offer nursing courses based on Nightingale's guidelines. Opened in 1872, the school offered a formal training program with a 1-year curriculum similar to the one Nightingale developed at St. Thomas Hospital School of Nursing. In addition to 12 hours of required lectures, students were taught to take vital signs and apply bandages. Interestingly, students were not allowed to know the names of medications given to patients and the medication bottles were labeled by numbers. In 1875, the curriculum was extended to 16 months (Davis, 1991). Linda Richards, considered to be America's first trained nurse, entered this school on the first day it opened and Mary Mahoney, the first African American nurse, was a graduate of the school (Davis, 1991).

In 1873, three more schools were opened that were supposedly patterned on the Nightingale model. The Bellevue Training School opened in New York City, the Connecticut Training School opened in Hartford, and Boston, Massachusetts was the site of the Boston Training School. These schools proposed to offer a desirable occupation for self-supporting women and provide good private nurses for the community (Kelly & Joel, 1996).

By the beginning of the 20th century, over 2,000 training schools had been opened. With few exceptions, Nightingale's principles of education and curriculum were ignored. Curricula focused on character traits and habits and school priorities were "service first, education second" (nursingeducationhistory.org, 2012). The 3-year program of most nursing schools consisted primarily of on-the-job training, courses taught by physicians, and long hours of clinical practice. Students, known as "pupils," provided nursing service for the hospital. In return, they received diplomas and pins at the completion of their training. Students entered the programs one by one as they were available and their services were needed. The patients were mostly poor, without families and/or homes to provide care. From the institution's standpoint, graduates were a byproduct rather than a purpose for the training school. "Trained nurses" generally gave private care in wealthy homes, oversaw pupils in a training school, or cared for the poor in their homes after graduation (Reverby, 1984).

If textbooks were available to students, they were primarily authored by physicians. The first nurse-authored text, *A Text-Book for Nursing: For the Use of Training Schools, Families and Private Students*, was written by Clara Weeks (later Weeks-Shaw), an 1880 graduate of the New York Hospital and founding super-intendent of the Paterson General Hospital School (Obituary, 1940). The posses-sion of such a text led to decreased dependence of graduates on their course notes, supplied information that would otherwise have been missed because of can-celled lectures or note-taking student exhaustion, reinforced the idea that nursing required more than fine character, and exerted a standardizing effect on training school expectations. The approximately 100 names in the comprehensive list of medicines, including ether, oxygen, topical agents, and multiple names for the same substance, subverted efforts to keep nurses ignorant of the names of medicines they were administering. By the third edition, Weeks-Shaw (1902) identified the pri-mary audience as "professional" nurses rather than "amateurs" and assumed an elementary acquaintance with subjects such as anatomy and physiology, "which is now a fundamental part of training."

Despite the founding of formalized education, the emergence of training schools and some public awareness of the need for "trained nurses," the social cli-mate of the late 1800s was not conducive to the advancement of women-centered issues. Society expected women to assume private, supportive roles rather than public, authoritative ones. The public perception of nursing was an extension of women's supportive and caring role in the home. Even Nightingale advocated against professional status for nurses through opposition of credentialing (or licen-sure) of graduate nurses (Palmer, 1985). The dependence of nursing education on hospitals perpetuated the private, supportive role of women, and precluded them from participation in substantive decisions related to health care policy within and outside of institutions (Ruby, 1999).

DIVERSITY IN EARLY NURSING EDUCATION

Diverse Schools

Mary Mahoney, the first African American nurse, entered the New England Hospital for Women and Children School of Nursing on March 23, 1878. Her acceptance at this school was unique at a time in American society when the majority of educational institutions were not integrated (Davis, 1991). This lack of integration, however, did not deter African American women from entering the profession of nursing. In 1891, Provident Hospital in Chicago was founded, which was the first training school for Black nurses (Kelly & Joel, 1996).

Howard University Training School for Nurses was established in 1893 to train African American nurses to care for the many Blacks who settled in Washington, DC after the Civil War. The school transferred to Freedman's Hospital in 1894 and by 1944 had 166 students (Washington, 2012). This rapid expansion was experienced by other African American nursing programs (Kalisch & Kalisch, 1978). Freedman's Hospital School transferred to Howard University in 1967 and graduated its last class in 1973. Howard University School of Nursing has offered a baccalaureate degree since 1974 and initiated a master's degree in nursing in 1980. After the *Brown vs Board of Education* decision in 1954, schools of nursing that served predominantly African American students began to decline and, by the late 1960s, nursing schools throughout the United States were fully integrated (Carnegie, 2005).

Sage Memorial Hospital School of Nursing opened in 1930 and was located in northeastern Arizona, at Ganado, 56 miles northwest of Gallup, New Mexico, in the heart of the Navajo Indian Reservation. It was part of Sage Memorial Hospital, built by the National Missions of the Presbyterian Church, which provided care for Native Americans (Kalisch & Kalisch, 1978).

The school of nursing operated through 1953; it was the only nursing school established for the sole purpose of training Native American women to be nurses. By 1943, students enrolled in the school came from widely diverse backgrounds including Native American, Hispanic, Hawaiian, Cuban, and Japanese. In the 1930s and 1940s, such training and cultural exchange among minority women was not found anywhere else in the United States. Students developed a camaraderie and commitment, while they completed coursework and tended the hospital floors 8 hours a day, 6 days a week (Pollitt, Streeter, & Walsh, 2011).

Men in Nursing Education

One little known legacy of the Civil War is the inclusion of men in nursing. Walt Whitman, known for his poetry, was a nurse in the Civil War. He cared for wounded soldiers in Washington, DC for 5 years and was an early practitioner of holistic nursing incorporating active listening, therapeutic touch, and the instillation of hope in patients (Ahrens, 2002).

There were, however, few nursing schools in the late 19th century that accommodated men; a few schools provided an abbreviated curriculum that trained men as "attendants." The McLean Asylum School of Nursing in Massachusetts was among the first to provide nursing education for men. Established in 1882, the 2-year curriculum prepared graduates to work in the mental health facilities of the time. Treatments in those facilities included application of restraints (such as strait jackets) and "tubbing" (placing the patient in a bathtub with a wooden cover locked onto the tub so only the patient's head was exposed) and it was believed the tubs required the physical power men possessed (Kenny, 2008).

The first true formal school of nursing for men was established at Bellevue Hospital in New York City in 1888 by Darius Mills. One of the best-known schools of nursing for men was the Alexian Brothers Hospital School of Nursing. It opened in 1898 and was the last of its kind to close in 1969 (LaRocco, 2011). Although the school admitted only religious brothers for most of its early history, in 1927 it began to accept lay students. In 1939, the school began an affiliation with DePaul University so students could take biology and other science courses to apply toward bachelor's degrees. By 1955, the school had obtained full National League for Nursing (NLN) accreditation and by 1962, 13 full-time faculty members and eight lecturers educated a graduating class of 42 students. This was the largest class in the school's history and one of the largest classes in any men's nursing school in the country (Wall, 2009). By the mid-1960s, men were being admitted to most hospital nursing programs and the school graduated its last class in 1969. In addition, by the 1960s, the ANA was encouraging prospective nurses to earn their baccalaureates in university nursing programs.

Reports and Standards of the Late 19th and Early 20th Centuries

The International Congress of Charities, Correction and Philanthropy met in Chicago as part of the Columbian Exposition of 1893. Isabel Hampton, the founding principal of the Training School and Superintendent of Nurses at Johns Hopkins Hospital, played a leading role in planning the nursing sessions for the Congress. At a plenary session, she presented a paper, "Educational Standards for Nurses," which argued that hospitals had a responsibility to provide actual education for nursing students; the paper also urged superintendents to work together to establish educational standards (James, 2002). At this time, curricula, standards for admission, and requirements for graduation varied dramatically among schools. Attempts at standardization had begun but were not common.

Hampton's paper included her proposal to extend the training period to 3 years in order to allow the shortening of the "practical training" to 8 hours per day. She also recommended admission of students with "stated times for entrance into the school, and the teaching year … divided according to the academic terms usually adopted in our public schools and colleges" (Robb, 1907). During the week of the Congress, Hampton instigated an informal meeting of nursing superintendents that laid the groundwork for the formation of the American Society of Superintendents of Training Schools (ASSTS) in the United States and Canada, which later, in 1912, was renamed the National League of Nursing Education (NLNE). Certainly a landmark event within nursing, this was also the first association of a professional nature organized and controlled by women (Bullough & Bullough, 1978).

The year 1893 marked the publication of Hampton's *Nursing: Its Principles and Practice for Hospital and Private Use*. The first 25 pages are devoted to a description of a training school, including physical facilities, contents of a reference library, a 2-year curriculum plan for both didactic content and planned, regular clinical rotations, and examinations. Hampton notably omitted reference to the pupil nurse residence as a character-training instrument in the training school system, though she noted the importance of the residence for the health and social development of students (Dodd, 2001). Clearly, she was pushing for a progressive professional education and a professional identity for nursing.

In 1912, the ASSTS became the NLNE and their objectives were to continue to develop and work for a uniform curriculum. In 1915, Adelaide Nutting commented on the educational status of nursing and the NLNE presented a standard curriculum for schools of nursing. The curriculum was divided into seven areas, each of which contained two or more courses. The total program of study was delineated including the general length, vacation time, daily hours of work, and the general scheme of practical work for 36 months of the program. There was a strong emphasis on student activity including observation, accurate recording, participation in actual dissection, experimentation, and giving of patient care (Bacon, 1987).

In 1925, the Committee on the Grading of Nursing Schools was formed. The function of the Committee was to study the ways and means for ensuring an ample supply of nursing service of whatever type and quality are needed for adequate care of the patients at a price within its reach. The Grading Committee worked from 1926 to 1934 to produce "gradings" based on answers to survey forms. Each school received individualized feedback about its own characteristics in comparison to all other participating schools (Committee on the Grading of Nursing Schools, 1931). The NLNE's 1927 *A Curriculum for Schools of Nursing* provided the implicit framework for the surveys and reports. Although the original hope was that the Committee would rank schools into A, B, and C categories as the Flexner report had, the Committee pointed out that the work and cost of visiting the many nursing schools (as compared to Flexner's 155) made this impossible.

Even without this actual "grading," it provided more data than nursing ever had about its schools. For example, it found that the median U.S. nursing school had 10 faculty members: the superintendent of the hospital, the superintendent of nurses, the night supervisor, the day supervisor, two heads of special departments—usually operating room and delivery room, one assistant in a special department, two other head nurses, and one instructor. This median varied by region from four to 17 faculty members. Forty-two percent of the faculty had not completed high school. Forty-five percent of the superintendents of nursing came to their positions more recently than the senior students' admission dates. Hospital schools in the inter-world-war period presented a highly variable picture. Some still offered only apprenticeship learning, but without "master craftswoman" nurses and with a social milieu more consonant with turn-of-the-century culture. This gave nursing a backward, rigid quality that was susceptible to caricature. Others were pushing their limits to provide stimulating learning and an environment more akin to other educational institutions (Egenes, 1998).

In 1917, 1927, and 1937, the NLNE published a series of curriculum recommendations in book form. The reaction to the title of the first, *Standard Curriculum . . .*, led to naming the second *A Curriculum ...* and the third *A Curriculum Guide. . . .* The first was developed by a relatively small group, but the second and third involved a long process with broad input, which, even apart from the product, served an important function. The published curricula were intended to reflect a generalization about what the better schools were doing or aimed to accomplish. As such they give a picture of change over the 20-year period, but cannot be regarded as providing a snapshot of a typical school. Each volume represents substantial change from the previous, and where the same course topical area exists in all three, the level of detail and specificity increases with each decade. Indeed, the markedly increased length and wordy style of the 1937 volume appropriately carries the title "Guide." Each *Curriculum* book increased the number of classroom hours and decreased the recommended hours of patient care, in effect making nursing service more expensive. Each *Curriculum* also increased the pre-requisite educational level: 4 years of high school (temporary tolerance of 2 years in 1917), 4 years of high school in 1927, and 1 to 2 years of college or normal school in addition to high school by 1937 (National League of Nursing Education, 1917, 1927, 1937). This was a selective standard, which was more easily met by students from urban homes. In 1920, only 16.8% of the age cohort graduated from high school; in 1930, 20%; and in 1940, 50.8% graduated (Tyack, 1974). It was not until the 1930s, with the depressed labor market and enforcement of child labor and mandatory attendance laws, that one-third of the age cohort nationally attended high school. With the beginnings of a nursing school accreditation mechanism before World War II and the post-war National Nursing Accrediting Service (NNAS), the function that the *Curriculum* books were intended to serve was now incarnated by consultants and supplanted by concise written standards (Committee of the Six National Nursing Organizations on Unification of Accrediting Services, 1949).

In 1951, the 42-year-old National Association of Colored Graduate Nurses merged with the ANA. The ANA took on new responsibilities through its Intergroup Relations Program, which was aimed at removing the remaining membership barriers in certain district and state associations (Kalisch & Kalisch, 1978).

THE 20TH CENTURY

Nursing Education Through Two World Wars

World War I

When the United States entered World War I, the need for nurses during national emergencies became clear. Admissions to nursing schools during 1917 and 1918 increased by about 25% (Bacon, 1987). The two phenomena that impacted nursing education during World War I were the development of the Vassar Training Camp and the founding of the Army School of Nursing.

The Vassar Training Camp for Nurses was established in 1918. Its purpose was to enroll female college graduates in a 3-month intensive course that addressed natural and social sciences and fundamental nursing skills. This 3-month intensive course replaced the first year of nursing school; following this course, students completed the final 2 years of school in one of 35 selected schools of nursing (Bacon, 1987). Of the 439 college graduates who entered the Vassar Camp, 418 completed the course, went on to nursing school, replaced nurses who had entered the armed services, and helped fill key leadership roles in nursing for the next several decades (Kalisch & Kalisch, 1978). Although short-lived, the Vassar Training Camp provided the opportunity to build nursing competencies on a college education foundation and contributed to the eventual move of nursing education into the university setting (Bacon, 1987).

In 1918, Annie W. Goodrich, president of the ANA, proposed the development of an Army School of Nursing. This was in response to extremely vocal groups who believed that, because of the war, the education preparation of nurses should be shortened. With the backing of the NLNE and the ANA in addition to nurse leaders such as Frances Payne Bolton, the Secretary of War approved the school and Annie Goodrich became its first dean. She developed the curriculum according to the *Standard Curriculum for Schools of Nursing* published by the NLNE in 1917 (Kalisch & Kalisch, 1978). The response to the Army School of Nursing was overwhelmingly positive and many more women applied than could be accepted.

World War II and the Cadet Nurse Corps

World War II, with its demands for all able-bodied young men for military service, mobilized available women for employment or volunteer service. Indeed, every resident was engaged in the effort by the mandates of food, clothing, and gasoline rationing, and by persuasion toward everything from tending victory gardens to buying savings bonds. From mid-1941 to mid-1943, with the help of federal aid, nursing schools increased their enrollments by 13,000 over the baseline year and 4,000 post-diploma nurses completed post–basic course work to enable them to fill the places of nurses who enlisted. Some inactive nurses returned to practice (Roberts, 1954). Despite the effort necessary to bring about this increase, hospitals were floundering and more nurses were needed for the military services.

Congress passed the Bolton Act, which authorized the complex of activities known as the Cadet Nurse Corps (CNC) in June 1943. It was conceived as a mechanism to avoid civilian hospital collapse, to provide nursing to the military, and to ensure an adequate education for student nurse cadets. The goal was to recruit 65,000 high school graduates into nursing schools in the first year (1943–1944) and 60,000 the next year. This represented 10% of girls graduating from high school and the whole percentage of those who would expect to go to college! The program exceeded the goals for both years (Kalisch & Kalisch, 1978).

Hospitals sponsoring training schools recognized that CNC schools would out-recruit non-CNC schools, thereby almost certainly guaranteeing their closure or radical shrinkage. Thus, they signed on, despite the fact that hospitals had to establish a separate accounting for school costs, literally meet the requirements of their state boards of nurse examiners to the satisfaction of the CNC consultants, and allow their students to leave for federal service during the last 6 months of their programs, when they would otherwise be most valuable to their home schools. Schools received partial funding from a separate appropriation for the modifications necessary to build classrooms and library space, and to secure additional student housing. Visiting consultants looked at faculty numbers and qualifications, clinical facilities available for learning, curricula, hours of student clinical and class work, the school's ability to accelerate course work to fit into 30 months, and the optimal number of students the school could accommodate (Robinson & Perry, 2001). Only high school graduates could qualify to become cadets (Petry, 1943). Schools were pressed to increase the size of their classes and number of classes admitted per year, to use local colleges for basic sciences to conserve nurse instructor time, and to develop affiliations with psychiatric hospitals, for educational reasons, and secondarily to free up dormitory space for more students to be admitted. Consultants could give 3-, 6-, or 12-month conditional approval to the schools while deficiencies were corrected (Robinson & Perry, 2001). Given the pressure to keep CNC-approved status, schools made painful changes.

Students, who were estimated to be providing 80% of care in civilian hospitals, experienced a changed practice context. They now had to decide what they could safely delegate to Red Cross volunteers and any paid aides available. Extra responsibility for nursing arose from the shortage of physicians. With grossly short staffing, nurses had to set priorities carefully. All of these circumstances altered student learning. The intense work of the consultants, who provided interpretation and linkage between the U.S. Public Health Service (USPHS) in Washington and each school, and their strategy of simultaneously naming deficiencies and identifying improvement goals, was a critical factor in the success of the programs as well as improvement in nursing education. Without the financial resources of the federal government to defray student costs, to assist with certain costs to schools, and to provide the consultation, auditing, and public relations/recruitment functions, the goals could not be met. Lucile Petry, the director of the Division of Nursing Education in the USPHS, combined a sense of the social significance of nursing with first-hand experience in nursing education, a humility that equipped her to work with all kinds of people, and generously give credit to everyone involved in the massive undertaking. Opinions differed on such questions as the cut-off point for irredeemably weak schools, but overall, the effort was pronounced a substantial success for nursing (Roberts, 1954).

The Remainder of the 20th Century

The nursing profession used the Depression years for major stock-taking and self-examination. For the first time registered nurses were available in hospitals for direct bedside care; patient care responsibility did not have to rest on students. Teachers and directors of nursing began to see the possibility of selecting patient care experiences for the student in relation to learning needs rather than to meet hospital service needs (Bacon, 1987). Increased expectations for cognitive learning by students were brought about by factors, which included hospital architecture, physician expectations, nursing efforts, and general culture change. With increased numbers of applicants during the Depression, schools were able to select capable students and grant diplomas that signified both cognitive learning and character.

By the 1940s, people routinely came to hospitals for care. In addition, patients who had formerly hired private nurses to care for them in the hospital were now admitted to wards, which were rooms that contained four to ten beds. Students were admitted as cohorts and attrition was hard to predict; the increased patient census made it necessary to hire graduate nurses (Vogel, 1980). These graduate nurses were often unemployed private duty nurses.

Experiments involving the housing of nursing programs in junior or community colleges were underway in the 1950s. Even the hospital-sponsored diploma programs, which decreased in numbers during the last part of the 20th century, were transformed into educationally focused efforts.

The development of coronary care and intensive care units in the 1960s required nurses to develop critical thinking and clinical reasoning skills and take action in a wider range of clinical situations than had formerly been within nursing's scope of practice. Educators were trying to sort out the implications for both undergraduate and graduate programs. Educators made decisions to focus on graduate preparation in nursing and by the 1960s, master's programs were beginning to prepare clinical nurse specialists and nurse practitioner roles were being described in the literature.

During the 1960s, there was vigorous debate about educational preparation for nurses. In May 1965, the NLN passed a resolution that supported college-based nursing programs. In January of 1966, the ANA released a position paper that recommended baccalaureate preparation for professional nurses and associate degree education for technical nurses. These two documents were seen by many as one of the highest peaks in the profession's history, one that reflected nursing's strength and unity. Sadly, conflict within the NLN and ANA and public opposition to college-based nursing programs (voiced primarily by nurses who graduated from diploma schools) doomed the premise that professional nurses required baccalaureate education (Fondiller, 1999).

The Evolution of Current Educational Paths of Nursing

Starting in the early 1900s, universities began to enfold disciplines such as education, business administration, and engineering, which had originally been taught in freestanding, single-purpose institutions (Veysey, 1965). By the interwar period, the university became the dominant institution for postsecondary education (Graham, 1978). From 1920 to 1940, the percentage of women attending college in the 18- to 21-year-old cohort rose from 7.6% to 12.2%. Men's college-going rates rose faster, so that the percentage of women in the student body dropped from 43% in 1920 to 40.2% in 1940 (Eisenmann, 2000; Solomon, 1985).

Nursing made overtures to a few colleges and universities prior to World War I. In 1899, the ASSTS developed the Hospital Economics course for nurses who had potential as superintendents of hospital and training schools. The program involved 8 months of study, using many courses existing in the Domestic Science department, but with a custom-designed course on teaching, and a Hospital Economics course that would be taught by nurses (Robb, 1907). This relationship with Teachers College grew and was cemented by the endowment in 1910 of a Chair in Nursing, occupied for many years by M. Adelaide Nutting. The nursing faculty at Teachers College continued to be influential in nursing education through the 1950s, as other educational centers began to share influence.

In the first decade of the 1900s, technical institutes such as Drexel in Philadelphia, Pratt in Brooklyn, and Mechanics in Rochester as well as Simmons College in Boston and Northwestern University in Chicago offered course work to nursing students (Robb, 1907). The designers of the 1917 *Standard Curriculum* ... gave some thought to the relationship of nursing education to the collegiate system. They suggested that the theoretical work in a nursing school was equivalent to 36 units, or about 1 year of college, and the clinical work another 51 units.

Few voices actively campaigned for the alignment of nursing education with institutions of higher learning even as late as the 1930s, despite the recommendation of the Rockefeller-funded Goldmark (1923) report, *Nursing and Nursing Education in the United States,* in the early 1920s. Initially, education at the university level was envisioned solely for the leaders of training schools.

Educators who wanted a university context for nursing, concentration on educational goals, and emancipation from dependence on the hospitals' student work–study schemes, looked hopefully at the Yale University School of Nursing, funded by the Rockefeller Foundation starting in 1924, and headed by the determined and respected Annie W. Goodrich. Similarly encouraging was the program at Case Western Reserve University, endowed by Francis Payne Bolton in 1923, following considerable prior work within the Cleveland civic community. Vanderbilt was endowed by a combination of Rockefeller, Carnegie, and Commonwealth funds in 1930. The University of Chicago established a school of nursing in 1925 with an endowment from the distinguished but discontinued Illinois Training School (Hanson, 1991). Dillard University established a school in 1942 with substantial foundation support and governmental war-related funds. Mary Tennant, nursing adviser in the Rockefeller Foundation, pronounced the Dillard Division of Nursing "one of the most interesting developments in nursing education in the country" (Hine, 1989). Although these were milestone events, endowments did little to dissipate the caution, if not hostility, toward women on American campuses. Neither did they cure all that was ailing in nursing education. They funded significant program changes, but even these would not meet the accreditation standards of later decades (Faddis, 1973; Kalisch & Kalisch, 1978; Sheahan, 1980).

According to the *Journal of the American Medical Association (JAMA)*, 25 universities granted bachelor's degrees to nurses by 1926 (*JAMA*, 1927). By the end of the 1930s a bewildering array of "collegiate" programs existed, partly because baccalaureate programs were being invented by trial and error within the combinations of opportunities and constraints presented in each local hospital and university pair (Petry, 1937).

BACCALAUREATE EDUCATION

The diverse baccalaureate curricula of the 1930s multiplied by the 1950s. As one educator wrote in 1954, "Baccalaureate programs still seem to be in the experimental stage. They vary in purpose, structure, subject matter content, admission requirements, matriculation requirements, and degrees granted upon their completion. Some schools offering baccalaureate programs still aim to prepare nurses for specialized positions. Others, advancing from this traditional concept, seek to prepare graduates for generalized nursing in beginning positions" (Harms, 1954).

Although a few programs threaded general education and basic science courses through 5 years of study, the majority structured their programs with 2 years of college courses before or after the 3 years of nursing preparation, or bookended the nursing years with the split 2 years of college work (Bridgman, 1949). Margaret Bridgman, an educator from Skidmore College who consulted with a large number of nursing schools, made favorable reference to the "upper division nursing major" in her volume directed toward both college and nursing educators (Bridgman, 1953). However, the paramount issues, she said, were whether or not (1) the academic institution and academic goals had meaningful involvement and influence in the program as a whole, and (2) degree-goal and diploma-goal students were co-mingled in nursing courses. Programs that failed the first test criterion were termed the "affiliated" type. In 1950, 129 of 195 schools offering a basic (pre-licensure) program were of the affiliated type. In 1953, 104 of the 199 schools still offered both degree and diploma programs (Harms, 1954) and probably co-mingled the two types of students in courses. To further complicate the situation, only 9,000 of the 21,000 baccalaureate students in 1950 were pre-licensure students. The remaining 12,000 postdiploma baccalaureate students were not evenly distributed among schools, so some programs found themselves with a sprinkling of pre-licensure students among a class of experienced diploma graduates.

Bridgman recommended that postdiploma students be evaluated individually and provisionally with a tentative grant of credit based on prior learning, including nursing schoolwork, and successful completion of a term of academic work. The student's program would be made up of "deficiencies" in general education and prerequisite courses and then courses in the major itself. Credit-granting practices varied considerably from place to place, so a nurse could easily spend 1½ to 3 years earning the baccalaureate (Bridgman, 1953). Bridgman provided "suggestions for content" using the categories of:

1. Knowledge from the physical and biological sciences
2. Communication skills
3. The major in nursing
4. Knowledge from social science [sociology, social anthropology, and psychology]
5. General education, all of which she thought should ideally be interrelated throughout the program

Of the 199 colleges and universities offering programs leading to bachelor's degrees in 1953, the NNAS accredited 51 basic programs.

Given the constant expansion of knowledge relevant to nursing, it was doubly difficult for programs with a history of a 5-year curriculum to shrink to 4 academic years in the 1960s and early 1970s. The expanded assessment skills expected of critical care nurses, together with the master's-level specialty emphases and certificate nurse practitioner programs, stimulated the inclusion of more sophisticated skills in baccalaureate programs in the early to mid-1970s (Lynaugh & Brush, 1996). In response to nursing service agitation to narrow the gap between new graduate skills and initial employment expectations, and much talk about "reality shock," baccalaureate programs structured curricula to allow a final experience in which students were immersed in clinical care to focus on skills of organization and integration.

Accreditation

From the standpoint of the ordinary nursing school, the possibility of actual accreditation became a reality in the 1950s. The NLNE developed standards for accreditation and made pilot visits from 1934 to 1938. By 1939, schools could list themselves to be visited in order to qualify to be on the first list published by NLNE. Despite the greatly increased work, turnover, and general disruption created by the war, 100 schools had mustered both the courage and energy required to prepare for accreditation evaluation and judged creditable by 1945. Many schools that had qualified for provisional accreditation, however, were due for revisiting by the end of World War II. The Association of Collegiate Schools of Nursing (ACSN), formed in 1932, exercised a kind of "accreditation" via its requirements for full and associate membership, but its standards primarily influenced schools that aspired to be part of this group or that attended conferences it co-sponsored. Only 26 schools were accredited by ACSN in 1949. The National Organization for Public Health Nursing (NOPHN) had been accrediting post–basic programs in public health since 1920 but more recently had considered specialty programs at both baccalaureate and master's level and the public health content in generalist baccalaureate programs (Harms, 1954). By 1948, these organizations, along with the Council of Nursing Education of Catholic Hospitals, ceded their accrediting role to the NNAS, which published its first combined list of accredited programs just 1 month before the survey-based interim classification of schools was published by the National Committee for the Improvement of Nursing Services (NCINS) in 1949 (Petry, 1949). The classification put schools in either Group I, the top 25% of schools, or Group II, the middle 50%, leaving other schools unlisted and unclassified.

The NNAS, much like the cadet nurse program before it, elected a strategy designed to entice schools with at least minimal strengths to improve. It published the first list of temporarily accredited schools in 1952, giving these schools 5 years to make improvements and qualify for full accreditation. During the intervening time, it provided many special meetings, self-evaluation guides, and consultant visits to the schools. By 1957, the number of fully accredited schools increased by 72.4% (Kalisch & Kalisch, 1978). Changes in hospital school programs were catalyzed and channeled by accreditation norms (Committee of the Six National Nursing Organizations on Unification of Accrediting Services, 1949). But ultimately, the forces that drove change were primarily external, ranging from public expectations of postsecondary education mediated through hospital trustees and physicians, to competition among programs for potential students, who now had access to information about accreditation and who were heavily recruited by schools, which still had substantial responsibility for nursing service. By 1950, all states participated in the State Board Test Pool examination, another measuring rod that induced improvement or closure of weaker schools.

Despite the influential Carnegie- and Sage-funded *Nursing for the Future* in 1948, which recommended a broad-based move of nursing education into general higher education, nursing's earliest centralized accreditation mechanism concentrated considerable energy on improving diploma schools, as had the Grading Committee before it (Brown, 1948; Roberts, 1954). Why this seeming mismatch between aspirations and effort? Partly, it sprang from realism: Students were in hospital schools, whether ideal or not, so they needed the best possible preparation because nursing services would reflect this quality. (Postgraduation learning via staff development or socialization into the traditions of a service was not considered a significant factor.) Further, the quality of many of the baccalaureate programs left a great deal to be desired and their capacity for more students was limited, so these could not be promoted as an immediate or ideal substitute for diploma programs. Although by 1957 there were 18 associate degree programs (Kalisch & Kalisch, 1978), no one foresaw the speed of their multiplication in the next decade. Finally, nursing's collective sense of social responsibility burdened it with finding ways to continue to provide essential services, both within the hospital and elsewhere, as its educational house moved from the base of the hospital to the foundation of higher education (Lynaugh, 2002).

Associate Degree Education

The NLNE held discussions during the middle and late 1940s with community colleges to discuss the possibility of associate degree nursing education (Fondiller, 2001). In 1945, the American Association of Junior Colleges (AAJC) showed an interest in nursing; at this point curriculum and recruitment were the two major challenges. In January 1946, a committee was established with representation from the ACSN to consider nursing education in community colleges. Between 1949 and 1950, the committee, along with NLNE and ACSN, discussed nursing education at this level. The focus was to be the "Brown" report, that is, *Nursing for the Future*, authored by Esther Lucille Brown, a social anthropologist with the Russell Sage Foundation (Brown, 1948). The immediate context for the committee, from the nursing side, was significant. In 1947, the Board of NLNE adopted the policy goal that nursing education should be located in the higher education system. Also in 1947, the faculty at Teachers College, Columbia University (TCCU) launched a planning process that involved Eli Ginzberg, a young economist, who asserted that nursing could be thought of as a whole set of functions and roles rather than a single role or type of worker. He posited that nursing needed at least two types of practitioners, one professional, and one technical (Haase, 1990). Starting in fall 1947, Brown began her conferences with nursing leaders and visits to more than 50 schools, completing her report so that it could be disseminated in September 1948. In one section of the report, she compared nursing to engineering with its highly valued technical workers. She believed that perhaps a "graduate bedside nurse" needed more preparation than a practical nurse, but less than a full-fledged professional nurse. In early 1949, NLNE sought funding for the joint work with community colleges, and found the Russell Sage and W.K. Kellogg Foundations responsive with substantial support (Haase, 1990).

The committee reported that junior (now known as community) colleges could develop one of two types of nursing programs: (1) a 2-year program that would be transfer oriented to a university program that offered a baccalaureate degree, or (2) a 3-year program leading to an associate of arts (AA) or an associate of science (AS). In 1951, Mildred Montag, whose dissertation had proposed a new type of technical nursing program embedded in junior colleges, joined the committee. She was subsequently appointed to the Joint Committee in 1951 and became the project director for the anonymously funded Cooperative Research Project (CRP) in Junior and Community College Education for Nursing in early

1952 (Haase, 1990). The CRP pilot programs were 2 years long, or 2 years plus a summer. Initially, they were one-third general education and two-thirds nursing, but they moved toward equal proportions of each by the end of the project. The curricula, although controlled by faculty in each school, tended to focus on variations in health in their first year, and then deviations from normal (physical and mental illness), in the second year. These "broad fields" were accompanied by campus nursing laboratory learning and by clinical learning experiences in a wide variety of settings, but with a major hospital component. Students in the pilot programs were somewhat older than diploma or baccalaureate students, and some were married (a nonstarter in many diploma programs), and had children. Men were a small percentage of the students, but tripled the representation in diploma programs. State Board Examination pass rates for graduates of the pilot group were comparable to those of other programs.

Montag intended, at that time, that this program would be self-contained, but stressed that graduates of this program could pursue baccalaureate education. She also recommended single licensure for nurses from all educational programs, although 25 years later, she rescinded that recommendation (Fondiller, 2001).

From the mid-1950s to the mid-1970s, when the associate degree program growth rate peaked, the number of programs doubled about every 4 years. By 1975, there were 618 associate degree programs in nursing, comprising 45% of basic nursing programs and graduating a comparable percentage of the new graduates each year. Diploma programs comprised 31% of basic programs, though given the recency of associate degree program development, the vast majority of nurses in practice still originally came from diploma programs (Haase, 1990; Rines, 1977). By 1959, W.K. Kellogg Foundation assistance to the expansion of associate degree nursing education totaled more than $3,000,000. The Nurse Training Act of 1964 and subsequent federal legislation funding nursing also contributed to program growth (Scott, 1972).

Over the ensuing years, elapsed time from enrollment to graduation lengthened, due in part to the expanding knowledge base needed to be "a bedside nurse," sometimes due to pressures from elsewhere on campus to expand general education, sometimes due to sequencing requirements of the nursing faculty, and on occasion due to the level of student preparation and ability or to student choice. Much time was devoted to communicating with hospital nursing service representatives to identify students' competencies at graduation so that new graduate orientations and staff development plans articulated with them. Curricular offerings were fine-tuned to ensure that these baseline competencies were met. When "the bedside" noticeably moved out of the hospital in the early 1990s, questions about preparation for practice in the home care context became urgent, but the familiar condition of the hospital "nursing shortage" laid these to rest.

Programs of the 1950s in university settings had to cope with the entrenched traditions of both hospitals and universities as they struggled to make changes. By contrast, associate degree nursing programs began with a clean slate. They were initially welcomed by community colleges. The lure of having an additional supply of nurses promoted at least grudging cooperation from clinical agencies, although hospital nursing staff and administrators in many places had misgivings about the curricular arrangements and limited clinical experience of students.

Associate degree–prepared nurses of the early 1980s found expectations and mechanisms for matriculating into baccalaureate programs much more clearly defined than described by Bridgman 30 years earlier and indeed, some baccalaureate programs were designed specifically for associate degree graduates. The ever-expanding body of nursing knowledge forced repeated decisions about which content was most essential and what clinical settings would bring about the best learning. By the 1990s, as hospital censuses plummeted and sick patients shuttled back and forth between home and ambulatory settings, programs were forced to consider increasing community-based clinical experience with its attendant challenges to find placements and provide geographically dispersed instruction.

A Nursing Education Civil War

The cultural upheaval that characterized the mid-1960s through the 1970s had its counterpart in nursing. Within nursing, a rift grew between those who believed an incremental approach would eventually get nursing education optimally situated and those who believed that the eventual goal should be clearly specified far in advance so that changes could take the goal into account. Nurses involved in day-to-day patient care and many diploma nurse educators tended to cluster in the first group, and those, particularly educators, who were in national or regional leadership positions were in the second group. The latter group focused on the professional end of the nursing continuum, working to achieve the fullest possible academic and professional recognition for nursing so that its advocacy and action would have broad credibility and influence.

From this perspective, the ANA 1965 position paper, "Educational Preparation for Nurse Practitioners and Assistants to Nurses," seemed like the next logical step (ANA, 1965). After all, for more than 15 years the NLNE, reconstituted and combined with the NOPHN, ACSN, and National Association of Industrial Nurses (NAIN) in 1952 to be the NLN, had been saying that education for nursing belonged in institutions of higher education. The idea that nursing was a continuum, composed of vocational, technical, and professional segments, had been talked about intermittently in those same circles during that entire period.

Unfortunately, the position paper dropped like a bomb on people who had never heard these conversations. It was said to ignore diploma schools and nurses altogether, classify associate degree-prepared nurses as technical nurses, and downgrade vocational/practical nurse preparation. Fundamental questions such as the "fit" of the three-part typology with the range of nursing work, the location and nature of the boundaries between the segments of the continuum, and the regulatory and licensure implications of such a plan could hardly be debated because of the emotionality that surrounded the specter of the loss of access to the RN title for associate and diploma nurses and what appeared to be the hijacking of the term "professional."

Regardless of nursing program background, the term "professional" had been applied to all that was good. General usage, likewise, cast "professional" in positive terms. A person who did a project or handled a situation "professionally" knew it was well done; a student who "looked professional" knew she had met certain standards (however little clean shoelaces may have had to do with actual professionalism); and a student who studied to be a "professional nurse" would qualify to take the state board examination, and in the years just before the position paper, thought she would give comprehensive, individualized care to patients. "Technical" just did not have the same ring to it; "technical" sounded limited and mechanical; "technical" sounded "less than." However knowledgeable, talented, and essential technical workers were in the discourse of educational macro-planners and economists, the word translated poorly to the world of nursing. Immense amounts of creative and emotional energy were diverted into this conflict.

The crisis was gradually defused, partly by action on the recommendations of the next committee to study nursing, "The National Commission for the Study of Nursing and Nursing Education" (1970), which was commonly known as the Lysaught Commission, which reported in 1970. Among the recommendations in *Abstract for Action* were (1) statewide planning for the number and distribution of nursing education programs, (2) career mobility for individual nurses, and (3) cooperation of nursing service and education in working to improve patient care. As the world around community colleges changed so that more and more people, particularly women, resumed formal education after a hiatus, and senior colleges had good experience with community college graduates who sought baccalaureate degrees, the concepts of "career mobility" and "articulation" came into nursing discourse. By 1972, the NLN prepared a collection titled "The Associate Degree Program—A Step to the Baccalaureate Degree in Nursing." However, according to Patricia Haase, a historian of associate degree programs, it was also true that "[i]t was assumed by some in baccalaureate education that the curricula of the two nursing programs were not related, that they occupied two separate universes" (Haase, 1990). Rapprochement was gradually achieved, but sensitivities, which have their roots in this conflict, exist to this day.

Master's Education

Master's programs were few and relatively small in the 1950s. The 1951 report of the NNAS Postgraduate Board of Review noted that in some instances, the same set of courses led to a master's degree for students who held a baccalaureate and to a baccalaureate for students who had no prior degree. Some of the clearly differentiated master's programs had so many prerequisites that few students qualified for admission without clearing multiple "deficiencies" by taking additional course work. The report opined that few programs focused on nursing "in its broadest sense," as contrasted to teaching and administration (National Nursing Accrediting Service Postgraduate Board of Review, 1951).

A Work Conference on Graduate Nurse Education, sponsored by the NLN Division of Nursing Education in fall of 1952, concluded that master's graduates needed competencies in interpersonal relations, communication skills, their selected functional area (e.g., teaching or administration), promotion of community welfare, and "sufficient familiarity with the principles and methods of research to conduct and/or participate in systematic investigation of nursing problems and evaluate and use research findings" (Harms, 1954). However, a 1954 study comparing six leading schools' master's curricula identified wide variability in actual practice. Program lengths were nominally 1 year for students without deficiencies; however, this actually ranged from 24 to 38 semester credits. Although research was an agreed-upon master's focus, only one of the six schools had one course that by title could be identified as addressing this area (Harms, 1954).

Given the relatively few students seeking admission, and the small size of programs, regional planning became important, particularly in the South and West United States. In regional activity that was the precursor to the formation of the Southern Council on Collegiate Education for Nursing (SCCEN), it was agreed in 1952 that six universities—Universities of Alabama, Maryland, North Carolina, Texas, Vanderbilt, and Emory University—would come together to plan five new master's programs to serve the South. This Regional Project in Graduate Education in Nursing garnered funding from both the W.K. Kellogg and Commonwealth Foundations. By 1955, all six programs were admitting students (Reitt, 1987).

In western states, the Western Conference of Nursing Education was convened in early 1956 by the Western Interstate Commission for Higher Education (WICHE). Nursing educators, nurse leaders in various other positions, and non-nurse representatives from higher education from the western states gathered to advise WICHE on the development of nursing education programs in the area. A 2-month study of nursing education in western states, conducted by Helen Nahm, laid the groundwork for the meeting. This report provided the group with the essence of hundreds of interviews conducted with educators in nursing and related fields in the eight states, as well as nurse manpower data by state for 1954. Respondents reportedly believed that graduate programs in nursing should contain more work in social science fields, advanced preparation in physical and biological science fields, strong foundations in education, courses basic to research, courses in philosophy, research in some area of nursing, and "graduate courses in a clinical nursing area which are truly of graduate caliber ... " (Western Interstate Commission for Higher Education, 1956). Subsequently, the Western Interstate Council for Higher Education in Nursing (WICHEN) sponsored joint work that developed early master's level clinical content and terminal competencies in the early and mid-1960s (Brown, 1978; WICHE, 1967).

Enrollment in master's programs almost doubled between 1951 and 1962, growing from 1,290 to 2,472 (Harms, 1954; Kalisch & Kalisch, 1978). During the 1960s, clinical area emphases replaced functional specializations as the organizing frames for curricula. This shift in focus to nursing itself not only clarified and enriched baccalaureate curricula in later decades (Lynaugh & Brush, 1996), but also freed doctoral level training to focus directly on nursing knowledge development.

Political pressure for access to care, interacting with the shortage and maldistribution of physicians and recognition that nurses could competently do a subset of physician work, led to federal support for the spread of nurse practitioner (NP) programs (Bullough, 1976; National Commission for the Study of Nursing and Nursing Education, 1971). Until the mid-1970s most nurse practitioner preparation was designed and offered as non-degree-related continuing education. The first national conference on family nurse practitioner curricula convened in January 1976. At that point, programs ranged from 4-month certificate level offerings to specialties set within master's programs, with divergent characteristics depending upon rural or urban settings. Certificate programs accounted for 71% of NP program grants funded by the Division of Nursing of the USPHS that year. Just 9 years later, in 1985, 81% of NP program grants went to master's level programs without any change in the authorizing law and presumably the award criteria (Geolot, 1987). Multiple factors drove or accommodated this change. Practice settings had higher expectations, fears of nurse educators about preserving the essence of nursing subsided, sufficient numbers of potential students saw value in a graduate degree, and faculty members who reconceptualized the curricula were persuasive. Not insignificantly, federal funds were available to assist with the costs of transition. Curricular trends over the 20-year period included a proportionate decrease in time spent on health assessment and medical management, movement of pharmacology from free-standing courses to integration in medical management courses—and back again to free-standing, increased emphasis on health promotion and chronic illness management, and development of common clinical core courses in schools where multiple NP specialty tracks existed (Geolot, 1987).

Most large master's programs had multiple specialties by the mid-1980s, but these only weakly correlated with the major specialty organizations and with certification mechanisms (Styles, 1989). The clinical expertise and interest of nursing faculty, links to local resources, community needs for a particular specialty, and federal/state/local voluntary organization financial initiatives to address specific health problems all drove the pattern of specialty development (Burns et al., 1993). Nursing specialty organizations, reflecting current practice perspectives, exerted a substantial shaping influence on specialty curricular content in their respective areas. The rapid expansion (27%) in the number of master's programs in the last half of the 1980s (Burns et al., 1993) may have spurred creative naming of specialties for purposes of student recruitment. Efforts to rationalize the relationships of the specialties to one another and where possible, to achieve common use of resources, were the natural response to this proliferation.

By the 1990s, permutations of what had been considered clinical specialist content were being combined with nurse practitioner approaches. Advanced practice nurses of both types were beginning to question whether the two roles were, after all, so different from one another (Elder & Bullough, 1990). Changes in health care financing and delivery were prompting clinical nurse specialist programs to include content to prepare graduates to deal with cost and reimbursement dimensions of care for populations (Wolf, 1990), and pressuring practitioner programs to prepare graduates to care for patients with less stable conditions. By the end of the first decade of the 21st century, this trend has coalesced into an advanced practice regulatory model that will have standardized graduate level educational requirements, if it is implemented as envisioned (Trossman, 2009).

In 2001, the Institute of Medicine (IOM) published a report calling for increased attention to the provision of safe patient care environments. In response to that report, in 2003 to 2004, the clinical nurse leader (CNL) was envisioned. The CNL is a role that provides leadership at the point of care. Advanced practice preparation and clinical leadership competencies, both acquired at the master's level, prepare this nurse leader to ensure the delivery of safe, evidence-based care that is targeted toward quality patient outcomes (Reid, 2011).

The Essentials of College and University Education for Professional Nursing (American Association of Colleges of Nursing [AACN], 1986), with its ambitious goals for a substantial liberal arts and sciences background, reflected both nursing's self-understanding and changing external circumstances. Applicant interest and professional vision converged to support the development of programs at the master's level for nonnurse college graduates. Students completed pre-licensure generalist preparation before focusing in a specialty or delimited area, leading to the master's as the first professional degree (Wu & Connelly, 1992). Very few such programs had existed in the prior two decades (Diers, 1976; Plummer & Phelan, 1976). *The Essentials of Master's Education for Advanced Practice Nursing* codified the broad areas of agreement about master's preparation among educators (AACN, 1996) and this, together with accreditation mechanisms and a shared external environment, nudged programs toward common curricular characteristics.

The 1986 *Essentials* document foreshadowed another turning point in the long evolution of organized nursing thinking about the placement of basic generalist professional preparation within the standard degree structures of higher education. Given projections of health care system demand for nurses over the next three decades, the need for more comprehensively prepared nurses at the microsystem level due to increased care complexity, and concurrent flagging applicant interest in bachelor's programs with contrasting brisk interest in first professional degree master's programs, it seemed that the time had come to begin to move basic generalist professional preparation to the master's level (AACN, 2002, 2003, 2007a). Early adopter programs began translating the curriculum template in the planning documents into the unique contexts of each school and cooperating nursing service provider(s). Variants were designed for both bachelor of science in nursing (BSN) and nonnurse college graduate applicants (AACN, 2007b). Accreditation and individual graduate certification reinforced curriculum similarity across institutions, and many hope that practice settings will adopt differentiated practice roles that will eventually support regulatory recognition (AACN, 2008, 2010). Concurrent with this consensus effort, the Carnegie Foundation for the Advancement of Teaching, as part of its multiyear comparative study of professional education in the United States, funded a study of education for nursing practice. Although this focuses more on the "delivery" of the curriculum, that is, on teaching-learning and the formation of nursing students, than on structures and content, the curricular implications both for basic programs and nurse teacher preparation are clear (Benner, Sulphen, Leonard, & Day, 2010).

Doctoral Programs

Educators began to focus on the hope of developing doctoral work in nursing in the midst of the chaotic educational diversity of the 1950s. The need for doctorally prepared faculty to teach master's students, who it was hoped would graduate and teach in the multiplying baccalaureate programs, fueled part of the interest in this topic. But for leaders already involved in higher education, it was painfully clear that nursing needed some capacity for its own research that would focus on questions related to nursing interventions to create a coherent body of tested knowledge and improve care.

Both Nursing Education Departments at TCCU and New York University (NYU) offered arrangements with their education departments for nurses to engage in doctoral level study before the 1950s; however, the numbers of graduates were small. TCCU revised its program in the 1950s but continued to grant the EdD. With Martha Rogers leading as chair of the Department of Nursing Education at NYU in 1954, the doctoral program was redirected to become a PhD in nursing. University of Pittsburgh established a PhD with a focus in pediatric or maternal nursing in 1954. In contrast to Martha Rogers's view that theory was the starting point that would lead to knowledge development in the "applied" field of nursing, Florence Erickson and Reva Rubin at Pittsburgh believed that extensive exposure to clinical phenomena, along with skilled faculty guidance, would develop a true nursing science (Parietti, 1979). In the West, in the early WICHE/WICHEN conversations, the temporary need for help from other disciplines for research training was posited as a mechanism to build nursing knowledge and a critical mass of investigators (WICHE, 1956). The journal *Nursing Research* became available in 1952 as a mechanism for systematic communication (Bunge, 1962).

In 1955, the Nursing Research Grants and Fellowship Program of the USPHS allocated $500,000 for research grants and $125,000 for fellowships, the first such funding for nursing. From 1955 to 1970, 156 nurses were supported by special pre-doctoral research fellowships for doctoral study, and from 1959 to 1968, 18 schools of nursing received federally funded faculty research development grants to stimulate research capacity. The nurse scientist graduate training programs, which provided federal incentive funding to disciplines outside of nursing to accept nurses as students and provided fellowships to the students, were designed to create a critical mass of faculty and a climate conducive to establishing doctoral programs in nursing (Grace, 1978). The program continued from 1962 to 1976 and funded more than 350 nurse trainees (Berthold, Tschudin, Schlotfeldt, Rogers, & Peplau, 1966; Murphy, 1981).

Three additional doctoral programs were established in the 1960s (Boston University, 1960, doctor of nursing science [DNS], psychiatric/mental health focus; University of California San Francisco [UCSF], 1964, DNS, multifocus; Catholic University, 1968, DNS, medical–surgical and psychiatric/mental health foci). The Boston program took a clinical immersion approach analogous to the University of Pittsburgh. UCSF's program was structured as a research degree, but identified clinical involvement as the base for knowledge development, influenced both by nurse faculty with a strong clinical identity and by the grounded theory perspectives of the several social scientists who were a part of the faculty.

A federally funded series of nine annual ANA-sponsored research conferences was initiated in 1965 and WICHEN sponsored the first of its annual Communicating Nursing Research conferences in 1968, thus creating space for face-to-face research exchange. Medical Literature Analysis and Retrieval System (MEDLARS) made its debut in 1964, the first in a series of databases that would aid dissemination. Essential components for school of nursing research centers were identified (Gunter, 1966). A series of three federally funded conferences in Kansas City, Kansas on nursing theory in 1969 to 1970 provided further opportunity to work through the divergent views of the relationships of theory, practice, and research to one another (Murphy, 1981).

In 1971, the Division of Nursing and the Nurse Scientist Graduate Training Committee (NSGTC) convened an invitational conference to address the type(s) of doctoral preparation. In this setting, Joseph Matarazzo, chair of the NSGTC, presented a paper arguing that nursing was ready as a discipline to launch PhD study, citing its body of knowledge and the qualifications of trainees (Matarazzo & Abdellah, 1971; Murphy, 1981). Comprehensive information about the state of nursing doctoral resources became available by the mid-1970s (Leininger, 1976) and by the late 1970s, national doctoral forums, open to schools with established programs, provided a mechanism for exchange of viewpoints about doctoral education. Three additional research journals began publication in 1978 (Gortner, 1991). "The discipline of nursing" (Donaldson & Crowley, 1978) was a milestone paper. It differentiated the discipline of nursing from the practice of nursing, but related the two as well, and proposed a productive interrelationship of research, theory, and practice. It shifted the terms of debate away from the dichotomous basic/applied categories.

The body of knowledge in nursing was still, relative to the old disciplines, rather modest in the late 1970s, but the progress in two decades had been amazing, and the infrastructure to support further development was substantial (Gortner & Nahm, 1977). Students were focusing their dissertation research on nursing clinical issues (Loomis, 1984). However, the DNS and PhD degrees, the two dominant degree titles, though differently named, were indistinguishable in their objectives and end products (Grace, 1978). Finally, themes related to the challenge of mentoring students who are dealing with what is not known and fostering "humanship" between students and faculty to encourage student growth were beginning to come to print at the end of this decade (Downs, 1978).

Fifteen additional doctoral programs opened their doors during the 1970s (Cleland, 1976; Parietti, 1979). From 1980 to 1989 the number of programs grew from 22 to 50, prompting editorial comment, "… as dandelions in spring, more and more doctoral programs are appearing" (Downs, 1984). Other observers surveying the situation recommended regional planning to sponsor joint programs, but conceded that the resources were in individual universities and states, and that the mechanisms for making such efforts were nonexistent. They predicted stormy waters for programs that launched without adequate internal and external supports in place (McElmurray, Krueger, & Parsons, 1982). At the end of the 1980s, doctoral educators were examining the balance between theory and research methods on the one hand and "knowledge" or "substance" in the curriculum (Downs, 1988).

Programs expanded from 50 to 70 from 1990 to 1999. By the early 1990s, as the research programs were more numerous and robust in the older and larger schools, greater emphasis on research team participation (Keller & Ward, 1993) and mentoring into the range of activities doctoral graduates became visible themes (Katefian, 1991; Meleis, 1992). Postdoctoral study became more feasible and attractive (Hinshaw & Lucas, 1993).

The perennial question from the 1960s to the 1980s, that is, whether nursing should adopt the PhD or the DNS, was answered by the hundreds of individual choices of applicants and the program choices of numerous schools: By 2000, only 12% of nursing doctoral programs conferred the DNS, or variants thereon (McEwen & Bechtel, 2000). Much less clear, however, was the difference between the two. Concerns about attention to "substance," that is, organized analysis of the body of nursing knowledge, the adequacy of research programs to provide student experience, and preparation for the teaching component of graduates' expected academic roles, occupied curriculum planners in research-focused doctoral programs at the end of the century (Anderson, 2000).

Questions about the desirability and feasibility of developing clinical or practice-focused doctoral programs in nursing were perennial but intermittent until the past decade (Mundinger et al., 2000), when the AACN in 2004 adopted a proposal that would move preparation for advanced practice nursing from the master's degree framework to the doctoral level by 2015 (AACN, 2004, 2009). Such programs are currently designed to articulate with both nursing baccalaureate and nursing masters (first professional degree and second). The four postbaccalaureate academic years include core areas for all students, as well as clinical specialty-focused study. The research-training component emphasizes the translation of research into practice, practice evaluation, and evidence-based practice improvement. Following from that, several possible forms of end-of-program practice-focused projects and project reporting formats demonstrate the student's synthesis and expertise, while laying the groundwork for future clinical scholarship (AACN, 2006). Currently (2014), there are 131 research-focused programs and 241 doctor of nursing practice (DNP) programs (AACN, 2014). What the long-term, steady state allocation of nursing's academic resources should be for the two types of programs is yet to be determined. And the development of combination programs, analogous to the MD-PhD, is also yet to be determined.

DISCUSSION QUESTIONS

1. The Nightingale model of nursing education was used to develop early nursing programs in the United States. What social and cultural phenomena were occurring in the United States during the 19th century that impacted the development of these, and subsequent, nursing education programs? Do similar phenomena impact nursing education today? If so, what are they and how do they impact education?
2. Associate degree programs were developed in the 1950s as a result of Mildred Montag's dissertation. Their intent was to prepare a different type of nurse than the one who was prepared at the baccalaureate level. That was not the reality however and debate continues (into the 21st century) about educational programs for entry-level nurses. What might nursing education, at both the associate degree and baccalaureate levels, look like today if Montag's plan for a different type of nurse had been followed?

LEARNING ACTIVITIES

STUDENT LEARNING ACTIVITY

Choose teams and debate the wisdom and feasibility of setting the doctoral degree as the minimum level of education for advanced practice nurses. Given hindsight gained from the efforts to transfer pre-licensure education into university settings, how would you go about assisting state boards of nursing with this transition?

NURSE EDUCATOR/FACULTY DEVELOPMENT ACTIVITY

Trace your school of nursing's history and link major curricular changes to events external to the nursing programs.

ACKNOWLEDGMENT

I would like to thank Dr. Marilyn Flood for providing such a rich discussion on which I was able to build.—*SME*

REFERENCES

Ahrens, W. D. (2002). Walt Whitman, nurse and poet. *Nursing, 32,* 43.

American Association of Colleges of Nursing. (1986). *Essentials of college and university education for professional nursing.* Washington, DC: Author.

American Association of Colleges of Nursing. (1996). *The essentials of master's education for advanced practice nursing.* Washington, DC: Author.

American Association of Colleges of Nursing. (2002). *Report of the task force on education and regulation for professional nursing practice I.* Retrieved from http://www.aacn .nche.edu/Education/edandreg02.htm

American Association of Colleges of Nursing. (2003). *Clinical nurse leader: Remarks delivered by AACN President Kathleen Ann Long.* Retrieved from http://www.aacn.nche .edu/cnl/history.htm

American Association of Colleges of Nursing. (2004). *AACN position statement on the practice doctorate in nursing October 2004.* Retrieved from http://www.aacn.nche.edu/ DNP/DNPPositionStatement.htm

American Association of Colleges of Nursing. (2006). *The essentials of doctoral education for advanced nursing practice.* Retrieved from http://www.aacn.nche.edu/DNP/pdf/ Essentials.pdf

American Association of Colleges of Nursing. (2007a). *Clinical nurse leader education models being implemented by schools of nursing.* Retrieved from http://www.aacn.nche. edu/cnl/pdf/CNLEdModels.pdf

American Association of Colleges of Nursing. (2007b). *White paper on the education and role of the clinical nurse leader February 2007.* Retrieved from http://www.aacn.nche. edu/Publications/WhitePapers/ClinicalNurseLeader07.pdf

American Association of Colleges of Nursing. (2008). *CNL frequently asked questions.* Retrieved from http://www.aacn.nche.edu/cnl/faq.htm

American Association of Colleges of Nursing. (2009). *Fact sheet: The doctor of nursing practice (DNP).* Retrieved from http://www.aacn.nche.edu/Media/FactSheets/dnp.htm

American Association of Colleges of Nursing. (2010). *Press release: Amid calls for more highly educated nurses, new AACN data show impressive growth in doctoral nursing programs.* Retrieved from http://www.aacn.nche.edu/Media/NewsReleases/2010/ enrollchanges.html

American Association of Colleges of Nursing. (2014). *DNP fact sheet.* Retrieved from http://www.aacn.nche.edu/media-relations/fact-sheets/dnp

American Nurses Association. (1965). *Educational preparation for nurse practitioners and assistants to nurses: A position paper.* New York, NY: Author.

Anderson, C. A. (2000). Current strengths and limitations of doctoral education in nursing: Are we prepared for the future? *Journal of Professional Nursing, 16,* 191–200.

Bacon, E. (1987). Curriculum development in nursing education, 1890-1952. *Nursing History Review, 2,* 50–66.

Benner, P., Sulphen, M., Leonard, V., & Day, I. (2010). *Educating nurses: A call for radical transformation.* San Francisco, CA: Jossey-Bass.

Berthold, J. S., Tschudin, M. S., Peplau, H. E., Schlotfeldt, R., & Rogers, M. E. (1966). A dialogue on approaches to doctoral preparation. *Nursing Forum, 5,* 48–104.

Bridgman, M. (1949). Consultant in collegiate nursing education. *American Journal of Nursing, 49,* 808.

Bridgman, M. (1953). *Collegiate education for nursing.* New York, NY: Russell Sage Foundation.

Brown, E. L. (1948). *Nursing for the future.* New York, NY: Russell Sage Foundation.

Brown, J. M. (1978). Master's education in nursing, 1945-1969. In J. Fitzpatrick (Ed.), *Historical studies in nursing* (pp. 104–130). New York, NY: Teachers College.

Bullough, B. (1976). Influences on role expansion. *American Journal of Nursing, 76,* 1476–1481.

Bullough, V., & Bullough, B. (1978). *The care of the sick: The emergence of modern nursing.* New York, NY: Prodist.

Bunge, H. L. (1962). The first decade of nursing research. *Nursing Research, 11,* 132–137.

Burns, P. G., Nishikawa, H. A., Weatherby, F., Forni, P. R., Moran, M., Allen, M. E., … Booten, D. A. (1993). Master's degree nursing education: State of the art. *Journal of Professional Nursing, 9,* 267–277.

Carnegie, M. E. (2005). Educational preparation of black nurses: A historical perspective. *The ABNF Journal, 16,* 6–7.

Cleland, V. (1976). Developing a doctoral program. *Nursing Outlook, 24,* 631–635.

Committee on the Grading of Nursing Schools. (1931). *Results of the first grading study of nursing schools.* Author.

Committee of the Six National Nursing Organizations on Unification of Accrediting Services. (1949). *Manual of accrediting educational programs in nursing.* Atlanta, GA: National Nursing Accrediting Service.

Davis, A. T. (1991, April). America's first school of nursing: The New England Hospital for Women and Children. *Journal of Nursing Education, 30,* 158–161.

Diers, D. (1976). A combined basic-graduate program for college graduates. *Nursing Outlook, 24,* 92–98.

Dodd, D. (2001). Nurses' residences: Using the built environment as evidence. *Nursing History Review, 9,* 185–206.

Donaldson, S., & Crowley, D. (1978). The discipline of nursing. *Nursing Outlook, 26,* 113–120.

Downs, F. S. (1978). Doctoral education in nursing: Future directions. *Nursing Outlook, 26,* 56–61.

Downs, F. S. (1984). Caveat emptor. *Nursing Research, 33,* 59.

Downs, F. S. (1988). Doctoral education: Our claim to the future. *Nursing Outlook, 36,* 18–20.

Egenes, K. J. (1998). An experiment in leadership: The rise of student government at Philadelphia General Hospital Training school, 1920–1930. *Nursing History Review, 6,* 71–84.

Eisenmann, L. (2000). Reconsidering a classic: Assessing the history of women's higher education a dozen years after Barbara Solomon. In R. Lowe (Ed.), *History of education: Major themes* (Vol. 1, pp. 411–442). New York, NY: Routledge & Falmer.

Elder, R. G., & Bullough, B. (1990). Nurse practitioners and clinical nurse specialists: Are the roles merging? *Clinical Nurse Specialist, 4,* 78–84.

Faddis, M. (1973). *A school of nursing comes of age.* Cleveland, OH: Howard Allen.

Fondiller, S. H. (1999). Nursing education in the 1960s: Revolt and reform. *Nursing and Health Care Perspectives, 20,* 182–183.

Fondiller, S. H. (2001). The advancement of baccalaureate and graduate nursing education: 1952–1972. *Nursing and Health Care Perspectives, 22,* 8–10.

Geolot, D. H. (1987). NP education: Observations from a national perspective. *Nursing Outlook, 35,* 132–135.

Goldmark, J. (1923). *Nursing and nursing education in the United States.* New York, NY: Macmillan.

Gortner, S. R. (1991). Historical development of doctoral programs: Shaping our expectations. *Journal of Professional Nursing, 7,* 45–53.

Gortner, S. R., & Nahm, H. (1977). An overview of nursing research in the United States. *Nursing Research, 26,* 10–33.

Grace, H. (1978). The development of doctoral education in nursing: An historical perspective. *Journal of Nursing Education, 17,* 17–27.

Graham, P. A. (1978). Expansion and exclusion: A history of women in higher education. *Signs, 3,* 759–773.

Gunter, L. M. (1966). Some problems in nursing care and services. In B. Bullough & V. Bullough (Eds.), *Issues in nursing* (pp. 152–156). New York, NY: Springer Publishing.

Haase, P. T. (1990). *The origins and rise of associate degree nursing education.* National League for Nursing. Durham, NC: Duke University.

Hanson, K. S. (1991). An analysis of the historical context of liberal education in nursing education from 1924 to 1939. *Journal of Professional Nursing, 7,* 341–350.

Harms, M. T. (1954). *Professional education in university schools of nursing.* Unpublished dissertation.

Hine, D. C. (1989). *Black women in white: Racial conflict and cooperation in the nursing profession, 1890–1950.* Indianapolis, IN: Indiana University.

Hinshaw, A. S., & Lucas, M. D. (1993). Postdoctoral education—a new tradition for nursing research. *Journal of Professional Nursing, 9,* 309.

James, J. W. (2002). Isabel Hampton and the professionalization of nursing in the 1890s. In E. D. Baer, P. O. D'Antonio, S. Rinker, & J. E. Lynaugh (Eds.), *Enduring issues in American nursing* (pp. 42–84). New York, NY: Springer Publishing.

Kalisch, P. A., & Kalisch, B. J. (1978). *The advance of American nursing.* Boston, MA: Little, Brown and Company.

Katefian, S. (1991). Doctoral preparation for faculty roles: Expectations and realities. *Journal of Professional Nursing, 7,* 105–111.

Keller, M. L., & Ward, S. E. (1993). Funding and socialization in the doctoral program at the University of Wisconsin-Madison. *Journal of Professional Nursing, 9,* 262–266.

Kelly, L. Y., & Joel, L. A. (1996). *The nursing experience: Trends, challenges, and transitions* (3rd ed.). New York, NY: McGraw-Hill.

Kenny, P. E. (2008, June). Men in nursing: A history of caring and contribution to the profession (Part 1). *Pennsylvania Nurse, 63,* 3–5.

LaRocco, S. (2011, February). The last of its kind: The all-male Alexian Brothers Hospital school of nursing. *American Journal of Nursing, 111,* 62–63.

Leininger, M. (1976). Doctoral programs for nurses: Trends, questions, and projected plans. *Nursing Research, 25,* 201–210.

Loomis, M. (1984). Emerging content in nursing: An analysis of dissertation abstracts and titles: 1976–1982. *Nursing Research, 33,* 113–199.

Lynaugh, J. E. (2002). Nursing's history: Looking backward and seeing forward. In E. D. Baer, P. O. D'Antonio, S. Rinker, & J. E. Lynaugh (Eds.), *Enduring issues in American nursing* (pp. 10–24). New York, NY: Springer Publishing.

Lynaugh, J. E., & Brush, B. L. (1996). *American nursing: From hospitals to health systems.* Cambridge, MA: Blackwell.

Major events in nursing and nursing education. Part 1: 1872 through the Great Depression. Retrieved from nursingeducationhistory.org

Matarazzo, J., & Abdellah, F. (1971). Doctoral education for nurses in the United States. *Nursing Research, 20,* 404–414.

McElmurray, B. J., Kreuger, J. C., & Parsons, L. C. (1982). Resources for graduate education: A report of a survey of forty states in the midwest, west and southern regions. *Nursing Research, 31,* 1–10.

McEwen, M., & Bechtel, G. A. (2000). Characteristics of nursing doctoral programs in the United States. *Journal of Professional Nursing, 16,* 282–292.

Meleis, A. I. (1992). On the way to scholarship: From master's to doctorate. *Journal of Professional Nursing, 8,* 328–334.

Mundinger, M. O., Cook, S. S., Lenz, E. R., Piacentini, K., Auerhahn, C., & Smith, J. (2000). Assuring quality and access in advanced practice nursing: A challenge to nurse educators. *Journal of Professional Nursing, 16,* 322–329.

Murphy, J. F. (1981). Doctoral education in, of, and for nursing: An historical analysis. *Nursing Outlook, 29,* 645–649.

National Commission for the Study of Nursing and Nursing Education. (1970). *An abstract for action.* New York, NY: McGraw Hill.

National Commission for the Study of Nursing and Nursing Education. (1971). *Nurse clinician and physician's assistant: The relationship between two emerging practitioner concepts.* Rochester, NY: Author.

National League of Nursing Education. (1917). *Standard curriculum for schools of nursing.* Baltimore, MD: Waverly.

National League of Nursing Education. (1927). *A curriculum for schools of nursing.* New York, NY: National League of Nursing Education.

National League of Nursing Education. (1937). *A curriculum guide for schools of nursing.* New York, NY: National League of Nursing Education.

National Nursing Accrediting Service Postgraduate Board of Review. (1951). Some problems identified. *American Journal of Nursing, 51,* 337–338.

Obituary. (1940). Mrs. Clara S. Weeks Shaw. *American Journal of Nursing, 40,* 356.

Palmer, I. S. (1985). Origins of education for nurses. *Nursing Forum, 22,* 102–110.

Parietti, E. S. (1979). *Development of doctoral education for nurses: An historical survey.* Ann Arbor, MI: University Microfilms International.

Petry, L. (1937). TBA. *American Journal of Nursing, 37,* 287–297.

Petry, L. (1943). U.S. Cadet Nurse Corps. *American Journal of Nursing, 43,* 704–708.

Petry, L. (1949). We hail an important first. *American Journal of Nursing, 49,* 630–633.

Plummer, E. M., & Phelan, J. J. (1976). College graduates in nursing: A retrospective look. *Nursing Outlook, 24,* 99–102.

Pollitt, P., Streeter, C., & Walsh, C. (2011). *Nurses journey. Minority nurse,* 1-6. Retrieved from http://www.minoritynurse.com/article/nurses-journey#sthash.cTtXookM.dpuf

Reid, K. B. (2011). The clinical nurse leader: Point of care safety clinical. *Online Journal of Issues in Nursing, 16*(3), 1–12.

Reitt, B. B. (1987). *The first 25 years of the Southern Council on Collegiate Education for Nursing.* Atlanta, GA: Southern Council on Collegiate Education for Nursing.

Reverby, S. (1984). "Neither for the drawing room nor for the kitchen": Private duty nursing in Boston, 1873–1914. In J. W. Leavitt (Ed.), *Women and Health in America* (pp. 454–466). Madison, WI: University of Wisconsin.

Reverby, S. M. (1987). *Ordered to care: The dilemma of American nursing, 1850–1945.* New York, NY: Cambridge University.

Rines, A. (1977). Associate degree education: History, development, and rationale. *Nursing Outlook, 25,* 496–501.

Robb, I. H. (1907). *Educational standards for nurses.* Cleveland, OH: E. C. Koeckert.

Roberts, M. M. (1954). *American nursing: History and interpretation.* New York, NY: Macmillan.

Robinson, T. M., & Perry, P. M. (2001). Cadet nurse stories: The call for and response of women during World War II. Indianapolis, IN: Center Press.

Ruby, J. (1999, January). History of higher education: Educational reform and the emergence of the nursing professorate. *Journal of Nursing Education, 38,* 23–27.

Scott, J. (1972). Federal support for nursing education, 1964–1972. *American Journal of Nursing, 72,* 1855–1860.

Sheahan, D. A. (1980). *The social origins of American nursing and its movement into the university: a microscopic approach.* Ann Arbor, MI: University Microfilms.

Solomon, B. (1985). *In the company of educated women.* New Haven, CT: Yale University.

Styles, M. M. (1989). *On specialization in nursing: Toward a new empowerment.* Kansas City, MO: American Nurses Foundation.

Trossman, S. (2009). APRN regulatory model continues to advance. *The American Nurse, 41*(6), 12–13.

Tyack, D. (1974). *The one best system: A history of American urban education.* Cambridge, MA: Harvard University.

Veysey, L. R. (1965). *The emergence of the American university.* Chicago, IL: University of Chicago.

Vogel, M. J. (1980). *The invention of the modern hospital: Boston 1870–1930.* Chicago, IL: University of Chicago.

Wall, B. M. (2009, May/June). Religion and gender in a men's hospital and school of nursing, 1866–1969. *Nursing Research, 58,* 158–165.

Washington, L. C. (2012). Preserving the history of black nurses. *Minority Nurse,* 28–31.

Weeks-Shaw, C. (1902). *A text-book of nursing: For the use of training schools, families, and private students* (3rd ed.). New York, NY: D. Appleton.

Western Interstate Commission for Higher Education. (1956). *Toward shared planning in western nursing education.* Boulder, CO: Author.

Western Interstate Commission on Higher Education. (1967). *Defining clinical content: Graduate programs, 1–4.* Boulder, CO: Author.

Wolf, G. A. (1990). Clinical nurse specialists: The second generation. *Journal of Nursing Administration, 20,* 7–8.

Wu, C.-Y., & Connelly, C. (1992). Profile of nonnurse college graduates in accelerated baccalaureate nursing programs. *Journal of Professional Nursing, 8,* 35–40.

Curriculum Development and Approval Processes in Changing Educational Environments

Patsy L. Ruchala

OBJECTIVES

Upon completion of Chapter 2, the reader will be able to:

1. Analyze facilitators for and barriers to effective curriculum development and redesign
2. Evaluate the effectiveness of a nursing curriculum
3. Apply knowledge of potential barriers to curricular innovations in obtaining approvals for innovative curricular redesign
4. Evaluate the impact of regulatory and accreditation agencies in the development and evaluation of nursing curriculum

OVERVIEW

Faculty members have ultimate responsibility for curriculum development, ongoing evaluation, and redesign; and must work together to determine what best practices must be implemented in nursing education so that students master the knowledge and skills necessary for them to become practicing nurses. The innate complexity of nursing education, the need for collaboration with other disciplines within the college or university, the ever-changing and complex health care systems, and the requirements of regulatory and accreditation agencies can position curriculum development and redesign as a daunting process. The use of technology has exploded in both education and health care settings. We are encountering a generation of students who embrace technology not only in education but also as ordinary methods of communication and social networking, and their expectations for the use of technology at an advanced level may far exceed the capabilities of many nursing faculty. In addition to navigating the internal approval processes for curriculum approval, meeting the requirements of regulatory and accrediting agencies can also impact the approaches taken when developing or redesigning nursing curricula. This chapter provides an overview of the preparation and support needed for curriculum development/change, issues, and challenges that can arise from and impact the curriculum development process, innovations in curriculum development, and approvals and accreditations related to nursing curriculum.

THE PROCESS OF CURRICULUM DEVELOPMENT

Preparation and Support for Curricular Change

Nursing education has evolved using a variety of theories from other disciplines as well as newer middle range theories developed specifically for their application to nursing practice. New roles for nurses have been developed to meet the needs of the practice setting as well as the increasing demand for more emphasis on education, primary prevention, and management of chronic diseases (American Association of Colleges of Nursing [AACN], 2013; Institute of Medicine [IOM], 2010; Pew Health Professions Commission, 1995). The need for change in health professions education is overwhelming, with an emphasis on evidence-based practice, quality improvement approaches, safety standards, competency frameworks, informatics, and interprofessional education (Andre & Barnes, 2010; Callen & Lee, 2009; Phillips et al., 2013; Spencer, 2012; Stephens-Lee, Der-Fa, & Wilson, 2013; Sullivan, 2010). Given the knowledge explosion in science and the emphasis on major reform of health care education, it is no wonder that Giddens and colleagues (2008) point out that curriculum redesign in nursing "is an overwhelming undertaking."

The support of both faculty and administration is imperative for curriculum change. According to Billings and Halstead (2012), curriculum change is inevitable. The need for curriculum change may be a result of community pressure, policy, or accreditation changes, programmatic funding, personnel changes, or the simple acknowledgement that the existing curriculum is no longer effective for current and future students. For effective change to take place, faculty must realize the need for change. This realization, however, may be more apparent to some faculty members and less apparent to others.

In addition to recognizing and embracing the need for curriculum change, faculty members need the knowledge and skills to engage in this endeavor. The engagement of faculty in ongoing curriculum development and change should begin with orientation to the university or college. It is routinely expected that faculty will update courses with cutting edge information each time a course is taught. Individual course updating over time, however, may impact the overall curriculum, resulting in "content gaps." Faculty members benefit from serving on their school's curriculum committee and engaging in ongoing dialogue about and evaluation of the curriculum with their faculty colleagues. New faculty or faculty who have not engaged in curriculum redesign benefit from mentoring by faculty with more experience in curriculum processes (Hagler, White, & Morris, 2011; Huybrecht, Loeckx, Quaey-haegens, DeTobel, & Mistiaen, 2011; Sawatzky & Enns, 2009; Slimmer, 2012). Support for curriculum change includes administrative assurance of needed resources: physical space, secretarial support, workload considerations, expert consultants, and internal administrative assurance and encouragement that the work toward curricular change is valued and needed by the organization and, most importantly, for successful student outcomes. Successful curriculum change requires support from all levels of the organization, including students. Students bring a unique perspective to curriculum committee discussions, particularly when faculty members are charged to design a rigorous program while creating an environment conducive to students' learning preferences (Mangold, 2007; Moch, Cronje, & Branson, 2010). In a study of faculty perceptions of implementation of curriculum change, Powell-Cope, Hughes, Sedlak, and Nelson (2008) found that administrators, other faculty, and students who were "champions for curricular change" were also identified as facilitators for successful implementation of the new curriculum.

Curriculum development and redesign always begin at the level of the school curriculum committee. This may be a formal committee within the school or for very small schools, it may consist of the entire nursing faculty. In most institutions of higher education, curriculum development and redesign must go through an extensive, multilevel approval process. Despite the number of levels in the approval process, a proposal for curriculum approval should be completed with the expectation that it will eventually be sent to the highest review body in the institution, keeping in mind all of the preceding levels of approval and the requirements and appropriate paperwork for routing of the proposal through each level. Although this process will vary at every institution, Figure 2.1 depicts an example for sequencing. Consideration should also be given as to whether or not this is a proposal for a graduate-level curricular change. If so, there may be another level of approval that would involve the graduate faculty of the school and/or the graduate school within the college or university. No matter what the individual process, completeness, accuracy, and acceptable institutional formatting are extremely important to successfully navigate all levels of curriculum approval.

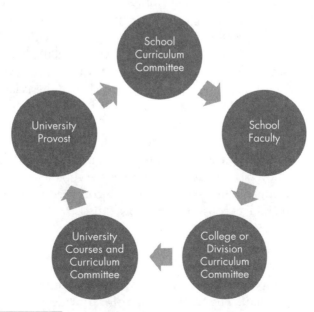

FIGURE 2.1   Example of curriculum approval process sequencing.

ISSUES RELATED TO CURRICULAR DEVELOPMENT OR REDESIGN

Faculty Development

Curriculum development is in itself a faculty development activity (Iwasiw, Goldenberg, & Andrusyszyn, 2009; Slimmer, 2012). To be successful in developing and implementing curricular change, Billings and Halstead (2012) indicate that faculty members who understand the problems inherent in the current curriculum and who can effectively evaluate strategies for solving the current problems should be the group initially involved in the change. Faculty members who have less experience in curriculum development may need to acquire the knowledge and skills necessary to engage in curriculum work. Working with more experienced faculty, engaging in group discussion and debate, knowing that their contributions to the process will be heard and valued, and providing ongoing administrative support are all part of mentoring less experienced faculty to learn the process for curriculum change.

Budgetary Constraints

Schmitt (2002) and Tanner (2004) postulate that the cost efficiency of clinical nursing education has not been properly assessed, yet nursing has always been considered one of the more costly programs in institutions of higher education. In recent years, the state of the national economy had a significant impact on all aspects of higher education, including nursing. Allen (2008) and Hinshaw (2008) both observed that the retirement of older faculty and the shortage of nurse educators stretch human, fiscal, and physical resources in nursing education. While the need for more nurses keeps growing, funding for many nursing programs has been significantly impacted. When developing or redesigning nursing curricula, assessment of current and future resources is crucial. Budgetary constraints in hiring faculty and other resources, such as the availability and use of high-fidelity simulation, will have a major impact on curriculum design/change and implementation of the curriculum (Adams, 2009; Bargagliotti, 2009; Lapkin & Levett-Jones, 2011; Nehring, 2008; Reese, Jeffries, & Engum, 2010). In 2014, over 53,000 qualified applicants were turned away from U.S. nursing schools due to insufficient numbers of faculty, clinical sites, classroom space, clinical preceptors, and budget constraints (AACN, 2014). Budget shortfalls and economic declines resulted in scarcer resources available for universities and colleges to support nursing programs, forcing programs to be much more creative in determining strategies to sustain nursing education. The creation of local and regional partnerships with nurse employers, foundations, and other stakeholders as a sustainability strategy needed by the nursing profession is highly encouraged in the current era of health care reform and budget constraints (AACN, 2012).

Amount of Curricular Content

Another issue impacting curriculum development and change is the management of curricular content. The nursing literature provides an overwhelming amount of evidence indicating that faculty and students are besieged with content (AACN, 2009; Giddens et al., 2008; Mailloux, 2011; Powell-Cope et al., 2008). As the information explosion in health sciences education continues to grow, an increasing amount of content is deemed essential to include in all nursing curricula (AACN, 2008; Accreditation Commission for Education in Nursing [ACEN], 2013a; Skiba, 2012). One example of essential knowledge content to include in nursing curricula relates to a series of reports issued by the IOM (Greiner & Knebel, 2003) that generated a great deal of attention to the need to improve the quality and safety of health care delivery. This led to dramatic changes in the practice of nursing, medicine, and other health disciplines. As nursing practice embraced the focus on improved quality and safety, it became clear that graduating nurses were missing critical competencies in this area. The result was a major national initiative, Quality Safety Education for Nurses, centered on patient safety and quality topics, with a primary goal to address the challenge of preparing future nurses with the knowledge, skills, and attitudes necessary to continuously improve the quality and safety of the health care systems in which they will work (Sullivan, 2010). As the amount of essential knowledge and content continues to increase, there seems, however, to be an inherent faculty perception that they must teach everything they possibly can to their students in the minutest of detail. Consequently, "content saturation" is a major problem in many nursing curricula. Giddens and Brady (2007) surmise that content saturation may be directly related to how faculty teach and that faculty should learn how to teach conceptually and, subsequently, minimize their emphasis on the *amount* of content students must learn.

Technology

Incorporating technology into the curriculum is a must to educate nurses in the 21st century (Skiba, 2012; Spencer, 2012). The advance of technology into our personal and professional lives marched into the arena of higher education, and the lecture method as the gold standard for teaching is rapidly being replaced by technology. The type of technology available for the classroom ranges from very low to very high fidelity (Thompson & Skiba, 2008). The methods of curriculum delivery and the use of technology must be addressed in any curriculum development or redesign, including the extent that technology will be used, resources to obtain and sustain technology, and faculty development to use technology effectively. For example, high-fidelity simulators are increasingly being used as an adjunct or replacement to some of the clinical experiences in nursing programs (Nehring, 2008; Reese et al., 2010). However, use of high-fidelity simulation requires a significant up-front investment as well as the cost for ongoing care, use and replacement of simulators, and staff for simulation centers. In addition, to effectively use high-fidelity simulation, a significant investment must be made for faculty development to use the equipment and for incorporation into the curriculum.

Hartman, Dziuban, and Brophy-Ellison (2007) identified a number of changes to which faculty must adapt as a result of diffusing technology into teaching and learning:

• Faculty who are the experts in their respective disciplines may experience a "balance-of-power shift" when confronted with technologically savvy students who know more about specific technologies than they do.

• Net Generation students use a range of technologies and information sources that are often unfamiliar to their faculty. When faculty communicate through technology, they are likely to use e-mail. Net Generation students communicate with peers through instant messages (IMs) and cell phone text messaging.
• Faculty are reporting a sharp decline in the quality of students' writing, which some attribute to the increasing popularity of IM and text messaging.
• Faculty see students as individual learners and regard students who complete assignments with others as cheaters. Net Generation students value social networking, working in groups, and experiential learning.
• Technology caused a shift in the way faculty use their time. Traditionally, faculty would be in class, their offices, or their labs, or they would be off campus and inaccessible to students. Students now expect faculty to be accessible via e-mail almost any hour of the day or night and to respond to e-mails within minutes.
• Faculty members think of technology as technology. Students think of technology as environment.
• A number of social networking and resource-sharing sites appeared over the past few years, including Facebook, Myspace, Flickr, YouTube, LiveJournal, Twitter, and Second Life. Students are using these sites as the nexus of their social and even academic universe. Faculty are beginning to use these sites as a means of getting to know their students, as a rapid and reliable way to reach students, and as a method for sharing faculty-produced and student-produced content.

Faculty Issues

The shortage of nurse educators has been discussed as an issue related to curriculum development and change, yet several other faculty issues arise that can impact curriculum development or redesign. In a study designed to determine nursing faculty perceptions regarding implementing a new curriculum, one of the two barriers determined by Powell-Cope et al. (2008) was the challenge of working with faculty colleagues who insisted on keeping the old curricular paradigm. Inherent in curriculum development and redesign is the human dimension of the nursing faculty and, subsequently, the interpersonal dynamics associated with every aspect of curriculum redesign.

Fear of and resistance to change are the most influential barriers to progress in curriculum development and redesign. While not an exhaustive list by any means, the following have been identified as barriers to successful curriculum development and redesign:

1. Differing faculty values about nursing education
2. Fear of losing control of certain aspects of the curriculum
3. Differing views about what needs to be done to the curriculum
4. Lack of embracing the need for curricular change
5. Uncertainty about how to begin the change process
6. Lack of resources
7. Desire to be vindictive so the curriculum committee chair, leader of curriculum change, or program dean or director looks bad

8. Lack of rewards
9. Feeling that the curricular change process is too overwhelming given the current resources or time constraints (Billings & Halstead, 2012; Cash, Daines, Doyle, & von Tettenborn, 2009; Iwasiw et al., 2009)

The work of faculty with the curriculum must take into account not only a rapidly changing health care environment, but also the pressures to maintain currency in both clinical expertise and teaching technologies (Gaza & Shellenbarger, 2010). Cash et al. (2009) identified these pressures as "tensions (that) underpin curriculum and the ways in which knowledge is constructed through the framing of educational (including clinical) experiences" (pp. 318–319). Most nursing faculty members are no longer employed in health care facilities, and, in many instances, this leads to an "education-practice gap." Although clinical supervision of students helps some faculty stay connected to practice, many nursing faculty find it challenging to balance their full-time roles as academicians with the need for ongoing clinical practice. Faculty may find it difficult to access clinical practice experiences even on a part-time basis to maintain current practice knowledge and skills, as complex health care systems and practices, cost implications, and risk management considerations further complicate faculty practice arrangements.

Cultural competence is identified as a critical component of the nursing curriculum. However, not only do students need to be versed in how to care for patients from many cultural backgrounds, due to the increased globalization of the nursing profession, faculty also needs to practice cultural competence in its teaching and in curriculum development. Over the past two or three decades, international experiences in higher education have become increasingly more commonplace. Cardwell, Hongyan, and Harding (2010) assert that nearly 2 million students worldwide are involved in formal education outside of their own country and that this figure is likely to reach 5 million over the next 20 years.

Implementation is a critical component to curriculum development and/or redesign. To ensure that the curriculum is implemented as planned, intense oversight is necessary. Rapid changes in technology and economics, along with the ever-increasing information explosion and the need for multiculturalism, dictate that ongoing review and redesign of nursing curricula must occur. One of the greatest challenges is to resist the temptation to make changes to the new curriculum too quickly before it has been thoroughly evaluated for effectiveness.

Innovations in Nursing Education

A major aspect of the nursing curriculum development and redesign process is the consideration of current and future resources and needs for implementation, including the nature of the health care environment in which future nurses will work. It is widely noted in the literature that due to the complexities of today's health care system and health care delivery, transformation of nursing education is a necessity (AACN, 2008; Bellack, 2008; Coonan, 2008; Greiner & Knebel, 2003; IOM, 2010; Phillips et al., 2013). Our traditional methods of nursing education need to give way to more innovative approaches to prepare graduates for the nursing practice of the future. The National Council of State Boards of Nursing (NCSBN) (2009a) defined innovation as "a dynamic, systematic process that envisions new approaches to nursing education." Innovations reported in the nursing litera-ture include the use of dedicated education units for clinical education (Moscato, Miller, Logsdon, & Chorpenning, 2007), pedagogical approaches such as "narra-tive pedagogy" and "deliberate discussion" (Brown, Kirkpatrick, & Mangum, 2008; Goodin & Stein, 2008), high-fidelity simulation as an adjunct to or replacement for clinical experiences (Nehring, 2008; Reese et al., 2010), and use of simulation and virtual reality to extend faculty (Cleary, McBride, McClure, & Reinhard, 2009). Other innovations in nursing education include partnering with clinical agencies or with other educational institutions to form a consortium for sharing resources for the delivery of nursing education.

While innovation in nursing education is a must to meet the future need for nurses and the demands of the health care environment, when planning an innovative curriculum, faculty should be aware of potential hindrances that may prolong or even become barriers to the approval and implementation of innovations. First and foremost are the barriers that educational institutions impose upon themselves such as multilevel institutional hierarchies and lengthy committee processes to obtain approval of curriculum changes (Bellack, 2008; Coonan, 2008). As a practice profession, nursing education's relationship with health care institutions is critical. Practice settings and educational institutions may not see eye to eye on innovative teaching strategies, and barriers may stem from centralized power bases and linear thinking found in practice (Unter-schuetz, Hughes, Nienhauser, Weberg, & Jackson, 2008). In addition, there may be real or perceived regulatory barriers to innovative nursing education. In 2008, the NCSBN established the Innovations in Education Regulation Com-mittee. The charge to this committee was to identify real and perceived regula-tory barriers to education innovations and to develop a regulatory model for innovative education proposals (NCSBN, 2009b). Potential regulatory barriers to innovative nursing education may include specified numbers of clinical or didactic hours in the nursing curriculum, faculty–student ratios, full- and part-time ratios of faculty, and simulation limitations (NCSBN, 2009a). Advance knowledge of potential barriers may assist faculty in negotiating with internal or external stakeholders to overcome these obstacles and create a curriculum that is innovative, resource-friendly, and forward-thinking in educating nurses for the future. Thinking about the consequences of and compliance with the individual state nurse practice act and state nursing regulations before planning innovative curricular changes is very important (Hargreaves, 2008). It is always advisable to consult with the respective state board at the beginning stages of planning for any innovative teaching strategy.

Program Approvals and Accreditation

After all institutional approvals are obtained for nursing program curriculum development or redesign, external approvals and accreditation processes are criti-cal for implementation and ongoing demonstration of quality and effectiveness.

State Boards of Nursing

Boards of Nursing are state governmental agencies that were established over 100 years ago to protect the public's health welfare. This is accomplished by overseeing and ensuring the safe practice of nursing through regulation of nursing practice. Each state determines the administrative responsibilities and oversight of the respective Board of Nursing (NCSBN, 2014). While most states in the United States only regulate entry-level nursing education programs, some states regulate advanced-practice programs. The NCSBN (2011) identified seven different models that are used by state boards of nursing across the country to approve nursing education programs (Table 2.1). Specific state board regulations for initial and ongoing approval of nursing programs vary, but generally include regulations related to program length, curriculum, number of didactic and/or clinical hours, qualifications of the nursing faculty and the program administrator, program resources, faculty–student ratios, and, more recently, high-fidelity simulation (NCSBN, 2009b; Savers, 2010).

TABLE 2.1   THE SEVEN APPROVAL PROCESSES USED BY BOARDS OF NURSING FOR PRELICENSURE NURSING EDUCATION PROGRAMS

1. Boards of Nursing are independent of the National Nursing Accreditors	These Boards of Nursing approve/accredit nursing programs separately and distinctly from the national nursing accrediting bodies. Initial approval processes are conducted before accreditation takes place.
2. Collaboration of Boards of Nursing and National Nursing Accreditors	Boards of Nursing share reports with the national nursing accrediting bodies, and/or make visits with them, sharing information. However, the final decision about approval is made by the Board of Nursing, independent of decisions by the national nursing accreditors. Initial approval processes are conducted before accreditation takes place.
3. Accept National Nursing Accreditation as meeting State Board of Nursing approval	Boards of Nursing accept national nursing accreditation as meeting state approvals, though they continue to approve those schools that don't voluntarily get accredited. The Board of Nursing is available for assistance with statewide issues; Boards of Nursing retain the ability to make emergency visits to schools of nursing, if requested to do so by a party reporting serious problems; and the Board of Nursing has the authority to close a school of nursing, either on the advice of national nursing accreditors or after making an emergency visit with evidence that the school of nursing is causing harm to the public. Initial approval processes are conducted before accreditation takes place.
4. Accept National Nursing Accreditation as meeting State Board of Nursing approval with further documentation	Similar to Process 3, these Boards of Nursing accept national nursing accreditation as meeting state approvals, but they may require more documentation, such as complaints, NCLEX results, excessive student attrition, excessive faculty turnover, or lack of clinical sites. Initial approval processes are conducted before accreditation takes place.

(continued)

TABLE 2.1	THE SEVEN APPROVAL PROCESSES USED BY BOARDS OF NURSING FOR PRELICENSURE NURSING EDUCATION PROGRAMS (*continued*)
5. Boards of Nursing require National Nursing Accreditation	Boards of Nursing require that their nursing programs become accredited by a national nursing accreditation body and will use Process 3 or 4 to approve them. Initial approval processes are conducted before accreditation takes place.
6. Boards of Nursing have no jurisdiction over programs that have national nursing accreditation	Nonaccredited programs are only initially approved by the Board of Nursing and under specific statutory requirements.
7. Boards of Nursing are not involved with the approval system at all	The Board of Nursing is not given the authority to approve nursing programs; this is done by another state/jurisdiction authority.

Adapted from NCSBN (2011).

ACCREDITATION

The Council for Higher Education Accreditation (2013) defines accreditation as a "... review of the quality of higher education institutions and programs. In the United States, accreditation is a major way that students, families, government officials, and the press know that an institution or program provides a quality education." According to Eaton (2009), accreditation is a "trust-based, standards-based, evidence-based, judgment-based, peer-based process" (p. 5). Institutional accreditation is conducted by regional, national faith-based, national private career, and/or programmatic accreditors. The roles of accreditation include ensuring quality, access to federal and state funds (i.e., student aid and other federal programs), engendering private sector confidence, and easing transfer of courses and programs among colleges and universities (Eaton, 2009). Higher education accreditation is a voluntary nongovernmental process and is complementary to federal and state mechanisms that promote quality in higher education. The U.S. Department of Education grants recognition to accrediting agencies that meet its criteria (Commission on Collegiate Nursing Education [CCNE], 2009).

Although steps in the accreditation process differ among agencies, typical steps in the process include:

- The accrediting agency establishes minimum accreditation standards.
- The institution or program seeking accreditation prepares a self-study.
- Volunteer representatives of the accrediting agency conduct site visit for on-site peer review of the institution or program applying for accreditation.
- The accrediting agency takes action regarding whether or not the institution or program meets the established accreditation standards.
- The accrediting agency publishes a list of institutions or programs accredited by the respective agency.
- There is ongoing monitoring of the institution or program for continuing compliance with the established accreditation standards (CCNE, 2009; Eaton, 2009).

Two national accrediting agencies currently provide accreditation for nursing education programs: the ACEN and the CCNE. The Commission for Nursing Education Accreditation (C-NEA) is a new accrediting division of the National League for Nursing (NLN) that is currently under development. Nursing education programs have, however, been accredited since the founding of the American Society of Superintendents of Training Schools for Nurses in 1893. This organization became the National League of Nursing Education (NLNE) in 1912, and in 1917 the NLNE published *A Standard Curriculum for Schools of Nursing* (Kalisch & Kalisch, 1978). In the early 1950s, the NLN evolved from the merging of the NLNE, the Association of Schools of Nursing, and the National Organization for Public Health Nursing. The NLN provided accrediting services until 1997, when the National League for Nursing Accrediting Commission (NLNAC) was formed as an arm of the NLN specifically for accreditation activities. In 2013, the NLNAC changed its name to the ACEN (2013b). ACEN accredits various types of nursing programs: practical nursing, diploma nursing, associate degree nursing, baccalaureate degree nursing and master's degree nursing, post-master's certificate, and clinical doctorate.

In 1995, the AACN appointed the AACN Task Force on Accreditation to examine the feasibility of AACN assuming accreditation activities for baccalaureate and higher degree nursing programs. Subsequently, in 1998 the CCNE was developed as an autonomous accrediting agency for baccalaureate and higher degree nursing programs. By the summer of 2008, 78% of institutions with baccalaureate and/or master's degree nursing programs in the United States were either accredited by or held new applicant status with CCNE. In the fall of 2008, CCNE conducted its first onsite evaluations of doctor of nursing practice programs (CCNE, 2009).

SUMMARY

Curriculum development and ongoing evaluation and redesign are core activities for nursing faulty. Determining how to best facilitate the process, working together as a group to identify and overcome potential barriers inherent in any nursing faculty, and being innovative to meet the challenges of educating future generations of practicing nurses are key elements for successful curriculum development or redesign. Ongoing challenges of the increasing volume of information in nursing and health sciences, the trend toward developing interdisciplinary curricula, the faculty–student gap in technological savvy, and meeting the requirements of regulatory and accrediting agencies are all important issues to address as we develop nursing curricula for the 21st century.

DISCUSSION QUESTIONS

1. What are ways in which nursing faculty can be motivated to engage in curriculum redesign?
2. What data can be used to convince faculty for the need for curriculum redesign?
3. What real or perceived barriers do regulatory agencies impose on curricular development or redesign?

LEARNING ACTIVITIES

STUDENT LEARNING ACTIVITIES

1. Review your State Board of Nursing regulations for nursing education programs. Describe how these regulations impact the process of curriculum development or redesign in a nursing program in your state.
2. As a small group activity, explore the process for student involvement in curriculum development and/or redesign in your program. In what ways would you change the current level of student involvement in curriculum development?
3. Determine how new or revised curricula of nursing programs are reviewed and acted upon by your local State Board of Nursing. Attend a State Board of Nursing meeting and describe how the process of nursing program approval relates to the board's mission of protection of the public's health welfare in your state.

NURSE EDUCATOR/FACULTY DEVELOPMENT ACTIVITIES

1. Review your curriculum to ensure incorporation of accreditation standards.
2. Describe two innovations in curriculum and/or teaching strategies for implementation of your curriculum. What constraints or barriers can you identify that would delay or prohibit you from implementing these innovations?
3. Develop a list of five key facilitators and five key barriers to curriculum development and/or redesign in your school of nursing. How can you as faculty assist your school or other faculty members to overcome the barriers you have identified?
4. Compare the benefits of having your baccalaureate or master's program accredited by the ACEN or by the CCNE.

REFERENCES

Accreditation Commission for Education in Nursing. (2013a). *ACEN accreditation manual.* Atlanta, GA: Author.

Accreditation Commission for Education in Nursing. (2013b). *Important update from ACEN.* Retrieved from http://acenursing.org

Adams, L. T. (2009). Nursing shortage solutions and America's economic recovery. *Nursing Education Perspectives, 30*(6), 349.

Allen, L. (2008). The nursing shortage continues as faculty shortage grows. *Nursing Economics, 26*(1), 35–40.

American Association of Colleges of Nursing. (2008). *The essentials of baccalaureate education for professional nursing practice.* Washington, DC: Author.

American Association of Colleges of Nursing. (2009). *The essentials of baccalaureate education for professional nursing practice: Faculty tool kit.* Washington, DC: Author.

American Association of Colleges of Nursing. (2012). *AACN-AONE task force on academic-practice partnerships: Guiding principles.* Washington, DC: Author.

American Association of Colleges of Nursing. (2013). *Competencies and curricular expectations for clinical nurse leader education and practice.* Washington, DC: Author.

American Association of Colleges of Nursing. (2014). (Press Release). *Enrollment growth slows at U.S. nursing schools despite calls for a more highly educated nursing workforce.*

Washington, DC: Author. Retrieved from www.aacn.nche.edu/news/articles/2014/slow-enrollment

Andre, K., & Barnes, L. (2010). Creating a 21st century nursing workforce: Designing a bachelor of nursing program in response to the health reform agenda. *Nurse Education Today, 30*(3), 258–263.

Bargagliotti, L. (2009). State funding for higher education and RN placement rates by state: A case for nursing by the numbers in state legislatures. *Nursing Outlook, 57*(5), 274–280.

Bellack, J. P. (2008). Letting go of the rock. *Journal of Nursing Education, 47*(10), 439–440.

Billings, D. M., & Halstead, J. A. (2012). *Teaching in nursing* (4th ed.). St. Louis, MO: Elsevier Saunders.

Brown, S. T., Kirkpatrick, M. K., & Mangum, D. (2008). A review of narrative pedagogy strategies to transform traditional nursing education. *Journal of Nursing Education, 47*(6), 283–286.

Callen, B. L., & Lee, J. L. (2009). Ready for the world: Preparing nursing students for tomorrow. *Journal of Professional Nursing, 25*(5), 292–298.

Cardwell, E. S., Hongyan, L., & Harding, T. (2010). Encompassing multiple moral paradigms: A challenge for nursing educators. *Nursing Ethics, 17*(2), 189–199.

Cash, P. A., Daines, D., Doyle, R. M., & von Tettenborn, L. (2009). Quality workplace environments for nurse educators: Implications for recruitment and retention. *Nursing Economics, 27*(5), 315 321.

Cleary, B. L., McBride, A. B., McClure, M. L., & Reinhard, S. C. (2009). Expanding the capacity of nursing education. *Health Affairs, 26*(4), w634–w645.

Commission on Collegiate Nursing Education. (2009). *Achieving excellence in accreditation: The first 10 years of CCNE.* Washington, DC: Author.

Coonan, P. R. (2008). Educational innovation: Nursing's leadership challenge. *Nursing Economics, 26*(2), 117–121.

Council for Higher Education Accreditation. (2013). *Information about accreditation.* Retrieved from http://www.chea.org/public_info/indes.asp

Eaton, J. (2009). *An overview of U.S. accreditation.* Retrieved from http://www.chea.org/pdf/2009.06_Overview_of_US_Accreditation.pdf

Gaza, E. A., & Shellenbarger, T. (2010). The lived experience of part-time baccalaureate nursing faculty. *Journal of Professional Nursing, 26*(6), 353–359.

Giddens, J. F., & Brady, D. (2007). Rescuing nursing education from content saturation: The case for a concept-based curriculum. *Journal of Nursing Education, 46*(2), 65–69.

Giddens, J., Brady, D., Brown, P., Wright, M., Smith, D., & Harris, J. (2008). A new curriculum for a new era of nursing education. *Nursing Education Perspectives, 29*(4), 200–204.

Goodin, H. J., & Stein, D. (2008). Deliberate discussion as an innovative teaching strategy. *Journal of Nursing Education, 47*(6), 272–274.

Greiner, A. C., & Knebel, E. (Eds.). (2003). *Health professions education: A bridge to quality.* Washington, DC: The National Academies Press.

Hagler, D., White, B., & Morris, B. (2011). Cognitive tools as a scaffold for faculty during curriculum redesign. *Journal of Nursing Education, 50*(7), 417–422.

Hargreaves, J. (2008). Risk: The ethics of a creative curriculum. *Innovations in Education and Teaching International, 45*(3), 227–234.

Hartman, J. L., Dziuban, C., & Brophy-Ellison, J. (2007). Faculty 2.0. *Educause Review, 42*(5), 62–76. [Online]. Retrieved from www.educause.edu/apps/er/_erm07/erm0753.asp

Hinshaw, A. S. (2008). Navigating the perfect storm: Balancing a culture of safety with workplace challenges. *Nursing Research, 57*(1 Suppl.), S4–S10.

Huybrecht, S., Loeckx, W., Quaeyhaegens, Y., De Tobel, D., & Mistiaen, W. (2011). Mentoring in nursing education: Perceived characteristics of mentors and the consequences of mentorship. *Nursing Education Today, 31,* 274–278.

Institute of Medicine. (2010). *The future of nursing: Leading change, advancing health.* Washington, DC: National Academies Press.

Iwasiw, C. L., Goldenberg, D., & Andrusyszyn, M. A. (2009). *Curriculum development in nursing education.* Sudbury, MA: Jones and Bartlett.

Kalisch, P. A., & Kalisch, B. J. (1978). *The advance of American nursing.* Boston, MA: Little, Brown.

Lapkin, S., & Levett-Jones, T. (2011). A cost-utility analysis of medium vs. high-fidelity human patient simulation manikins in nursing education. *Journal of Clinical Nursing, 20*(23/24), 3543–3552.

Mailloux, C. F. (2011). Using the Essentials of Baccalaureate Education for Professional Nursing Practice (2008) as a framework for curriculum revision. *Journal of Professional Nursing, 27*(6), 385–389.

Mangold, K. (2007). Educating a new generation: Teaching baby boomer faculty about millennial students. *Nurse Educator, 32*(1), 21–23.

Moch, S. D., Cronje, R. J., & Branson, J. (2010). Part I: Undergraduate nursing evidence-based practice education: Envisioning the role of students. *Journal of Professional Nursing, 26*(1), 5–13.

Moscato, S. R., Miller, J., Logsdon, K., & Chorpenning, L. (2007). Dedicated education unit: An innovative clinical partner education model. *Nursing Outlook, 55*(1), 31–37.

National Council of State Boards of Nursing. (2009a). *Innovations in education regulation committee: Recommendations for boards of nursing for fostering innovations in education.* Retrieved from https://www.ncsbn.org/Recommendations_for_BONS.pdf

National Council of State Boards of Nursing. (2009b). *Innovations in education regulation report: Background and literature review.* Retrieved from https://www.ncsbn.org/Innovations_Report.pdf

National Council of State Boards of Nursing. (2011). *A preferred future for prelicensure nursing program approval.* Retrieved from http://www.ncsbn.org/Report_on_Future_of_Approval.pdf

National Council of State Boards of Nursing. (2014). *Boards of nursing.* Retrieved from https://www.ncsbn.org/boards.htm

Nehring, W. (2008). U.S. boards of nursing and the use of high-fidelity patient simulators in nursing education. *Journal of Professional Nursing, 24*(2), 109–117.

Pew Health Professions Commission. (1995). *Critical challenges: Revitalizing the health care professions for the twenty-first century.* San Francisco, CA: UCSF Center for the Health Professions.

Phillips, J. M., Resnick, J., Boni, M. S., Bradely, P., Grady, J. L., Ruland, J. P., & Stuever, N. L. (2013). Voices of innovation: Building a model for curriculum transformation. *International Journal of Nursing Education Scholarship, 10*(1), 1–7.

Powell-Cope, G., Hughes, N. L., Sedlak, C., & Nelson, A. (2008). Faculty perceptions of implementing an evidence-based safe patient handling nursing curriculum module. *Online Journal of Issues in Nursing, 13*(3), 6.

Reese, C. E., Jeffries, P. R., & Engum, S. A. (2010). Using simulations to develop nursing and medical student collaboration. *Nursing Education Perspectives, 31*(1), 33–37.

Savers, C. (2010). Trends and challenges in regulating nursing practice today. *Journal of Nursing Regulation, 1*(1), 4–8.

Sawatzky, J., & Enns, C. L. (2009). A mentoring needs assessment: Validating mentorship in nursing education. *Journal of Professional Nursing, 25*(3), 145–150.

Schmitt, M. H. (2002). It's time to revalue nursing education research. *Research in Nursing & Health, 25*, 423–424.

Skiba, D. (2012). Technology and gerontology: Is this in your nursing curriculum? *Nursing Education Perspectives, 33*(3), 207–209.

Slimmer, L. (2012). A teaching mentorship program to facilitate excellence in teaching and learning. *Journal of Professional Nursing, 28*(3), 182–185.

Spencer, J. A. (2012). Integrating informatics in undergraduate nursing curricula: Using the QSEN framework as a guide. *Journal of Nursing Education, 51*(12), 697–701.

Stephens-Lee, C., Der-Fa, L., & Wilson, K. E. (2013). Preparing students for an electronic workplace. *Online Journal of Nursing Informatics, 17*(3), 1–10.

Sullivan, D. T. (2010). Connecting nursing education and practice: A focus on shared goals for quality and safety. *Creative Nursing, 16*(1), 37–43.

Tanner, C. A. (2004). Nursing education research: Investing in our future. *Journal of Nursing Education, 43,* 99–100.

Thompson, B. W., & Skibaa, D. J. (2008). Informatics in the nursing curriculum: A national survey of nursing informatics requirements in nursing curricula. *Nursing Education Perspectives, 29*(5), 312–317.

Unterschuetz, C., Hughes, P., Nienhauser, D., Weberg, D., & Jackson, L. (2008). Caring for innovation and caring for the innovator. *Nursing Administration Quarterly, 32*(2), 133–141.

CHAPTER 3

The Role of Faculty in Curriculum Development and Evaluation

Sarah B. Keating

Sarah B. Keating

OBJECTIVES

Upon completion of Chapter 3, the reader will be able to:

1. Participate in faculty development activities to increase knowledge and skills in curriculum development and evaluation
2. Analyze the role and responsibilities of faculty in curriculum development and evaluation including:
   a. Assessment of the relationship of course content and learning activities to the mission, philosophy, framework, goals, and student learning outcomes of the curriculum
   b. Implementation of the curriculum
   c. Identification of needs for curricular revision or new programs
   d. Participation in program evaluation and accreditation activities
3. Participate in or generate research relating to curriculum development and evaluation in nursing education

OVERVIEW

Chapter 3 discusses the critical role that faculty plays in curriculum development and evaluation. Since faculty is the ultimate developer, implementer, and evaluator of the curriculum, knowledge of the processes for development and evaluation is necessary. Seeing the curriculum as a whole and its purpose helps to direct the faculty's activities to carry out the plan, assess its implementation, and recognize the need for revision of the current program, or perhaps, development of a new program. Both novice and experienced teachers collaborate with students and colleagues in the health care system to ensure the integrity of the curriculum and to identify when changes are needed. Faculty responsibilities to bring about curricular change from the course level to governance and administrative approval are reviewed. Additionally, the role of faculty related to program evaluation and accreditation activities is discussed. Suggestions for research leading to evidence-based practice in education are provided.

LEVEL OF INDIVIDUAL FACULTY MEMBER'S KNOWLEDGE OF CURRICULUM DEVELOPMENT AND EVALUATION

New Faculty

With the current and projected nursing faculty shortage (American Association of Colleges of Nursing, 2014), schools of nursing are recruiting new faculty from health care institutions and recent graduates of master's or doctoral programs. Many of these faculty members have little or no experience in academe and although they may have clinical expertise, they have little or no formal education in instructional design and strategies and in curriculum development and evaluation. It becomes the responsibility of the school administrator and faculty members to orient new faculty members to the curriculum and the processes of learner-centered education.

Orientation

Orientation programs usually take place prior to the first week of scheduled classes for new faculty to attend institutional meetings set up to familiarize them with human resources and personnel policies as well as to the mission and philosophy of the overall institution and the home college or department within which the nursing school resides. The nursing program has parallel activities and reviews faculty governance such as committee structures and membership, administrative organization, expectations for participation in meetings and other related activities, and introduction of the curriculum, program of study, and overviews of the courses that carry out the curriculum. Relative to the latter, the course and level assignments are reviewed along with teaching and reporting responsibilities. New faculty members meet with course and/or level coordinators to go over grading policies, testing and clinical supervision policies, and other course-related activities. The following studies describe some orientation programs that have been successful. However, for the most part, they describe strategies for orientation and do not necessarily link them to the importance of orienting new faculty to the total curriculum.

Mangum (2013) created an orientation program for experienced clinicians assuming the role as clinical faculty in an associate degree program in nursing. The Structured Orientation Development System program was based on the National League for Nursing (NLN) Core Competencies of Faculty (NLN, 2005) and Benner's (1984) from Novice to Expert model. Faculty participated in pre- and post self-assessments of their competency in teaching. Although the study was limited to a small sample size and one geographical location, it provides a model for orientation of faculty to the NLN core competencies for nursing educators.

Horton (2013) conducted a qualitative study to investigate the perceptions of adjunct faculty in an associate degree program on orientation, mentoring, and faculty development programs. Through a survey, focus group, and interviews of faculty representing various disciplines at the college she found recurring themes. Part-time teachers wanted to be paid for orientation attendance since many had other jobs and family responsibilities and they indicated a desire to have an official mentor to help guide them in honing their teaching skills, and for managing students and their learning. Although the study was limited in number and geographical location, it has implications for administrative support for paying for faculty time for orientation and faculty development activities, and for the need for formal mentoring programs with experienced faculty members.

Forbes, Hickey, and White (2010) studied over a hundred adjunct faculty's orientation needs in a school of nursing. They found that faculty members indicated that they felt the need for and would attend orientation sessions. An added incentive was to offer continuing education (CE) credits for attendance; however the majority indicated they would attend the sessions even if CE was not offered. One hundred percent (n = 60+) of those answering open-ended questions indicated they felt the need for and would attend formal courses on education. The survey listed topics of interest to them that included teaching diverse learners, test construction, technology (e-mail, BlackBoard, personal digital assistant [PDA]), developing a lesson plan, handling student issues, and evaluation and grading. Based on the study the orientation sessions were lengthened to 3-hour workshops and offered each semester. Useful information on the content of orientation programs for faculty is included in the authors' recommendations.

A planned orientation, mentoring, and instructional design and support services for faculty is essential for new and experienced faculty that are teaching online for the first time. Vaill and Testori (2012) describe in detail the program used at their college for faculty development, which applied adult and constructivist learning theories. Faculty who planned to teach online for the first time attended an online course the semester prior to the course. Through planned sessions online, participants developed an online course ready for presentation the following semester. Experienced online teachers acted as mentors for the learners and support for developing the course. How to utilize related technology was offered during the experience. A cohort-style program was developed owing to the large number of courses converting to online format and the need for increased numbers of faculty prepared for online teaching. The program has been successful and faculty reported high satisfaction with the experience.

A national survey of part-time faculty in baccalaureate nursing programs was conducted to determine what effects orientation, integration, and evaluation have on *intent to stay in teaching*. Results revealed that planned orientation, evaluative student feedback, adequacy of pay, mentor support, and completion of an education course were significant factors in the intention to continue teaching (Carlson, 2012). While not the purpose of the study, Carlson noted that a significant number of the respondents had baccalaureates (31%) as the highest degree and 37% had a master of science in nursing (MSN). Since recommendations are that faculty has at least a master's degree, this is worrisome and bears attention to find solutions to the nursing faculty shortage and faculty's educational preparation.

Mentorship

A planned orientation program for new faculty is highly recommended. Although reading faculty handbooks and reviewing each policy can be tedious, orienting the new faculty members to the most critical policies is essential and should be shared in formal or informal meetings with all new members and selected experienced faculty members. Individual mentoring for new faculty members provides a resource for discussing everyday teaching activities, relationships with students and peers, and organizational hierarchy. Planned meetings should be part of the mentor's and mentoree's calendar even if there are no pressing issues to discuss. This gives them the opportunity to share teaching experiences and issues and troubleshoot. Vital to the mentorship and orientation is the necessity to review the curriculum, the courses in which the new member teaches, and the relationship of the courses to the overall program of study. The orientation plan may assign mentors to new faculty on a one-on-one basis or several according to the needs of the faculty members and the program. Many times, as new faculty adjust to the new role, they will self-select a mentor according to academic or individual needs. These relationships usually last over time even after planned meetings are no longer indicated as they evolve into professional, collegial relationships with shared interests in academic and research/scholarship activities.

Barksdale et al. (2011) present a faculty orientation, mentoring, and development model for supporting faculty members in their teaching role and professional growth. At their institution, there is a formal program for faculty development participation. Faculty satisfaction with the program was high. Examples of the program include a formal assignment of a mentor for new faculty members with the option to change mentors as needed, meetings in which participants share ideas for scholarship and research, and workshops for developing and improving teaching and learning strategies.

EXPERIENCED FACULTY

Leadership

The role of experienced faculty in curriculum development and evaluation is multifaceted. The primary role is that of effective teaching and role modeling through the application of learner-centered theories, instructional design and strategies, and learner and program assessment. Based on experienced faculty members' activities in helping to develop and implement the curriculum, it is their responsibility to ensure that the curriculum remains intact and, at the same time, current with changes and trends in education and the health care system that call for curriculum assessment and revision. Experienced faculty members serve in leadership roles within the curriculum including participation on curriculum and other academic committees, accreditation and program review assignments, institutional service that relates to curriculum development and evaluation, and service as course coordinators or level and specialty leaders. Additionally, it is expected that they serve as official or unofficial mentors for new faculty members.

Young, Pearsall, Stiles, and Horton-Deutsch (2011) interviewed nurse leaders to study how they became faculty leaders and found three major themes, *being thrust into leadership, taking risks, and facing challenges.* The descriptions of these factors indicate that experienced faculty members are often thrust into leadership positions without seeking them. For example, the need for developing a new track in a program resulted in the two experienced clinical experts assuming the leadership for developing the program. An example of taking risks was developing a new method for promoting student learning and skills that led to challenges from other faculty but proved to be an effective instructional strategy. Facing challenges by faculty led to the realization that overcoming challenges meant consensus building on the part of the leader and faculty. These themes illustrate how faculty members can become leaders, whether planned or not, in their role in curriculum development and evaluation.

Currency of Curriculum

Experienced faculty members observe changes in nursing and health care through their activities when reviewing the literature for current trends in their specialty, professional organization activities, academic responsibilities, and in clinical practice situations. Working with colleagues in the practice setting, supervising students or conducting research, and attending professional meetings and conferences are sources for identifying changes and future implications. These activities contribute to the faculty's ability to assess the curriculum for its currency and to identify revisions that might be indicated. New faculty members are usually immersed in assuming the new role of educator and thus may not have the time or experience to observe these implications for curriculum development and evaluation. At the same time, experienced faculty can take the opportunity to mentor new faculty and demonstrate the importance of assessing trends and changes in the health care system or education that influence the curriculum. As mentioned previously, the role of mentor to new faculty is a responsibility of practiced faculty and can be an expected formal assignment as part of an orientation plan or, informally, as part of the expectations for faculty.

Samples of how faculty are involved in ensuring a current and relevant curriculum are available in the literature. Implementing the knowledge and skills related to evidence-based practice across the curriculum and into the practice setting to promote its use by nurses is an example (Moch, Cronje, & Barnson, 2010). The authors conducted an extensive review of the literature to identify evidence-based practice in nursing curricula and its implementation in the practice setting. They found little information on how this practice is shared with nurses in the practice setting where students are assigned. They identified the need for collaboration between education and practice to integrate evidence-based practice into the health care setting.

Faculty Development for Curriculum Development and Evaluation

It is the responsibility of the administrators and faculty in the school of nursing to build in faulty development activities to ensure the integrity of the curriculum and the quality of instruction in its implementation. These activities ultimately lead to the realization of the program goals and student learning outcomes that ensure a quality program in the preparation of professional nurses for the health care system. While orientation to the curriculum was mentioned previously as the first step for faculty development in a school of nursing, other topics include the provision of knowledge on faculty governance related to curricular activities;

the processes of curriculum development, program evaluation, and accreditation; application of learning theories, instructional design, and strategies including technology; and student assessment methods. To meet the role expectations of service and scholarship, workshops can be offered to review service opportunities within the institution and in the community and skills for writing grants and preparing manuscripts for publications. Ideas that apply specifically to research related to curriculum development, program evaluation, and evidence-based practice in education can be shared in faculty meetings, workshops, and conferences that focus on the needs of the curriculum.

A comprehensive model for nursing faculty development is described by Drummond-Young et al. (2010). The model was initiated by a faculty work group to provide orientation, mentorship, and ongoing developmental activities based on the concept of teaching as scholarship (Boyer, 1990). The model presupposed the need for faculty members to link courses in which they teach to the curriculum and its plan of study. The model contains four developmental outcomes for faculty, that is, teaching, wisdom, discovery, and excellence. Within the outcomes are instructional, leadership, organizational, and professional development characteristics. Central to the components are exploring, reflecting, focusing, applying, mentoring, and evaluating activities that promote educational vitality.

ROLES AND RESPONSIBILITIES OF FACULTY

Implementation of the Curriculum

Implementation of the curriculum is the responsibility of the faculty. Therefore, all faculty members should be thoroughly familiar with the total curriculum specifically, its mission, philosophy, organizational framework, student learning outcomes, and plan of study. Full-time faculty should have a working knowledge of these components for all levels of education within their program including undergraduate and graduate programs. While teaching activities may focus on graduate studies or undergraduate, it is necessary for faculty to know how they relate to one another and build upon the other. Part-time faculty may not need the details of the curriculum when compared to full-time faculty, but they should understand the relationship of the course(s) in which they teach to the curriculum and its framework and goals.

Schools of nursing curricula generally have one organizational framework that acts as the guide for all levels of degree work and demonstrates the rationale for preparing professional nurses at various levels. While it is not necessary to know the details of the courses that implement the curriculum, it is critical to its integrity for faculty to identify the place that the courses in which they teach has in the framework. Thus, the temptation to change course objectives and/or content is less likely to occur. The role of course coordinator is to assume the responsibility for new faculty's orientation to the course and its relationship to the curriculum and also to periodically assess the delivery of the course to ensure its germaneness to the curriculum. Periodic meetings of faculty members in the courses to review teaching strategies, learning activities, and learning outcomes are vital to the implementation of the curriculum and to overall quality control.

Need for Revision or New Programs

As the curriculum is implemented, faculty members observe and assess the effectiveness of learning activities, teaching methods, student learning outcomes, and the relationship of courses to the curriculum. When gaps or problems are detected, it is the instructors' responsibility to report the observations to the course leader, or level coordinator. Together, faculty should investigate the situation and, with input from students and other stakeholders, bring the matter to the curriculum committee (or academic committee that has responsibility for curricular change) for their consideration. Suggestions for remediation of the problem should accompany the report to facilitate the expedient processing of the need for curricular revision, if indicated. Many times, faculty and students observe the need for new programs based on their experiences and interactions with the public and other professionals in the health care system. The processes for bringing the possibility to the attention of the curriculum committee are the same, that is, a summary of the need with documentation and possible plans for the development of a new track/program.

Davis (2011) reports on a conceptual model developed by an associate degree program faculty when it identified the need for a curricular revision. Faculty believed that a change to learner-centered instruction was indicated owing to the NLN's call for nursing education transformation and declining National Council Licensure Examination (NCLEX) results. In order for all faculty members to be involved, the conceptual model helped them to organize their work to review the current curriculum, revise it according to needs identified, and design the new curriculum. The conceptual model was built upon learning as central with the curriculum, faculty, students, and resources interacting to achieve program outcomes. It proved successful with faculty using the model as a guide, which led to a plan to assess the curriculum every 3 years using the same model.

D'Antonio, Brennan, and Curley (2013) describe a 3-year process for re-designing a baccalaureate curriculum. The undergraduate curriculum committee acted as a steering committee for mapping the curriculum from the mission and vision to the organizational framework and courses. All faculty members were involved in each step of the process and constituents were invited to participate as well. The authors report that the process generated excitement, enthusiasm, and commitment of the faculty to the program. They offer it as a model for other faculty considering curriculum revision.

Another model for involving faculty in curriculum revision and for faculty development was the cognitive tools scaffolding model used to revise an undergraduate curriculum (Hagler, Morris, & White, 2011). The levels of function for the cognitive tools included those of Erkens, Prangsma, and Jasper (2006), that is, task, metacognitive, and sociocommunicative levels, and served to involve faculty in the process for developing the new courses. Tables and models to facilitate the use of the cognitive tools provided the guide for faculty. The involvement of cross-specialty, full-time and part-time faculty, and teamwork caused faculty to increase their knowledge and interest in instructional design and in formative and summative evaluation activities.

Activities Related to Curriculum Development, Evaluation, and Accreditation

Many of the roles and responsibilities of faculty in curriculum development have been reviewed. They include, on an individual level, familiarization with the components of the curriculum; developing and carrying out instructional designs and strategies that are congruent with the curriculum; observation, assessment, and reporting of needs for either curricular revision or development of new programs; participation on curriculum/academic/evaluation/accreditation committees; and developing or participating in scholarly activities that relate to curriculum development and evaluation. As a group, faculty members should participate in the orientation of new faculty members to ensure the integrity of the curriculum, review faculty governance structures to maintain faculty ownership of the curriculum, form research/scholarly groups to identify trends and issues in curriculum development and evaluation, generate research ideas, identify program development grants, and build on ideas for evidence-based educational practice.

Accrediting agencies such as the Accreditation Commission for Education in Nursing (2014) and the Commission on Collegiate Nursing Education (2014) standards/criteria include the educational preparation and qualifications for nursing faculty. As part of their role, faculty members should be familiar with these expectations and assure that they meet the qualifications and expectations for the role of faculty. A model for tracking faculty accomplishments can be found in the article by Pettus, Reifschneider, and Buruss (2009). The model provides for the maintenance of current information on faculty members resulting in documentation of faculty achievements as well as a record for accreditation purposes.

Participation in accreditation activities and program evaluation activities is expected for all faculty members. Leadership roles include chairing committees for program review and accreditation and coordinating and presenting evaluation and accreditation reports for the nursing faculty as a whole and with other approval bodies on the institutional level, for example, graduate school, senate committees, academic administrators, and so on. Program evaluation for the academic institution usually takes place every 5 years, while accreditation takes place from every 5 to 10 years, depending upon the program's history and type of program. For example, new graduate programs receive initial accreditation for 5 years and renewed accreditation every 10 years. Exceptions also depend upon the accreditation status such as full accreditation, placed on warning, or denied accreditation. Faculty members' roles in evaluation and accreditation include knowing the curriculum components such as the mission, vision, philosophy, organizational framework, student learning outcomes, and the program of study. They should be able to articulate where the courses in which they teach fall into the curricular model. Identifying needs for revision and bringing it to the attention of faculty and curriculum committees is an important role for all teachers and, finally, participation on committees that evaluate and develop the curriculum is an additional responsibility. Chapters 16 and 17 discuss evaluation and accreditation for academic nursing programs in detail.

RESEARCH IN CURRICULUM DEVELOPMENT AND EVALUATION

Issues and Trends

Major issues and trends in nursing education as they apply to the nursing faculty role in curriculum development and evaluation are as follows:

1. A current and looming nursing faculty shortage
2. Increasing ratios of part-time to full-time faculty
3. Fewer faculty members with formal preparation in education
4. Increasing numbers of doctoral prepared graduates, especially doctor of nursing practice (DNP) graduates, who may not have the pedagogy required for the faculty role
5. Rapid changes in teaching formats including online platforms, simulations, and other technological advances affecting instructional design and the implementation of the curriculum
6. Health care system changes that influence the preparation of nurses and therefore the role of faculty in keeping the curriculum current and ready for the future

Roberts and Glod (2013) address some of these issues in their paper regarding the dilemmas in nursing faculty roles. They trace this history of nursing education from diploma programs with a focus on the development of clinical skills in the care of patients to its move into the academic setting with a focus on the sciences, social sciences, and liberals arts integrated into the science and clinical skills of the profession. As a result, nursing found itself with many dilemmas as to faculty role in order to meet the academic expectations of scholarship and the professional requirements for clinical practice. More recently, institutions that are research-focused expect tenured/tenure-track faculty to generate research that helps to support their research as well as fund their teaching positions. This results in increasing numbers of clinical faculty who usually are part-time and who have a minimized role in faculty governance activities and scholarship. Yet, these instructors are the workhorses of the prelicensure programs in delivering clinical supervision, while tenure-track or tenured faculty deliver the didactic courses and teach in graduate level courses that result in lower teaching loads to provide time for research activities. This is a major issue in nursing education and has implications for how education will be delivered and curricula maintained to keep current with changes in the health care system.

Research Implications for Evidence-Based Curriculum Development and Evaluation

Nursing faculty members have boundless opportunities for educational research as it relates to curriculum development and evaluation. There is a dearth of recent research related to nursing education owing to nursing's move to its own doctoral education either on the nursing science PhD/doctor of nursing science level or the applied/translational research, professional practice degree (DNP). Previous generations of nurse educators received doctoral degrees in education, social sciences,

sciences, administration, and so on with their dissertations and research focused on the disciplines in which they earned the degree and its application to nursing. This author, for example, earned a doctorate in education and compared two types of curricula to discover their differences in influencing graduates' choice of practice arena.

Owing to this recent phenomenon, much of nursing research focuses on practice issues and health care policy, which is beneficial for the profession, health care, and the public. However there is a neglect of research studying education and its processes and outcomes. Throughout this text, the reader will find many issues and needs for investigation as they relate to curriculum development and evaluation. For example, comparisons of types of programs (accelerated, entry-level, online-based, etc.), program evaluation models specific to nursing education, and student learning outcomes compared to intended outcomes. NLN (2014) has an updated list of research priorities for nursing education on its website: www.nln.org/researchgrants/researchpriorities.pdf.

SUMMARY

Chapter 3 reviewed the roles and responsibilities of faculty in curriculum development and evaluation. Orientation and faculty development activities were discussed as they relate to tying instructional design and learning activities to the curriculum's mission, vision, philosophy, and organizational framework. Other faculty responsibilities were described including participation and leadership in curriculum development and evaluation and accreditation activities. Trends, issues, and research needs in curriculum development and evaluation were summarized.

DISCUSSION QUESTIONS

1. Why do you think faculty has the ultimate responsibility for curriculum development and evaluation? List at least five reasons for this responsibility.
2. Based on a current issue in nursing education, develop a research question for investigation into the issue and possible solutions. Explain why you chose the issue and what implications it has for the future of nursing education.

LEARNING ACTIVITIES

STUDENT LEARNING ACTIVITIES

1. Imagine yourself in the role of a new faculty member in a school of nursing. List the topics that you believe you need to know in order to be an effective teacher. Prioritize the list and explain the rationale for the order of priority.
2. Describe the process you would take to change a learning activity in a course that you teach or will teach. How will you relate it to the curriculum?

NURSE EDUCATOR/FACULTY DEVELOPMENT ACTIVITIES

1. Assess your school's orientation and faculty development programs. Identify any gaps in the programs as they relate to curriculum development and evaluation. How would you develop or change the programs to meet the needs of new and experienced faculty?

2. Recall your experience as a mentor or mentoree in nursing education. What were the positive aspects to the experience? What would you change to improve the experience?

REFERENCES

Accreditation Commission for Education in Nursing. (2014). *Accreditation manual.* Retrieved from http://www.acenursing.net/manuals/SC2013.pdf

American Association of Colleges of Nursing. (2014). *Nursing shortage.* Retrieved from http://www.aacn.nche.edu/media-relations/fact-sheets/nursing-shortage

Barksdale, D. J., Woodley, L., Page, J. B., Bernhardt, J., Kowlowitz, V., & Oermann, M. H. (2011). Faculty development: Doing more with less. *The Journal of Continuing Education in Nursing, 42*(12), 537–544.

Benner, P. (1984). *From novice to expert: Excellence and power in clinical nursing practice.* Menlo Park, CA: Addison-Wesley.

Boyer, E. L. (1990). *Scholarship reconsidered: Priorities of the professoriate.* Princeton, NJ: The Carnegie Foundation for the Advancement of Learning.

Carlson, J. S. (2012). *The influence of orientation, integration and evaluation on intent to stay in part-time clinical nursing faculty* (Unpublished doctoral dissertation). Simmons College, Boston, MA.

Commission on Collegiate Nursing Education. (2014). *Standards, procedures, and resources.* Retrieved from https://www.aacn.nche.edu/ccne-accreditation/standards-procedures-resources/overview

D'Antonio, P. O., Brennan, A. M. W., & Curley, M. A. Q. (2013). Judgment, inquiry, engagement, voice: Reenvisioning an undergraduate nursing curriculum using a shared decision-making model. *Journal of Professional Nursing, 29*(6), 407–413.

Davis, B. W. (2011). A conceptual model to support curriculum review, revision, and design in an associate degree nursing program. *Nursing Education Perspectives, 32*(6), 389–394.

Drummond-Young, M., Brown, B., Noesgaard, C., Lunyk-Child, O., Maich, N. M., Mines, C., & Linton, J. (2010). A comprehensive faculty development model for nursing education. *Professional Nursing, 26,* 152–161.

Erkens, G., Prangsma, M., & Jaspers, J. (2006). Planning and coordinating activities in collaborative learning. In A. O'Donnell, C. Hmelo, & G. Erkens (Eds.), *Collaborative learning, reasoning & technology.* Mahwah, NJ: Erlbaum.

Forbes, M. O., Hickey, M. T., & White, J. (2010). Adjunct faculty development: Reported needs and innovative solutions. *Journal of Professional Nursing, 26*(2), 116–124.

Hagler, D., Morris, B., & White, B. (2011). Cognitive tools as a scaffold for faculty during curriculum redesign. *Journal of Nursing Education, 50*(7), 417–422.

Horton, D. (2013). *Community college adjunct faculty perceptions of orientation, mentoring, and professional development* (Unpublished doctoral study). Walden University, Minneapolis, MN.

Mangum, D. R. (2013). *A structure orientation development system for nursing* faculty (Unpublished capstone project). Gardner-Webb University, School of Nursing, Boiling Springs, NC.

Moch, S. D., Cronje, R. J., & Branson, J. (2010) Undergraduate nursing evidence-based practice education: envisioning the role of students. *Journal of Professional Nursing, 25*(1), 5–13.

National League for Nursing. (2005). *Core competencies of nurse educators.* New York, NY: Author. Retrieved from http://www.nln.org//beta/facultydevelopment/pdf/corecompetencies.pdf

National League for Nursing. (2014). *NLN Research priorities in nursing education 2012-2015.* Retrieved from http://www.nln.org/researchgrants/researchpriorities.pdf

Pettus, S., Reifschneider, E., & Buruss, N. (2009). Faculty achievement tracking tool. *Journal of Nursing Education, 48*(3), 161–164.

Roberts, S. J., & Glod, C. (2013). Dilemmas in faculty roles. *Nursing Forum, 48*(2), 99–105.

Vaill, A. L., & Testori, P. A. (2012). Orientation, mentoring and ongoing support, a three-tiered approach to online faculty development. *Journal of Asynchronous Learning Networks, I16* (2), 111–119.

Young, P. A., Pearsall, C., Stiles, K. A., & Horton-Deutsch, S. (2011). Becoming a nursing faculty leader. *Nursing Education Perspectives, 32*(4), 222–228.

Learning Theories, Education Taxonomies, and Critical Thinking

Sarah B. Keating

OVERVIEW

Section II introduces learning theories, education taxonomies, and the application of critical thinking to evidence-based practice as they apply to curriculum development. Chapter 4 discusses classic and newer learning theories and concepts, while Chapter 5 reviews classic and updated education taxonomies and their application to nursing education in addition to the integration of critical thinking skills. These major theories, concepts, and models serve to guide educators as they develop mission and philosophy statements for the program and build the curriculum plan. They are considered again in detail as faculty applies them to the implementation of the curriculum through the processes of instructional design and strategies, and student evaluation.

LEARNING THEORIES

As discussed in Chapter 3, faculty holds the ultimate responsibility for curriculum development. In that role, faculty members must reach consensus on their beliefs about the learning processes their students undergo to master the knowledge and skills necessary for practicing as nurses. Identification of beliefs about teaching and learning processes is one of the earliest activities that faculty members take when revising or developing the curriculum. Although this text does not focus on instructional design and strategies, identification of applicable learning theories helps to guide the development of the courses that carry out and evaluate the curriculum.

Learning theories are often identified by major categories and include classic theories and newer applications of them to the learning environment. Chapter 4 discusses some of the major learning theorists and their postulates as they apply to the teaching and learning processes, specifically in nursing. Many times faculty are unaware of the learning theories that provide the foundation for such teaching strategies as lecturing, demonstrating skills, supervising students, and so on. Yet, an analysis of the teaching/learning situation can reveal the utilization of a theory or amalgamation of several theories. Such an analysis and the learning theories' relevance to the evaluation of intended learning outcomes (objectives) can lead to changes that improve the educator's teaching skills as well as increase student learning.

EDUCATION TAXONOMIES

Chapter 5 reviews the traditional education taxonomies and domains of learning as they apply to nursing education. While nursing adopted and continues to use modified models of educational taxonomies and behavioral models for goals and objectives to organize the curriculum, there is a need to examine newer taxonomies that foster critical thinking processes. The continuing issue that faces nursing educators is its reliance on behaviorist theories of learning that focus on the teacher as transmitter of knowledge instead of the learning needs and characteristics of the learner. Behaviorist models of learning are appropriate for students to gain basic knowledge and skills; however, to facilitate the critical and creative thinking skills necessary for clinical decision making and evidence-based practice, newer models of educational taxonomies and learning theories are necessary. The application of the new taxonomies recognizes the role of the teacher as facilitator, the learner as the focus, and the interactions between the two. They lift the objectives from rote or recall memorization on the part of the learner to higher orders of understanding, conceptualization, and application. To facilitate the development and evaluation of a curriculum, Chapter 5 offers a model for the *contextual approach to navigate delivery of outcomes* for curriculum alignment with its stated goals.

CRITICAL THINKING

An essential part of curriculum planning is the recognition by faculty of critical thinking and the role it plays in the development of clinical decision-making skills and evidence-based nursing practice. Thus, critical thinking must be part of faculty's planning for the curriculum and how it will be integrated into courses and their instructional designs. Critical thinking is a necessity for students as they apply prerequisite and nursing knowledge to the development of complex thinking skills. The modalities of problem solving, critical and creative thinking, and decision making are suited to the current evolving health care system. There is a need for professionals who can respond to health care needs and system changes with strategies that use evidence-based and innovative solutions to health care problems and that help to develop policies that foster health promotion and the prevention of disease.

CHAPTER 4

Learning Theories Applied to Curriculum Development

Coleen Saylor

OBJECTIVES

Upon completion of Chapter 4, the reader will be able to:

1. Evaluate learning theories as possible foundations to guide nursing and health care program curricula including learning objectives, strategies, and outcomes
2. Compare learning theory strengths, weaknesses, and relevancy as a conceptual basis for teaching and learning strategies within a nursing or health care curriculum
3. Analyze various learning theories for appropriateness and congruency with the philosophy and mission of educational institutions, schools of nursing, or health care agencies
4. Select a learning theoretical approach as an overall guide for developing teaching and learning strategies in a specific curriculum program or course

OVERVIEW

Educators who revise and develop a curriculum deal with many difficult questions. How can the program balance expectations between ideal and practical considerations? How can philosophical beliefs be congruent throughout the curriculum? Which instructional strategies are most relevant for these particular learners? How much flexibility should be included? Selecting relevant content, appropriate clinical placements, the difficulty level of assignments, and budget and time constraints provide even further critical issues.

As curriculum planners wrestle with these and many other concerns, a conceptual or theoretical foundation for learning provides a consistent rationale for their decisions, particularly those about instructional strategies (Dennick, 2012). That is, learning theories and concepts provide explanations of how learners learn and how educators can facilitate the best educational outcomes. Each of these approaches to learning suggests applications in the form of teaching and learning strategies that can be emphasized in the curriculum. Just as clinical nursing actions may be based on an understanding of physiological and pharmacological principles, for example, so learning strategies are based on principles or concepts of how people learn. Nurses are expected to provide rationale for their actions, and similarly, educators rely on learning theory and principles as rationale for curriculum decisions. The choice of assumptions of how learners learn also guides the consistency among course objectives, assessment and evaluation strategies, and program outcomes.

An essential part of the curriculum development process is a discussion among the curriculum planners of their perspectives about how learning occurs. As educators with varied backgrounds and experiences, curriculum planners bring a range of viewpoints about the best way for a curriculum to facilitate learning. In addition, nurse educators and students span the generations and embrace different worldviews and philosophical beliefs (Hunt, 2013). In order to produce the best curriculum for a particular program, its faculty, and learners, educators consider assumptions and beliefs, discuss previous experiences, and identify the appropriate explanations for learning, as they are relevant to the program under revision.

This collegial discussion, although sometimes difficult, provides a unique opportunity for learning as educators describe why a particular theoretical perspective is appropriate or not, in their view. The inclination to jump quickly to choose teaching strategies should be resisted as it would cut short this process of using a theoretical foundation as rationale for the later decisions.

The choice of relevant perspective about how learning occurs guides the consistency among goals, course objectives, assessment, and evaluation. Learning outcomes demonstrate whether or not the goals and objectives have been met, and provide feedback on the educational processes. In addition, the graduates' professional performance provides critical measurement of the educational program.

An underlying philosophy of one perspective, constructivism, guided a curriculum redesign by emphasizing aspects of that perspective: inclusion of all faculty, promotion of cognitive apprenticeships, and strengthening communities of practice during the redesign process. These priorities were also demonstrated in learning objectives, strategies, and outcomes (Hagler, White, & Morris, 2011).

In addition to the differences among educators, professional literature does not provide consistent categories of theories, concepts, models, or principles relevant to nursing programs. For example, the constructivist perspective may or may not be included, or it may be seen as a subcategory of the cognitive theory, also called social constructivism. Gardner's (1983) view of multiple intelligences is sometimes included as a distinct theory. Humanism may be called a theory or an educational framework (Braungart, Braungart, & Gramet, 2014; Candela, 2012). The various educational theories contain related ideas, concepts, and frameworks from psychology, sociology, and neuroscience (Dennick, 2012). A discussion of what defines a theory versus a principle or concept is beyond the scope of this chapter. However, the inconsistent list and variety of theories provide even further confusion for educators and clinicians attempting to base program strategies on a theoretical foundation.

Without attempting to rank or rate the myriad educational models, concepts, principles, and theories, this chapter includes six perspectives and two related concepts that are commonly used and have proved useful in academic and health care settings. Although there is inconsistency among these perspectives, educators recognize the importance of learning theory. In addition to the inconsistency of the models, they may be used in combinations. Many times, educators use combinations of theories according to diverse learner needs and the topic under study. In any case, educators are encouraged to examine their beliefs and knowledge about how people learn to provide an appropriate theoretical foundation for the learning strategies within their program.

This chapter reviews learning theories from the behaviorist, social cognitive, cognitivist, constructivist, adult, and humanistic perspectives. In addition, the concepts of metacognition and transformative learning are included within the cognitive perspective.

Learning is defined in this chapter as a "change in behavior (knowledge, attitudes, and/or skills) that can be observed or measured and that occurs … as a result of exposure to environmental stimuli" (Bastable & Alt, 2014, p. 14). Changes caused by maturation, such as growing taller, do not qualify. Temporary changes from fatigue or drugs do not qualify.

The learning paradigm shifted its emphasis over time from teacher to learner. The earlier instructional paradigm describes the faculty as giving out knowledge and students as passive recipients (filling the empty vessel). In contrast, the contemporary learning paradigm emphasizes the learner, while faculties are responsible for creating the learning experiences. Most importantly, the outcomes of the learning experience are of primary importance (Candela, 2012).

A *learning theory* is defined as a "coherent framework of integrated constructs and principles that describe, explain or predict how people learn" (Braungart et al., 2014, p. 65). Learning theories and concepts have much to offer in the practice of health care and nursing education, whether used alone or in combination. In the real world of complex clinical sites and busy classrooms, educators draw from a variety of learning theories for the teaching strategies that are appropriate for a particular course, learner, and content. Educators may utilize a variety of approaches to learning due to diversity in learners (Hunt, 2013). Although everyone has favorite theoretical approaches, many of them have the potential to contribute strategies to teaching and learning situations.

Rewards and reinforcement (behaviorism), role modeling (social cognitive), organization of content (cognitivism), the unique perspective of the learner (constructivism), and positive regard for students (humanism) all have important benefits. An educator can use strategies from several theoretical models at the same time. For simplicity, this chapter discusses each learning paradigm separately, but remember that the boundaries between theoretical paradigms are somewhat artificial. Further, as stated earlier, within and between each paradigm there is often controversy and disagreement, and newer researchers may argue for a different point of view, all of which are outside of the scope of this discussion.

Finally, in no way does this overview take the place of a more thorough understanding of the many researchers and schools of thought that have contributed to knowledge of how people learn and how educators can utilize those theoretical understandings for improved learning outcomes. There are many print and electronic resources available for further study in each of these paradigms and others that not included here.

BEHAVIORIST LEARNING THEORY

Behaviorism is a group of learning theories, often referred to as stimulus–response, that view learning as the result of the stimulus conditions and the responses (behaviors) that follow. Behaviorism is primarily concerned with observable and measurable associations made by the learner (Hunt, 2013). Early work associated behavior with response to rewards and reinforcement. Although there are differences among the behaviorists, they generally view learning as the result of the stimulus conditions and the responses (behaviors) that follow, essentially ignoring what goes on inside the learner. For this reason, the theories are often referred to as stimulus-response or behavioristic (Braungart et al., 2014; Candela, 2012). This perspective asserts that behaviors, rather than thoughts or emotions, are the focus of study since behavior is affected by its consequences. To change people's responses, this perspective changes either the environmental stimulus conditions or what happens after the response occurs. Currently behavioral educational perspectives are more likely to be used in combination with other learning theories, especially cognitive theory, instead of being used alone; and they are an effective adjunct to these other points of view about learning.

Behaviorist principles have been widely incorporated into nursing education and education in general, due to the work since the 1950s of widely acknowledged educators (Candela, 2012). Tyler (1949) addressed the learning setting; Bloom, Englehart, Furst, Hill, and Krathwohl (1956) developed a taxonomy of the cognitive domain, and Mager (1962) developed a model for writing behavioral objectives. Educators should not shy away from these classic books that provide the history of much that is current in nursing education.

CLASSICAL CONDITIONING

Respondent conditioning, also called *classical* or *Pavlovian conditioning*, emphasizes the stimulus and associations made with it in the learning process, depending on associations that are often unconscious. In this model, prior to the conditioning (learning), a neutral stimulus, with no particular value to the learner, is paired with a naturally occurring unlearned (unconditioned) stimulus leading to the elicited (unconditioned) response. Ivan Pavlov, the Russian physiologist, noticed that the dogs in his lab began to salivate before their feeding when they saw the keeper or heard his feet, and before they could see or smell the food. To explain this, Pavlov's following experiment paired a bell, a neutral stimulus that would not ordinarily lead to salivation, with the dog food, the unconditioned stimulus that led to salivation, which is the unconditioned response. If repeated enough, the bell alone began to elicit salivation, showing that conditioning (learning) had occurred. After conditioning, the bell was the conditioned stimulus; salivation in response to the bell was the conditioned response (Braungart et al., 2014; Candela, 2012). Those with well-trained dogs have many examples of this type of conditioning.

Classical conditioning, especially of emotional reactions, occurs in all schools mostly through unconscious processes in which students come to like or dislike school, subjects, and teachers. A particular school subject is neutral, evoking little emotional response in the beginning. But the teacher, the classroom, or some other stimulus in the environment that is repeatedly associated with the subject can become a conditioned stimulus (Braungart et al., 2014).

One of the processes in classical conditioning is *generalization*, that is, a conditioned response that spreads to similar situations. After Pavlov's dogs learned to salivate to one particular sound, they would also salivate after hearing other higher or lower sounds. The conditioned response of salivating *generalized* or spread to similar situations (Braungart et al., 2014). These findings have implications for teachers and all educational settings. Students with previous unpleasant or embarrassing educational experiences may well be reminded of them in a new classroom.

OPERANT CONDITIONING

Within behaviorism, *operant conditioning* is a second, much larger and more important, class of behavior. In classical conditioning, responses are brought about by a stimulus and could become conditioned to other stimuli. But the principles of classical conditioning account for only a small portion of learned behaviors (Braungart et al., 2014). These responses are *elicited responses* and the behavior *respondent* because they occur in response to a stimulus. The second class of behaviors is not elicited by any known stimuli, but they are simply *emitted responses*. These classical conditioning responses are called *operants* because they are operations performed by the individual. In the case of respondent behavior, the person is reacting *to* the environment, whereas in operant behavior the person acts *on* the environment. Another distinction is that respondent behaviors are largely involuntary, while operants are voluntary (Woolfolk, 2010). *Operant conditioning* is rewarding a desired behavior or random act to strengthen the likelihood of it being repeated. Praise and encourage patients' efforts to ambulate the first time after surgery; rewarding that behavior will improve the chances that it will continue (Braungart et al., 2014). Similarly, teachers' positive responses can reinforce students' attempts to answer tough critical thinking questions.

REINFORCEMENT AND PUNISHMENT

Reinforcement is commonly understood to mean *reward*, but in this case it means any consequence that strengthens the behavior it follows. Whenever a behavior persists or increases, one can assume that its effects are reinforcing for the individual involved. However, individuals vary greatly in their perceptions of whether consequences are rewards or not. Students who repeatedly misbehave may be indicating that the consequence is reinforcing, even if it hardly seems desirable to another (Braungart et al., 2014; Woolfolk, 2010). *Positive reinforcement* is a (usually) pleasant stimulus presented following a particular behavior, such as a good grade or praise for an excellent project. However, inappropriate behavior can also be positively reinforced if, for example, an inappropriate student comment elicits laughter in the classroom. *Negative reinforcement* involves the removal of an unpleasant stimulus. If a behavior allows a student to avoid something unpleasant, that is a negative reinforcement. A common example is the car seatbelt buzzer.

As soon as the seatbelt is buckled, the annoying noise stops. Both types of reinforcement strengthen behavior (Woolfolk, 2010).

In contrast to reinforcement, *punishment* decreases or suppresses behavior; therefore, behavior followed by a punishment is less likely to be repeated. In *presentation punishment*, the appearance of the stimulus following the behavior suppresses or decreases that behavior. Extra work assigned following unacceptable classroom work is an example. In contrast, *removal punishment* removes a stimulus following the behavior in question. Taking away privileges after inappropriate behavior decreases the likelihood of that particular behavior (Braungart et al., 2014; Woolfolk, 2010).

Instructional implications of the work on reinforcement focus on the belief that learning results from correct responses being rewarded. Therefore, schools and teachers should provide many opportunities for the desired responses and subsequent reinforcements. Students respond to satisfying experiences. Generally, rewards include teacher attitudes, acknowledgement of good questions, praise of work well done, grading policies that reward effort and excellence fairly, flexibility in assignments, a safe classroom emotional climate, regard for the students and their goals (Braungart et al., 2014), and positive comments on returned papers in any color of ink besides red.

Behaviorist perspectives recommend that teachers be sensitive to this phenomenon and minimize the unpleasant aspects of their courses, the subjects, and of being a student as much as possible (Woolfolk, 2010). Increasing the number of parking facilities may not be possible, but the teacher's awareness of student inconveniences goes a long way in establishing a more positive experience. Look carefully for assignments seen as "busywork," as each assignment that requires student time and effort should have a clear purpose in meeting the course objectives.

In addition to reinforcement, contracts and behavior modification provide common behaviorist techniques. Contracts can be used to change specific behaviors such as not completing an independent project or meeting clinical assignments. The contract is mutually agreed upon and signed by all relevant parties. Behavior modification is simply changing the consequences of behavior by applying positive rewards systematically in order to improve performance. Reinforcement of the behavior pattern then continues until the student establishes a pattern of success, at which time the reinforcement is gradually decreased and stopped. In contrast, ignoring an undesirable behavior tends to lead to extinction, according to this perspective (Braungart et al., 2014).

Behaviorism is relatively easy to understand and can be effectively utilized with other learning paradigms. However, some criticisms include this being a mechanistic, teacher-centered model in which learners are considered to be passive and easily manipulated. Complex mental processes, such as critical thinking are not emphasized in this perspective. Further, the rewards are usually external ones rather than promoting intrinsic satisfaction (Candela, 2012).

SOCIAL COGNITIVE THEORY/SOCIAL LEARNING THEORY

Social cognitive theory emphasizes the importance of observing and modeling the behaviors, attitudes, and emotional responses of others. This theory is largely attributed to Bandura (1986), who described how learning takes place with consideration of personal learner characteristics, behavior patterns, and the social environment. Over time, Bandura changed the name of his theory from social learning to social cognitive to distance it from the social learning theories of that time, and to emphasize the importance of cognition in people's behavior (Boston University School of Public Health, 2013; Braungart et al., 2014). This chapter does not differentiate between social learning and social cognitive theory and, for simplicity, uses the term social cognitive theory.

According to the social cognitive theory, people are not driven by inner forces nor controlled by external stimuli. Rather, human functioning is explained in terms of interaction among cognitive, behavioral, and environmental influences, and it stresses the idea that much learning occurs in a social environment. People learn rules, skills, beliefs, attitudes, and strategies by observation. They learn from models and act in accordance with beliefs about their skills and the possible result of their behaviors (Burke & Mancuso, 2012).

Initially, behaviorist features and the imitation of role models were emphasized in this explanation for learning. In some texts, the earlier social learning theory was included within the behaviorist category, as it was based partially on behaviorist principles of reinforcement. In later constructions, however, the focus was on attributes of the self and internal processing. More recently, the theory focused on social factors and the social context for learning, but it clearly encompasses both cognitive and behavioral frameworks. The self-regulation and control that the learner exercises are considered more critical and more reflective of cognitive principles (Braungart et al., 2014; Burke & Mancuso, 2012).

This theory and its evolution emphasize the agency of the learner, and therefore, it is important to understand what learners perceive and interpret. This perspective views people as able to organize and reflect on their behavior, and therefore, regulate themselves, rather than simply reacting to environmental forces. The model emphasizes intentionality, self-regulation, self-efficacy, and self-evaluation in the learning process (Purzer, 2011). Learners can make things happen by their actions because they possess a measure of control over their thoughts, feelings, and actions. Thus individuals are both products of and producers of their own environments (Braungart et al., 2014).

With the three essential components of this theory, personal factors, behavior, and environmental influence, teachers can influence learning by strategies focused on any or all of these. They can work to improve students' self-beliefs and habits of thinking (personal factors), improve academic skills and self-regulatory practices (behavior), and change the classroom procedures that might encourage student success (environmental factors) (Bandura, 1986; Burke & Mancuso, 2012).

SELF-EFFICACY

One of the most useful constructs of Bandura's theoretical work is the concept of *self-efficacy*. Perceived self-efficacy is defined as "people's judgments of their capabilities to organize and execute courses of action required to attain designated types of performances" (Bandura, 1986, p. 391). Research shows that beliefs about one's self-efficacy influence persistence, effort, and choice of tasks, all of which influence behavior. This concept is particularly important in academic settings, because progress toward the desired goal and positive feedback from teachers and peers both influence the perception of self-efficacy, further raising persistence and effort (Purzer, 2011; Townsend & Scanlan, 2011).

A strong sense of efficacy enhances individual accomplishment and personal well-being in many instances. People who realistically believe that they will be successful sustain their efforts and quickly recover their sense of efficacy after setbacks, since they assume that failure can be corrected with more effort or acquired skills or knowledge. This high self-efficacy approach of individuals produces more successful outcomes and reduces stress (Bandura, 1986).

Beliefs about one's efficacy are developed through four main sources. Mastery experiences are the most effective source of beliefs in one's capabilities, as success builds a strong belief that one can be successful in the future. Experiences in overcoming obstacles through sustained effort, perhaps after setbacks, serve to create a strong sense of self-efficacy (Townsend & Scanlan, 2011; Woolfolk, 2010).

The second source of self-beliefs of efficacy is through the vicarious experiences of others. Seeing similar others succeed by sustained effort increases beliefs that an individual is able to master similar activities. Persuasion by a realistic and authentic person, perhaps a teacher or peer, is a third source of efficacy. As a result, an individual may exert greater effort and persistence than they would have otherwise (Purzer, 2011; Townsend & Scanlan, 2011).

The fourth source of self-beliefs of efficacy is the perception of stressful bodily and emotional states. Students with a lower sense of self-efficacy may consider a stress reaction a predictor of poor academic performance. In contrast, those with higher self-efficacy beliefs may interpret the stress as an energizing facilitator of performance. "Butterflies" in the stomach can be interpreted as a sign that one has a lot of energy and will give a good oral performance in class, rather than a sign that one will fail. A growing body of evidence suggests that self-efficacy is important not only in educational pursuits, but also in other human accomplishments. Ordinary social realities are filled with problems, adversities, and setbacks, and a strong sense of self-efficacy helps to sustain efforts to succeed, as long as the sense of one's abilities is accurate and not overestimated (Bandura, 1986).

ROLE MODELING

People learn not only from their own experience, but also by observing others; therefore, modeling is a critical component of this theory. Role modeling refers to behavioral, cognitive, and affective changes resulting from observation of others. Thus, learning is often a social process, and significant people provide examples or role models for how to think, feel, and act. Bandura (1986) believed that social learning occurs principally by imitation. This type of learning is considered to be one of the important capabilities of the human species and includes the following steps (Braungart et al., 2014).

1. Attention is the observation of the relevant actions of a model
2. Retention involves processing and organizing the information so that the learner can reproduce the behavior

3. Production or reproduction refers to engaging in the observed behavior
4. Motivation is required to adopt and repeat the behavior if it produces valued results

Modeling serves many functions, particularly in academic settings. One of these is *response facilitation,* or providing social prompts for observers to behave in a certain way. The first students to arrive in the classroom or lab can be directed to a desired behavior, such as examining a model or relevant object the instructor has provided. When other students enter the room, they will follow the lead of the earlier students. Another function, *inhibition,* occurs when models receive negative feedback for performing certain actions, such as calling attention to students whose cell phones ring, and *disinhibition* occurs when these behaviors do not result in negative consequences (Burke & Mancuso, 2012).

Cognitive modeling includes explanation and demonstration, while verbalizing the model's thoughts and reasons for a particular activity. Case studies are only one instance in which teachers can model their problem-solving approach. "What are the most relevant factors with this client?" "What further information do I need right away?" Educators can "think aloud" while they discuss the case study, ethical dilemma, or other critical thinking example.

Nursing educators often use nurses in clinical settings, guest speakers, and the instructors themselves as role models to demonstrate procedures and content knowledge. However, these professional role models also demonstrate attitudes and values. What does it mean to "think like a nurse"? How does a competent nurse say that he or she doesn't know the answer? How does one handle disagreement with other team members? Experienced teachers and nurses often have lasting memories of nurses they saw as role models early in their career. Providing the best possible examples for students to observe in their educational experience is a critical part of professional development.

COGNITIVE LEARNING THEORY

Cognitivism is defined as a group of learning theories focused on cognitive processes such as decision making, problem solving, synthesizing, and evaluating. Historically, educational researchers focused on behavioral objectives and programmed learning from the behavioral perspective, as discussed in a previous section. As that influence declined, however, the focus expanded to the learner and instructional variables in educational settings. In contrast to the behaviorist approach, cognitivist approaches to learning focus on the human information processing system as it affects cognitive processes during learning and stresses their importance. Some argue that this focus means a shift from seeing learners as passive products of incoming stimuli from the environment to seeing learners as active agents who have goals, ideas, plans, and actively attend to, select, and organize information (Braungart et al., 2014; Candela, 2012).

The key to learning, according to the cognitive perspective, is the learner's perception, thinking, memory, and information processing and organization. Learning involves the formation of mental connections that may not necessarily be demonstrated in overt behavior changes. This viewpoint has often been compared to computer information processing, with a focus on how people process information from the environment, perceive the stimuli around them, put those perceptions into memory, and retrieve that knowledge (Candela, 2012; Hunt, 2012).

Educators generally agree that many of these cognitive processes such as concept learning, problem solving, transfer, and metacognition are central to learning. Within these cognitive processes, this theory acknowledges the wide variation in individual learners' perceptions, information processing, and other mental activities as part of the learning process (Hunt, 2012). Although there are individual variations that are important, the influence of instructional and motivational variables on learners' cognition, creative thinking, critical thinking, and cognitive development is also paramount (Braungart et al., 2014).

Cognitive theorists emphasize content organization, as it contributes to memory processing and retrieval of information. Using the cognitive processes, this perspective suggests that memory is enhanced by organizing information and making it meaningful. How learners organize and interpret information is very important. If learners already have some knowledge that is similar, showing connections to previous experience or content makes the new information more easily remembered (Hunt, 2012). Faculty can create structures for content, such as cause and effect, time sequence, and pros versus cons (Candela, 2012). Similarly, the actual content organization or structure may be remembered. The categories of pharmacology provide an excellent example of this kind of information organization as nursing students learn categories of drugs in which to place new drugs throughout their career, making that learning easier.

In addition to using these cognitive based strategies in classes, one can also teach the strategies to learners to enhance their own studying. One important factor about the use of cognitive study strategies is that they can be learned through educational intervention, in contrast to inherent student traits or abilities. The use of learning strategies based on cognitive principles is important to student success and efficiency (Candela, 2012).

The following is a sequence of nine specific events for learning using this information-processing model of memory (Braungart et al., 2014).

1. Gain attention
2. Inform of the objective and expectation
3. Stimulate recall of prerequisite learning
4. Present material
5. Provide learning guidance
6. Elicit performance
7. Provide feedback about correctness
8. Assess performance
9. Enhance retention, transfer, and recall

METACOGNITION

Metacognition is an important concept that plays a critical role in successful learning. It may be placed within cognitive theory (Braungart et al., 2014) or in constructivist theory (Candela, 2012). It consists of one's ability to assess one's own skills, knowledge, or learning. This process monitors the learning progress by checking the level of understanding, evaluating the effectiveness of efforts, planning activities, and revising as necessary. It is called *metacognition* because it is cognition about cognition, or thinking about thinking. This activity refers to the deliberate control of thinking activity, or the study of how one develops knowledge about one's own cognitive system. This reflective process of monitoring one's own thinking is a good example of the kind of critical thinking necessary in nursing (Rowles, 2012).

Educators can acknowledge, cultivate, and enhance metacognitive capabilities of learners by becoming facilitators of learning rather than simply teachers of content. A metacognitive approach to teaching helps students monitor their progress in learning, estimate the time required, plan study time, organize materials, and evaluate performance as a few of the possible activities. Explicitly teaching study strategies in content courses has been shown to improve learning. Some metacognitive strategies focus on helping students tackle particularly difficult assignments, avoid oversimplified thinking about complex situations, and see this as part of learning rather than just an obstacle (Chick, 2013).

Metacognition can affect motivation because it affects how well and how long students study, an important factor in how much they learn. It increases students' abilities to transfer learning to new situations. Students with poor metacognition skills believe that they have mastered course content too soon. Teaching students effective ways of preparing for exams and projects, suggesting valid assessment of readiness, and providing fair, consistent, and transparent grading policies are important metacognitive strategies to promote motivation (Chick, 2013).

TRANSFORMATIVE LEARNING

A description of how learners construct, validate, and reformulate their understandings of their experience makes up *transformative learning*. This concept is included here as it uses cognitive processes and metacognition, with the specific purpose of transforming one's perspectives. In this perspective, the learner's assumptions are disoriented with some kind of dilemma, leading to self-examination and resulting in a new perspective or revised interpretation (Candela, 2012). Using reflective learning experiences, such as service learning activities, students make their own interpretations rather than act on the judgments and beliefs of others (University of Central Oklahoma, 2013). Experience and critical reflection are central to the individual's constructing their own beliefs and judgments, rather than uncritically assimilating those of others. Many sensitive issues within health care, such as social justice, ethnicity, poverty, inequality of access, and physical abuse, provide examples in which learners' perspectives may be transformed with expanded experiences and information.

General implications of cognitive learning approaches emphasize mental processes and the role of the teacher in terms of effective teaching strategies that facilitate learning. For example, presenting information in an organized manner reflecting students' previous knowledge and its relation to new content helps students understand and make connections, as new information is most easily learned when associated with previous knowledge. Teachers can encourage reflection, and sequencing and present materials using as many modalities as possible (Candela, 2012).

Ultimately, this perspective acknowledges that learners determine what is learned, not the teacher. However, teachers can facilitate learning outcomes by using many of the cognitive teaching strategies alone or in combination with strategies associated with other learning perspectives.

CONSTRUCTIVIST LEARNING THEORY

Constructivism is a learning perspective arguing that individuals construct much of what they learn and understand, producing knowledge based on their beliefs and experiences. Although there is not just one constructivist theory of learning, most agree on two assumptions: (Learners are active in constructing their own knowledge, and social interactions are important in this process) (Dennick, 2012; Kala, Isaramalai, & Pohthong, 2010). According to this perspective, knowledge is subjective and personal, emphasizing the importance of culture and context. The emphasis on constructivism follows the shift away from environmental factors toward human factors as explanations for learning. Although cognitive theories emphasize learners' information processing, some think that these theories fail to capture the complexity of human learning (Candela, 2012).

The constructivist perspective has a basic assumption that active learners construct knowledge as they try to make sense of their experiences. Learners are not passive, "empty vessels waiting to be filled" (Woolfolk, 2010, p. 314). These learners develop mental models and revise them to make sense of their educational experience. These representations are the unique perspective of the learner and, therefore, are unique to the learner. In addition, this type of learning cannot be separated from its context (Dennick, 2012). The way learners interact with their worlds transforms their thinking, and this is known as *situated cognition*. An instructional implication of this idea is that teaching strategies should be consistent with the desired learning outcomes for a particular situation. If the objective is to teach inquiry skills, the curriculum must incorporate inquiry activities (Kala et al., 2010). This expectation fits well with nursing courses, as clinical activities provide the necessary situations for learning (Hampton, 2012).

Although constructivism is a more recent perspective, it underlies such educational thinking as the integrated curriculum in which learners study a topic from multiple perspectives. In addition, this perspective emphasizes learner-centered principles such as structuring the learning situation so that learners become actively involved with the content through manipulating materials or social interaction. This theory has been suggested as a relevant conceptual basis for student centered learning and for e-learning courses. Observing phenomena, collecting data, generating hypotheses, and working collaboratively, even online, are recommended strategies, as examples of hands-on, project-based activities suggested by this approach (Candela, 2012; Hampton, 2012; Kala et al., 2010).

Woolfolk (2010) presents five conditions for learning from the constructivist perspective. The first is to provide complex, realistic, and relevant learning environments. Students should not be given "stripped down, simplified problems and basic skills drills" (p. 315) instead of realistic projects, complex situations with many parts, and problems that might have several solutions. Tasks should be authentic, the kind of tasks that learners will confront in the real world. For some of these procedures, students can initially be supported through a process called *instructional scaffolding*, a procedure of controlling task elements that are initially beyond the learners' capacity. For example, the teacher might do much of the work in the beginning, after which the learner does an increasing role, leading to independence.

The second condition is to provide for social interaction and social responsibility as part of learning. Peer collaboration, either in person or online, is therefore valued; peers working cooperatively create social interactions that provide an instructional function. One goal of teaching may be to develop students' abilities to establish their own positions and defend them, yet respect other points of view. In the United States, considered to be individualistic and competitive, peer collaboration may be more of a challenge, yet some constructivists believe that higher order mental processes develop through these social interactions (Kala et al., 2010).

The third condition for learning from the constructivist perspective is to encourage multiple perspectives and representations of content. Complex content requires more than a simple explanation or one particular approach. Nurturing self-awareness in understanding how knowledge is constructed is the fourth constructivist condition for learning. Finally, the fifth condition is to facilitate student ownership of learning. This might include encouraging learners to make their own thinking processes explicit through dialogue, writing, or other representations (Woolfolk, 2010).

Problem-based learning is another strategy consistent with the constructivist learning perspective that initially grew out of research on expert knowledge in medicine. Using this strategy, learners are confronted with a problem that initiates their inquiry and collaboration to find solutions. Students analyze the problem, generate ideas, identify missing information, apply new knowledge, and evaluate the solutions (Hampton, 2012). During this process the teacher supports them with *scaffolded* information, if necessary. In true problem-based learning, the problem is real and the students' actions matter (Kala et al., 2010; Woolfolk, 2010). Teachers who wish to incorporate constructivist pedagogy in their program face the challenges of providing the necessary complex, collaborative, and relevant learning environments balanced with the practical considerations of a content-heavy curriculum and real-life limits on time and energy.

ADULT LEARNING THEORY

Malcolm Knowles is the central figure in U.S. adult education. First interested in *informal education,* he used the term to refer to informal programs in associations or clubs, pointing to the friendly and informal climate, flexibility of the process, and the enthusiasm and commitment of learners and teachers. He initially differentiated these informal programs at community centers, industries, and churches from the formal programs established by educational institutions (Knowles, 1978; Teaching Excellence in Adult Literacy [TEAL] Center Staff, 2011).

Androgogy or *adult learning* is a perspective focused on understanding how adults learn. Knowles (1978) was convinced that adults learn differently from children and his earlier work on informal adult education provided the foundation for his later work on the adult education movement. He assumed that adult learners are different from child learners in self-concept, experience, readiness to learn, orientation to learning, and motivation. Knowles's conception of *andragogy* was the adult equivalent of pedagogy and assumed that individuals become adults when they develop a self-concept and are capable of self-direction and responsibility for their lives. His concept of andragogy included the strategies of helping adults learn (Candela, 2012; TEAL Center Staff, 2011). Therefore, when an adult individual is in a situation in which self-direction is not possible, a tension arises. Knowles observed that when students enter a professional school, they have usually made a big step toward becoming self-directing and identifying with the adult role (Knowles).

Another difference of this perspective is that adults are not content centered, but problem centered. This viewpoint states that adult learners do best when they can utilize their experience and use new knowledge to solve real-world problems. These learners are more likely to learn if, in their view, the course material is relevant and viewed as important to them (Candela, 2012).

Knowles's (1978) concept of andragogy was an attempt to build a comprehensive, integrated theory or model of adult learning out of the isolated concepts, insights, and research findings regarding adult learning. However, some believe that Knowles simply provided a set of guidelines for practice rather than a theory. Therefore, his assumptions can be read as descriptions of the adult learner rather than a conceptual framework (TEAL Center Staff, 2011). This perspective is relevant to nursing instructors, and in addition, it is clear and easy to understand. Staff development or continuing education provides another example in which these learning principles are particularly helpful. In addition, the principles or assumptions of learning and learner characteristics fit nicely with other, more comprehensive theories, such as cognitivism or constructivism, thereby providing instructors with many ideas for projects and assignments with enough flexibility to be interesting and relevant to the adults in their classes. Thus, the ideas that began as related to informal education settings can be appropriate strategies within formal academic settings of all kinds.

These adult teaching principles and assumptions based on Knowles's model are as follows (Bastable & Myers, 2014; Candela, 2012; TEAL Center Staff, 2011).

1. The learning experience values and respects learner knowledge, feelings, ideas, and life experiences by connecting them to the learning experience and acknowledging their value
2. The course assists learners in developing learning objectives, learning contracts, activities, and evaluation. Working cooperatively with participants to choose projects or objectives meets their need for self-direction
3. Faculty and learners work together to establish relevant, immediate problems that may be solved by course material. The ability to apply knowledge and skills for the solution of immediate problems is one of the prime motivators for adults

4. The course and its activities create a comfortable and cooperative psychological and physical environment that encourages participation, while holding appropriately rigorous standards

Using this adult learning perspective, faculty often act as facilitators, as they consider the learners' perspectives about topics and projects. However, instructors have the final responsibility, using their content expertise to determine what matters in this particular area and, perhaps, articulate why certain knowledge is essential.

(In addition, this perspective reminds instructors that learning is a continuing process through life, one particularly relevant for nursing education.)Most nurses will act as teachers at several points in their lives. Client education, professional development, preceptor relationships, and faculty role all provide instances in which nurses teach throughout their professional careers.

This perspective provides additional difficulties in that the suggestions are more ambiguous than in traditional classrooms. Learners may be uncomfortable establishing their own goals and objectives. Learners who are inexperienced in this particular content will have difficulty with the increased expectations of participation and collaboration. These methods may not be suitable for all situations even though the learners are adults, particularly when the content or procedures are unfamiliar to the learners (Candela, 2012).

Further, allowing learners to develop goals and projects requires the in-depth content knowledge of the faculty. Inexperienced teachers or those without deep content knowledge will be much more comfortable with a more scripted course. In time, however, teachers will develop a bigger repertoire of handling different points of view and a variety of student activities. Finally, however, faculty has the responsibility for evaluation of the learning.

In general, adults have special needs and requirements as learners, according to this adult learning perspective. Adults desire an organized, well-defined program that is relevant to their personal goals. Effective teaching involves understanding how to use the characteristics of mature learners to the best advantage in a particular learning situation. Knowles (1978) reminds us that the accumulated experience of a mature individual provides a rich resource for learning as well as a broader base to which the learner can relate new information. Adults tend to have a problem-centered orientation to learning and want to apply information to today's problems. The more relevant the course work is to the learner's real world, the more important and motivating the material is for a nursing student.

HUMANISTIC LEARNING THEORY

Finally, this chapter discusses the *humanistic* perspective. *Humanism* is an approach to teaching that assumes people are inherently good and possess unlimited potential for growth; therefore, it emphasizes personal freedom, choice, self-determination, and self-actualization. Its approach to education in recent times is attributed to Abraham Maslow (1954), who was concerned with the study and development of self-actualization as fully functioning persons (Candela, 2012).

Maslow (1954) is perhaps best known for his hierarchy of needs, an important part of motivation. Maslow believed that humans strive to satisfy their needs, which are hierarchical. Lower order needs, such as physiological and safety needs, must be satisfied before higher order needs can influence behavior. The highest level need is self-actualization or the desire for self-fulfillment. Self-actualization can be expressed in many different ways according to the individual: the desire to be an ideal parent, to be an athlete, or to attain academic achievement. Therefore, the humanistic perspective is largely a motivational theory. The motivation originates in each person's needs and subjective feelings (Braungart et al., 2014; Dennick, 2012).

Carl Rogers (1954) also contributed to humanistic theory. His theory emerged primarily as a reaction against the dominant views of the 1940s, Freudian theory, and behaviorism. Rogers believed that individuals instinctively value positive regard, love, affection, and attention. His approach allows individuals to grow in self-esteem, self-discovery, and self-directed learning, with the goal of self-actualization, a person's basic overriding tendency. Rogers asserted that individuals are the center of their own personal experience. He stressed the importance of the teacher–student relationship and encouraged teachers to be facilitators rather than the traditional transmitters of information (Dennick, 2012).

Proponents of the humanistic approach to teaching object to what they perceive as mechanistic approaches to education, such as the use of drill and practice strategies. This perspective has its roots in the existential philosophy that wondered about the nature and purpose of humanity, sees humans as basically good, and asserts that teachers place far too much emphasis on measurable outcomes such as standardized tests. It assumes that individuals are unique and have a desire to grow in a positive way toward self-actualization (Braungart et al., 2014). Humanistic interpretations emphasize affective outcomes of education, promoting creativity and human potential. In addition to the student uniqueness, this view emphasizes the teacher's attitudes toward the learners. Humanism is compatible with nursing's emphasis on caring, an orientation that is challenged by the increasing emphasis on technology, cost efficiency, and time pressure (Braungart et al., 2014; Candela, 2012).

This actualizing tendency is the source of hunger and thirst, but also of personal growth, autonomy, and freedom according to this approach. Mastering information and facts is not the central objective of this approach to learning; rather fostering curiosity, enthusiasm, and responsibility are more important and should be the goal of the educator. Humanists believe that self-concept and self-esteem are necessary considerations in any learning situation, and what people want is unconditional positive regard, the feeling of being loved without strings attached. Experiences that are coercive or threatening diminish the learning outcomes for individuals. Humanistic principles have been a cornerstone of self-help groups, wellness programs, and palliative care. In professional education, the goal is to provide psychologically safe classrooms and clinical settings where humanistic principles can be demonstrated through a variety of instructional strategies (Braungart et al., 2014; Dennick, 2012).

Preparation of a humanistic teacher devotes as much attention to teacher attitudes as to subject matter and instructional strategies. Spontaneity, the importance of emotions, an individual's choices, and creativity are critical aspects of a humanistic approach to learning, which has the fulfillment of one's potential as its purpose. Students perceive meaningful learning as relevant because they believe it is important and will enhance their lives. This perspective recommends that humanistic educators act as facilitators who help students clarify and achieve their goals and establish a classroom climate oriented to significant learning. In this perspective, individual contracts and flexible procedures are preferable to lockstep sequences (Braungart et al., 2014; Dennick, 2012).

This theory has its weaknesses as well as strengths, as critics assert it is more of a philosophy than a science, and that it is practically impossible to maintain positive self-regard toward all learners (Braungart et al., 2014; Dennick, 2012). Moreover, information, facts, memorization, drill, and the tedious work sometimes required to master knowledge may well be necessary for knowledge building as even the most self-actualized nursing student still needs to know how to take care of patients safely, function as part of a health care team, and pass professional exams.

As before, strategies that arise from humanism and instructional strategies from other approaches such as behaviorism or cognitivism are often compatible to some extent. In the real world, teachers can demonstrate humanistic approaches and still use the strategies offered by other approaches. This statement reinforces the notion that in busy classrooms or clinical settings, the boundaries between applications of the theories discussed in this chapter are arbitrary and somewhat blurred. In addition, most educators do not fall neatly into one perspective or another; but combine strategies from several approaches as relevant for their work.

Important discussions can take place among nursing educators regarding the need to balance preparing professionals for the real world of complex health care settings with the humanistic goal of personal development. Within the content-heavy courses required for accreditation and clinical settings, how much is it possible to add a degree of student choice about assignments, increase the feeling of safety within classrooms, and encourage self-esteem and personal growth? How well can educators demonstrate positive regard, empathic understanding, and genuineness with the heavy demands of academic or professional programs? The focus on helping people maximize their potential provides an important addition to any theory's strategies, while presenting challenges to teachers and courses with high work demand.

SUMMARY

This chapter presented an overview of six perspectives on how learning occurs. As educators revise or create new curricula, they are encouraged to consider the potential contributions of all of the different explanations of learning processes. They provide the foundation for alternative teaching strategies that are relevant and applicable to particular classrooms, content, and students.

Ⓘ Behaviorism emphasizes the importance of environmental stimuli (the bell, the food) rather than internal thinking processes of the learner. Reinforcement of the resulting behaviors increases the likelihood of that particular behavior being repeated. Associations are formed with positive and negative stimuli that often generalize to new situations (Braungart et al., 2014; Candela, 2012). Within the classroom and clinical situation myriad examples of rewards and punishment provide opportunities for application of these principles.

Social cognitive theory moves the emphasis to the context of learning, emphasizing the importance of the interaction among personal characteristics, behaviors, and the social environment. Learning, according to this perspective, occurs in a social environment using observation, often of role models. Personal beliefs such as self-efficacy are important contributions to this perspective, providing the foundation for powerful teaching strategies that strengthen persistence and effort. Role modeling and other kinds of observational learning provide common and influential teaching strategies relevant for nursing students (Burke & Mancuso, 2012; Townsend & Scanlan, 2011).

Cognitivism focuses attention on internal, mental processes such as thinking, memory, information processing, and information organization. This perspective suggests many strategies for presenting content in ways that foster memory and understanding for the learner. Metacognition, or thinking about thinking, provides an essential part of inquiry, ethical dilemmas, and critical thinking generally and thereby occupies an important place in nursing classrooms. Transformative learning involves constructing or reformulating one's understanding of an experience (Chick, 2013; Hunt, 2012).

The constructivist perspective assumes that learners construct their own version of what they learn and understand. That means that learners produce knowledge based on their beliefs and experience, and social interactions are a critical aspect of this process. This perspective argues for teaching content from multiple perspectives and providing real-life problems in all their complexity and realism. Apprenticeships, in which learners work in authentic situations with experts, and problem-based learning are two strategies supported by this approach, since they embrace complex situations, perhaps with more than one good approach (Kala et al., 2010).

The adult learning perspective reminds instructors that adult students bring a reservoir of experiences and knowledge plus a focus on real-world, relevant, practical issues. Relevancy in course work and clinical assignments is particularly important for these mature students. In addition, adults prefer the flexibility to focus on their own goals and want respect for their accumulated experiences (Candela, 2012). Faculty must balance these flexibility concerns with the real world of course and time demands.

Finally, the humanistic perspective focuses on development of the individual, with self-actualization as the highest level. Facilitating the learner's positive attitude, self-esteem, responsibility, and enthusiasm are goals of this approach. Teaching strategies in a humanistic classroom consider the desire of all people for unconditional positive regard (Dennick, 2012).

Conceptual models and theories provide the foundation for many curricular decisions, especially the critical choice of teaching strategies. Management of curricular content and pedagogical innovations is necessitated by several factors including the rapid expansion of knowledge, content-saturated curricula, and changes to the health care delivery system. The learning theories discussed here predate recent technology and electronic educational issues, such as large online courses. Education may need newer paradigms or continue to use traditional models. Time, empirical research, and thoughtful discussion will determine whether traditional theories remain relevant to tomorrow's classrooms and academic issues, and whether new paradigms will emerge.

A curriculum plan provides guidelines for a specific educational program to be implemented. Today's nursing programs have constraints on resources, clinical settings that may be less than perfect, and too little time. These factors create enormous downward pressure on programs to simplify, eliminate, and generally make things easier. Learning theories remind planners about the importance of complex content, challenging cognitive tasks, self-efficacy, professional role models, information organization, and regard for students. These theories help provide counteracting "upward" pressure for faculty to design appropriately challenging, yet practical, curricula for today's health care practitioner.

DISCUSSION QUESTIONS

1. Evaluate learning theories as possible foundations to guide nursing program curricula in schools of nursing and health care settings.
2. Analyze various learning theories for appropriateness and congruency with the philosophy and mission of educational institutions, schools of nursing, or health care agencies.

LEARNING ACTIVITIES

STUDENT LEARNING ACTIVITIES

1. Compare learning theory strengths and weaknesses as a conceptual basis for teaching and learning strategies within a nursing or health care curriculum.
2. Contrast two learning theories for relevance with a health care organization's values or mission statement.

NURSE EDUCATOR/FACULTY DEVELOPMENT ACTIVITIES

1. Select one learning theoretical approach as an overall guide for developing teaching and learning strategies in a curriculum program or course.
2. Evaluate a learning theory as a foundation for a nursing program's objectives, strategies, and outcomes.

REFERENCES

Bandura, A. (1986). *Social foundations of thought & action. A social cognitive theory.* Englewood Cliff, NJ: Prentice-Hall.

Bastable, S., & Alt, M. (2014). Overview of education in health care. In S. Bastable (Ed.), *Nurse educator: Principles of teaching and learning for nursing practice* (4th ed., pp. 3–30). Burlington, MA: Jones & Bartlett.

Bastable, S., & Myers, G. (2014). Developmental stages of the learner. In S. Bastable (Ed.), *Nurse educator: Principles of teaching and learning for nursing practice* (4th ed., pp. 166–216). Burlington, MA: Jones & Bartlett.

Bloom, B., Englehart, M., Furst, E., Hill, W., & Krathwohl, D. (1956). *Taxonomy of educational objectives, the classification of educational goals—Handbook I: Cognitive domain.* New York, NY: McKay.

Boston University School of Public Health. 2013. *The social cognitive theory.* Retrieved from http://sphweb.bumc.bu.edu/otlt/MPH-Modules/SB/SB721-Models/SB721-Models5.html

Braungart, M., Braungart, R., & Gramet, P. (2014). Applying learning theories to health care practice. In S. Bastable (Ed.), *Nurse educator: Principles of teaching and learning for nursing practice* (4th ed., pp. 63–110). Burlington, MA: Jones & Bartlett.

Burke, H., & Mancuso, L. (2012). Social cognitive theory, metacognition, and simulation learning in nursing education (electronic version). *Journal of Nursing Education, 51*(10), 543–548.

Candela, L. (2012). From teaching to learning: Theoretical foundations. In D. Billings & J. Halstead (Eds.), *Teaching in nursing: A guide for faculty* (4th ed., pp. 202–243). St. Louis, MO: Elsevier Saunders.

Chick, N. (2013). *Metacognition.* Retrieved from http://cft.vanderbilt.edu/teaching-guides/pedagogical/metacognition/

Dennick, R. (2012). Twelve tips for incorporating educational theory into teaching practices (electronic version). *Medical Teacher, 34,* 618–624.

Gardner, H. (1983). *Frames of mind.* New York, NY: Basic Books.

Hagler, D., White, B., & Morris, B. (2011). Cognitive tools as a scaffold for faculty during curriculum redesign (electronic version). *Journal of Nursing Education, 50*(7), 417–422.

Hampton, M. (2012). Constructivism applied to psychiatric-mental health nursing: An alternative to supplement traditional clinical education (electronic version). *International Journal of Mental Health Nursing, 21,* 60–68.

Hunt, D. (2013). The new nurse educator: Mastering academe. New York, NY: Springer Publishing.

Hunt, E. (2012). Educating the developing mind: The view from cognitive psychology (electronic version). *Educational Psychology Review, 24,* 1–7.

Kala, S., Isaramalai, S., & Pohthong, A. (2010). Electronic learning and constructivism: A model for nursing education (electronic version). *Nursing Education Today, 30,* 61–66.

Knowles, M. (1978). *The adult learner: A neglected species* (2nd ed.). Houston, TX: Gulf Publishing.

Mager, R. (1962). *Preparing instructional objectives.* Palo Alto, CA: Fearon Publishers.

Maslow, A. (1954). *Motivation and personality.* New York, NY: Harper and Row.

Purzer, S. (2011). The relationship between team discourse, self-efficacy, and individual achievement: A sequential mixed-methods study. *Journal of Engineering Education, 100*(4), 655–679.

Rogers, C. (1954). *Client-centered therapy.* Boston, MA: Houghton Mifflin.

Rowles, C. (2012). Strategies to promote critical thinking and active learning. In D. Billings, & J. Halstead (Eds.), *Teaching in nursing: A guide for faculty* (4th ed., pp. 258–284). St. Louis, MO: Elsevier Saunders.

Teaching Excellence in Adult Literacy Center Staff. (2011). Adult learning theories, U.S. Department of Education. Retrieved from https://teal.ed.gov/tealGuide/adultlearning

Townsend, L., & Scanlan, J. (2011). Self-efficacy related to student nurses in the clinical setting: A concept analysis. *International Journal of Nursing Education Scholarship, 8*(1), 1–15.

Tyler, R. W. (1949). *Basic principles of curriculum and instruction.* Chicago, IL: University of Chicago.

University of Central Oklahoma. (2013). *Transformative learning.* Retrieved from http://www.uco.edu/central/tl/index.asp

Woolfolk, A. (2010). *Educational psychology* (11th ed.). Upper Saddle River, NJ: Merrill.

Using Contextual Curriculum Design With Taxonomies to Promote Critical Thinking

Lori Candela

OBJECTIVES

Upon completion of Chapter 5, the reader will be able to:

1. Examine the evolution of educational taxonomies in curriculum development and evaluation
2. Explore updates in and revisions to educational taxonomies
3. Analyze the development of critical thinking in the context of educational taxonomies
4. Categorize objectives to progress cognitive, affective, and psychomotor skills through nursing education levels
5. Produce learning activities and objectives that demonstrate structured, higher order thinking skills and exemplify dispositions of critical thinking
6. Explore the use of models to align curriculum design

OVERVIEW

Taxonomy refers to classification. An educational taxonomy provides a way for educators to view, develop, and evaluate learning objectives via a classification system. It is suitable for use at course and curricular levels. For more than 60 years, educators have turned to taxonomies to provide the terminology for objectives that could be behaviorally measured. Initially, educational taxonomies focused on the cognitive or thinking aspects of learning. Later, the affective (values) and psychomotor (physical skills) domains of learning were more fully developed.

The role of critical thinking is directly applicable to educational taxonomy. Even in its earliest version, taxonomy developers acknowledged the need to assess reasoning and problem solving abilities of students. Some argue that only the upper levels of the taxonomy include critical thinking, while others see all levels as influential in the development process.

Central to the development of critical thinking skills is the degree to which the student engages with the content. This can best be achieved through the use of well thought out, structured active learning strategies.

Curriculum developers must consider the global context in which students learn and develop their critical thinking abilities This requires consideration of multiple factors including the learners and educators, program framework and underlying philosophy, resources, larger institution alignment, the community, local and global health care environments, and the dynamic nature of society at large. The ability to consider these factors in a logical way can be enhanced through the understanding of the contextual nature in which learning occurs. A contextual model to assist in thinking through curriculum design that uses a taxonomy was developed by this author and is presented for consideration in this chapter.

THE USEFULNESS OF EDUCATIONAL TAXONOMIES

Taxonomy provides a common language and framework for classifying, categorizing, and defining educational goals. The use of taxonomy over the past several decades facilitated a shift in focus from what is taught to what students are expected to learn. Educators at every level use taxonomy to develop, communicate, and evaluate learning objectives. Curriculum developers and evaluators use taxonomy as a method for mapping the progression of student learning toward larger program outcomes.

OBJECTIVES AND OUTCOMES

The use of objectives in education can be traced back to when Ralph Tyler (1949) published a little book with great influence titled *Basic Principles of Education and Instruction.* Tyler argued that education should center on the learner and that changes in learner behavior be measured by statements or objectives. Prideaux (2000) noted that Tyler had a "broad view of the nature of objectives . . ." (p. 168). Ralph Mager later advocated that those learner behaviors needed to be stated in very specific terms. These became known as behavioral objectives that replaced verbs such as "understand" with verbs like "identify" (Pridaeaux).

Many terms have been used over the years to describe how and what students should learn. Terms such as learning objectives, learning targets, behavioral objectives, instructional objectives, and learning outcomes have inadvertently caused confusion among educators (Marzano, 2013). Some have argued that there is no difference between objectives and outcomes (Harden, 2002). Even today the verbiage used varies among nursing programs.

Particular confusion seems to exist regarding the use of the term learning "outcome" versus "objective." The outcome-based education movement of recent years advanced the need for clearly articulated intended learner goals. But many educational programs merely tinkered with small word or title changes instead of truly considering the differences. A quick review of 25 bachelor of science in nursing (BSN) programs on the Internet revealed the use of "terminal objectives," "learning objectives," "end-of-program objectives," and "learning outcomes." Harden (2002) argued that there are definite differences between objectives and outcomes.

Both describe products of learning but objectives are more specific and detailed, delineated into learning domains (knowledge, skills, attitudes), stated as intentions, and are more owned by individual instructors. Simply put, "Outcomes relate directly to professional practice; objectives relate to instruction" (Glennon, 2006, p. 55).

It may be clearer to consider an outcome as the essential, significant learning that the student achieves at the *end* of a course or at the *end* of the program (most often, the term *outcome* is used at the program vs. course level). Objectives are the behaviors (knowledge, skills, and attitude) that are to be demonstrated at the end of a unit of instruction (such as a learning module or course). What is most important is that each nursing program has clarity and consistency in whatever term is decided upon in order to avoid confusion or reluctance when educators attempt to distinguish and align curriculum outcomes or objectives to courses (Noble, 2004).

THE CONNECTION OF OBJECTIVES TO LEARNING THEORY

Most educational objectives are rooted in behaviorism. The behavioral view posits that learning does not occur if the desired behavior produced by education is not observable or measurable. This served nursing education well, particularly in terms of skill acquisition. However, the complexity and pace of new information assures that not every skill can be taught. Students must learn to construct new knowledge throughout their lives in order to adapt and thrive in unknown, ambiguous situations.

The constructivist view is that reality is built, or constructed, by the person. New information that is taken in is then integrated within the context of previous knowledge, experiences, and perceptions to form new learning and insight (Goudreau et al., 2009; Hagstrom, 2006). Constructivist, behavioral, or other theories of learning can be readily adapted for use with educational taxonomy.

DOMAINS OF LEARNING WITHIN TAXONOMIES

Without question, the work of Benjamin Bloom and his colleagues in the late 1940s and 1950s to develop a common taxonomy will forever be viewed as one of the most important achievements in education in the 20th century (Granello, 2001). Bloom's taxonomy is certainly the most familiar and, most likely, one of the most common educational taxonomy frameworks in use by educators today. It has been translated into every language for use in in academic settings from elementary through postsecondary schools (Wineburg & Schneider, 2010). The ideas behind the taxonomy were first discussed by Bloom and a group of colleagues attending the American Psychological Association conference in 1948 (Bloom, 1994). The group was looking to develop a common framework to promote sharing of ideas for examination materials, research on the examinations, and their connection to education. The group determined that this framework could best be achieved if it included "a system of classifying the goals of the educational process using educational objectives" (Bloom, 1994, p. 2).

The group continued meeting regularly for the next several years. It became apparent that the best way to develop a comprehensive taxonomy suitable for the evaluation of learning was to consider it through three categories (domains) that affect the *process* of learning: cognitive behavior, affective behavior, and psychomotor behavior (Halawi, Pires, & McCarthy, 2009). Each domain was conceived as a category and the categories were arranged in a simple to complex hierarchical order. Mastery of behaviors in each lower category was prerequisite to mastery of the next level. Also, every level was a part of the next higher level. This early work was considered as an aid for "studying, understanding, and solving educational problems" (Krathwohl & Anderson, 2010, p. 64). The first and most complete work occurred in the cognitive domain. This was logical as it was most closely related to the types of examinations occurring at that time (Bloom, 1994). The work of the group culminated with the publication of *The Taxonomy of Educational Objectives, Handbook 1: Cognitive Domain* (Bloom, 1956).

THE COGNITIVE DOMAIN OF BLOOM

The first level of the taxonomy is knowledge. For Bloom (1956) and his group, knowing was considered to be foundational to all other levels. It is remembering what is known and demonstrating it by recitation or recall. The second level is comprehension. Comprehension goes beyond knowledge as the person is able to grasp, understand, and make some sense of information. The understanding may not be complete but is indicative of being able to do something with what you know. Bloom (1994) points out three types of comprehension: (1) translation (putting the information into a different language "in your own words"), (2) interpretation (reordering the information, considering the importance of the concepts, summarizing, generalizing), and (3) extrapolation (making predictions or forecasts).

The third level of the six-tier taxonomy is application. At this level, the student can solve a problem or issue that is new by applying what is known and understood from other experiences. Bloom points out that application is different and more complex than extrapolation at the comprehension level. Extrapolation is based on "what is given" versus the abstraction necessary in application, such as applying a general rule or principle to a new situation. The fourth level is analysis, in which one knows, understands, and can apply information well enough to then break it down into component parts, examine how it is organized and the relationships that exist among the parts. Bloom considered this analysis as a necessary "prelude" to being able to evaluate the sixth and final level.

The fifth level is synthesis. This involves the ability to take parts, such as pieces of information and put them together to form something that was not "clearly present" before. This level is most closely linked with creativity. However, it is not viewed as complete freedom of expression since there are generally some set guidelines or restrictions.

The sixth and final level of the taxonomy is evaluation. This level incorporates all of the previous levels in order to judge (quantitatively and/or qualitatively) the value of what is being studied. Criteria or standards are used in making such judgments. This clearly differentiates it from opinions, which may exist without full awareness or conscious use of logical criteria. Bloom did not see evaluation as the last step of the cognitive levels but as the real connection to the affective domain, which is concerned with values. Sousa (2005) noted the connection between the affective and cognitive domains as a way of developing the higher order thinking skills of students.

According to Sousa (2005), the lower three cognitive levels involve convergent thinking in which learners apply what they remember and understand to solving new problems. The upper three levels use more divergent or higher order thinking to develop new insights (Sousa, 2005). Bissell and Lemons (2006) believe that higher order thinking is also present at the application level.

Bloom's taxonomy is widely used in primary, secondary, and postsecondary education to both establish and evaluate learning (Athanassious, McNett, & Harvey, 2003; Cochran, Conklin, & Modin, 2007). McNeill, Gosper, and Hedberg (2011) describe the use of Bloom's taxonomy in connecting course outcome indicators to program level evaluation. The taxonomy is used across various educational levels and disciplines (Manton, English, & Kernek, 2008). It has been translated into at least 22 languages (Krathwohl, 2002) and is referenced in citations nearly 100 times per year (Bloom, 1994). The taxonomy provides a structure for educators to consider learning and the products of learning.

One of the more recurring criticisms of the original taxonomy is that it is simplistic (Kuhn, 2008). The hierarchal structure of the taxonomy is unidirectional and presumes that each simpler category, such as, comprehension, must be "mastered" before the next level; in this case, application (Krathwohl, 2002; Paul, 1993). It has been argued synthesis may not necessarily be more complex than evaluation (Asim, 2011). Another criticism of the taxonomy revolved around the category of knowledge. The verbs associated with the knowledge category, such as recall and recite, suggested that knowledge was simplistic, little more than memorization (Booker, 2008; Paul, 1993).

As the use of learning theories such as constructivism became more prominent, the entire notion of how a student learns by building on previous learning to structure new knowledge may not fit neatly into the hierarchical format of the taxonomy. New information and research into the areas of learning and cognition led to a significant revision to the original taxonomy (Anderson & Krathwohl, 2001).

The Revised Taxonomy

In 2001, Anderson and Krathwohl published a significant revision to Bloom's taxonomy. Rationale for the revision included the need to again think of the impact of the original taxonomy on education and how visionary it was at the time. Second, there was a need to revise as new knowledge regarding thinking and learning became available (Bumen, 2007). Even as the original handbook was being published, Bloom advocated for updates and changes to the taxonomy as new knowledge became available. Bloom actually collaborated with others to revise the taxonomy prior to his retirement (Pickard, 2007).

The original taxonomy was one-dimensional (cognitive process), while the revised taxonomy was considered to be two-dimensional: knowledge and cognitive process and differed in three areas. The first change was one of terminology. The knowledge category was renamed remember; comprehension was renamed understand. The second change was to move the synthesize level to the top and rename it "create." The third change was to add a second dimension. The revised taxonomy retained the cognitive process dimension and added a knowledge dimension (Anderson & Krathwohl, 2001). The knowledge dimension consists of factual, conceptual, procedural and metacognitive levels (Roberts & Inman, 2007). The revision allowed for the cognitive category to focus on the noun aspect of an objective "principles of sterile technique," while the knowledge dimension focused on the verb portion "remember" (Krathwohl, 2002).

Factual knowledge includes the basics that students need to know to be acquainted with the discipline such as knowledge of terminology or specific details. Conceptual knowledge involves understanding the interrelationships of parts within a structure (knowledge of classifications or categories, principles and generalizations, theories and models). Procedural knowledge includes knowing how to do something such as knowledge of criteria for determining which procedure to use, proper steps in performing a procedure, or developing algorithms/concept maps for patient-specific care. Metacognitive knowledge is knowledge of cognition in general as well as having a personal awareness and knowledge of cognition, such as strategic knowledge, knowledge about cognitive tasks within different contexts, and self-knowledge (Krathwohl, 2002).

The first level of the cognitive dimension, remember, involves retrieving relevant knowledge. This is typified by verbs such as recall and recognize. The second level is to understand or be able to discern the meaning of information. Verbs in this category include interpreting, classifying, summarizing, comparing, explaining, inferring, and exemplifying. At the apply level, the learner is able to use what he or she remembers and understands to carry out an action in a given situation (verbs: execute, implement). To be able to analyze (level 4) is to be able to break something down into parts, examine relationships between, them and determine how each part relates to the whole (verbs: differentiate, organize, attribute). The fifth level, evaluate, represents the ability to make judgments based on criteria and includes verbs such as checking and critiquing. The final level is create and includes the ability to put elements together to form new, original products (verbs: generate, plan, produce) (Krathwohl, 2002).

OTHER EDUCATIONAL TAXONOMIES

The Affective Domain of Krathwohl

Krathwohl, who was a member of the original taxonomy group, further delineated the affective domain of the taxonomy. The affective domain is concerned with feelings or emotions that are expressed as values and interests. This domain includes ethical and moral behaviors and features five levels. According to O'Neill (2010, p. 2), "learners move from being aware of what they are learning to a stage of having internalized the learning so that it plays a role in guiding their actions."

Receiving involves being conscious of phenomena and to another's expression of ideas or beliefs. Verbs such as attends, shares, selects, prefers, describes, follows, names, observes, and replies are typical in this category. Subcategories include awareness (becoming aware of something), willingness to receive (ability to suspend judgment or maintain neutrality), and controlled or selected attention in which one is able to differentiate and make selections regarding various stimuli, such as, alertness to human values and judgments about living wills.

Responding is the verbal and nonverbal reactions that indicate a response to a phenomenon ranging on a continuum from compliance to satisfaction. The subcategories range from acquiescence (compliance) in responding to a willingness to respond (voluntarily responding without fear of recrimination) to satisfaction with the response (expressing satisfaction with the response). An example objective for this is, "The first level nursing students express enjoyment when participating in student nurse association activities" (Krathwohl, 2002).

In valuing, students make choices and internalize the value of that choice. It implies that something has worth. Subcategories include acceptance of a value by being able to consistently describe its worth; preference of the value by seeking it out to fulfill a desire for it; and commitment, which is activated when the learner develops deep convictions about the value to the point of trying to convince others of the value, for example, "right to life" or "right to choose." The final level is organizing, in which the learner is able to examine values, determine the most significant values, and organize them, even if some conflict with others (Krathwohl, 2002).

By the time a person reaches the highest level of the affective domain, he or she has internalized values and placed them into an internal organized system. Behaviors are consistent and in tune with those values. This is a gradual process and may take a lifetime to achieve. One method to help educators assess learner progression is through writing activities, such as articulating a life philosophy. If done early in the program, it could then be repeated near the end of the program to examine development and differences of thought.

The Psychomotor Domain of Simpson, Dave, and Harrow

There are three psychomotor taxonomies in education. The first was proposed by Simpson (1966) and consists of:

- Perception: tuning into sensory cues (verbs: distinguish, identify, select)
- Set: readiness to act (verbs: assume a position, demonstrate, show)
- Guided response: occurs early in the skill and indicates that the learner is capable of completing the steps (verbs: attempt, initiate, try)
- Mechanism: can perform a complex skill at an intermediate stage (do, act upon, complete)
- Complex overt response: involves correctness in performing the skill (verbs: operate, carry out, perform)
- Adaptation: can modify skills in a new situation (verbs: adapt, change, modify)
- Origination: creative ability to develop an innovative, unique skill that replaces one that was learned (verbs: create, design, invent) (Oermann, 1990)

Harrow (1972) developed a taxonomy based on reflex movement, basic fundamental movements, perceptual abilities, skilled movements, and nondiscursive communication. The taxonomy is organized by degree of coordination. At the lowest level, reflex movements include automatic reactions. The next level, basic fundamental movement, involves simple movements that can build to more complex sets of movements. At the perceptual level, environmental cues are used to adjust movements. Perceptual abilities at this level are described as tactile, visual, kinesthetic, visual, auditory, and coordinated, whereas physical abilities are described as agile, flexible, endurance, and strength. The level of nondiscursive communication is expressive and interpretive, as in the use of body language.

Dave (1970) published a taxonomy on constructivism including imitate, manipulate, precision, articulation, and naturalization. The taxonomy was based on neuromuscular movement and coordination and underlies criteria proposed by Reilly and Oermann (1990), which were based on a developmental approach to competency. The criteria for each level, according to Reilly and Oermann, are:

- Imitation level: occasional errors are apparent in the necessary actions of the skill and are accompanied by some weakness of gross motor actions, and the time required to complete the skill is dependent on the learner's need (verbs: attempt, copy, duplicate, imitate, mimic)
- Manipulation level: coordination of movements occurs with some variation in the time required to complete the actions of the skill (verbs: complete, follow, play, perform, produce)
- Precision level: a logical sequence carries activities through to completion, almost free of errors in noncritical actions, although the speed of completion continues to be a concern (verbs: achieve automatically, excel expertly, perform masterfully)
- Articulation level: logic is evident in the coordinated actions, few, if any errors are noted, and the time required to execute the skill is considered reasonable (verbs: customize, originate)
- Naturalization level: professional competence is noted in the skill performance that is automatic and well coordinated (verbs: naturally performs and perfectly performs)

The Holistic Taxonomy of Hauenstein

Hauenstein (1998) proposed a taxonomy that synthesized cognitive, affective, and psychomotor learning into a fourth domain he called "behavior domain." He felt the original taxonomy lacked integration and connection, both of which he considered necessary in order to achieve a holistic curriculum that focused on student understanding, skills and dispositions. He reduced the categories of the first three domains from six to five. The cognitive domain involved the process of knowing and the development of intellectual abilities and skills. The affective domain is directed toward developing dispositions in relation to feelings, values, and beliefs. The psychomotor domain is defined as the development of physical abilities and skills that result from the input of information and content.

The behavioral domain is the "tempered demeanor" that one displays as a reaction to a social stimulus, or an inner need, or both. The behavioral domain consists of acquisition, assimilation, adaptation, performance, and aspiration. The acquisition objective is the process of understanding, perceiving, and conceptualizing new information. Assimilation involves comprehending concepts in relation to prior knowledge and explaining it in his or her own terms. Adaptation involves the ability to modify knowledge, skills, or dispositions to conform to an established standard or criterion. Performance is the ability to analyze, qualify, evaluate, and integrate information with personal values and beliefs so that it becomes ingrained and able to be repeated in either new or routine situations (Hauenstein, 1998).

Sipos, Battisi, and Grimm (2008) used the Hauenstein taxonomy to develop a transformative sustainability learning (TSL) unifying framework. The authors used the metaphors of head (cognitive), hands (psychomotor), and hearts (affective) to describe a curriculum in sustainability education. Course objectives and learning activities were developed using all three domains to promote learning, skill acquisition, and a sense of values that could result in "societal transformation."

Fink Taxonomy of Significant Learning

The Fink taxonomy (2003) grew from the work of Bloom but added major considerations in the areas of motivation and human interaction. The taxonomy is circular versus hierarchical and is composed of six categories: foundational knowledge, application, integration (making connections), human dimension (student learning about themselves and others—why one does what one does), caring, and learning how to learn. The taxonomy sees learning as multidirectional and that significant learning requires alignment among learning goals, learning activities and learning assessment (Levine et al., 2008).

Biggs SOLO Taxonomy

The Biggs (1996) Structure of Observed Learning Outcome (SOLO) distinguishes five levels of learning by their cognitive processes. It offers a way to view the progression of learning from surface to deep. This is accomplished by moving through cognitive processes that grow in complexity: prestructural (not knowing about the concept or area), unistructural (knowing one facet of the concept or area), multistructural (knowing several aspects of the concept or area), relational (integrating those aspects into a whole), and extended abstract (knowledge can be generalized to other areas) (Boulton-Lewis, 1995; Brabrand & Dahl, 2009).

The Fink and SOLO taxonomies have been most frequently used at the course level. The SOLO taxonomy in particular is often used in the evaluation of writing development. However, the utility of each could be a basis for progression through a curriculum of study such as nursing, which is concerned with learner development in areas including human interaction, motivation, and communication.

A New Taxonomy

In 2007, Marzano and Kendall published *The New Taxonomy of Educational Objectives* (2nd ed.). The book provides a detailed description of the theories behind and the use of a two dimensional taxonomy: levels of processing and domains of knowledge. One of the criticisms of the original taxonomy was the hierarchical nature of cognition that indicated the increasing difficulty with each ascending level. Marzono and Kendall disagreed, noting a common psychological principle that even the most difficult mental processes become simple as they become more familiar. The number of steps needed to carry out the mental process and the relationships between steps may not change but the speed at which one can perform them does. For example, a student nurse may take 15 minutes or more to match medications to a medication administration record (MAR) and draw up an injection. That same nurse would likely be able to carry out the task in less than 2 minutes if he or she had performed it many times.

The new taxonomy features six horizontal levels of processing and three vertical rows of knowledge domains. The first four levels of processing are within the cognitive system: retrieval (recognizing, recalling, executing), comprehension (integrating, symbolizing), analysis (matching, classifying, analyzing errors, generating, specifying), and knowledge utilization (decision making, problem solving, experimenting, investigating). The next level is the metacognitive system, which specifies and monitors knowledge in terms of goals, processes, clarity, and accuracy. Self-system thinking is the sixth level of processing. This level is concerned with how motivated a person is in learning a new task given the importance, efficacy, and emotional responses attached to it. Emotions can hinder or facilitate learning (Sousa, 2001). Shulman (2002) discussed the influence of engagement and motivation as both a purpose of education and a ""proxy" for subsequent learning.

It is the self-system that decides whether to engage in a new learning task. Examples of internal questions that affect motivation to learn are: How important is this to learn? How much do I believe I can learn it? How positive or negative do I feel about this new task? Once the self-system decides to engage, the metacognitive system is activated followed by the cognitive system. "All three systems use the student's store of knowledge" (Marzano & Kendall, 2007).

The three domains of knowledge are information, mental procedures, and psychomotor procedures. The information domain (declarative knowledge) is represented as hierarchical. The lower three are described as details (vocabulary terms, facts, time sequences), while the higher levels are organizing ideas (principles, generalizations). The mental procedures domain (procedural knowledge) contains two categories: a skills category that uses algorithms, tactics, and single rules, and a processes category of macroprocedures. Unlike the procedures in the skills category that can be learned so well as to require little or no conscious thought, macroprocedures are highly complex and require conscious control. The psychomotor domain involves a skill category of simple combination and foundational procedures as well as a processes level of complex combination procedures.

The new taxonomy builds on the work of Bloom's original taxonomy and the Anderson revised taxonomy. According to the authors, new taxonomy differs because it: (1) addresses cognitive, affective, and psychomotor learning domains very specifically; (2) places the metacognitve system above the cognitive system; and (3) considers the self-system at the top of the six processing levels. For a more detailed discussion of the new taxonomy, readers are encouraged to consult the Marzano and Kendall (2007) book.

Bloom's Digital Taxonomy

Revisions to Bloom's taxonomy continue to focus on specific areas of skill development. One example is the work of Andrew Churches, an educator in an elementary/secondary school in New Zealand. Using the revised taxonomy, he created "Bloom's Digital Taxonomy." The taxonomy depicts each increasingly complex level of cognitive ability with technology to ascending levels of higher order thinking—from accessing and finding information, to using and analyzing it, to designing it. This all occurs within the context of developing communication through the use of technology (Churches, 2007, 2008).

Churches does not work with college-level students. However, there is relevance in his work to nursing programs. Many nursing programs include a program outcome related to the use of technology in patient care. Both the Accreditation Commission for Education in Nursing (ACEN) and the American Association of Colleges of Nursing (AACN) contain verbiage regarding the use of technology as a competence for students in prelicensure nursing programs (AACN, 2014; ACEN, 2014). Creative uses of taxonomy such as the one proposed by Churches may be helpful in progressing the competence level of students in the use of technology throughout the curriculum.

Curriculum Alignment Using a Taxonomy Table

The use of a taxonomy table is beneficial to ensure that there is alignment between curricular objectives, instruction, and assessment (Anderson, 2002). Educators who assess both cognitive and knowledge dimensions are able to discern a more complete understanding of intended learning (Su, Osisek, & Starnes, 2004). Misalignment of the curriculum may result in assessments and/or objectives that do not reflect instruction (Airasian & Miranda, 2002).

Virtually any objective, activity, or assessment can be plotted into any taxonomy table and can be reviewed and updated regularly to assure the curriculum is aligned and incorporates concepts that are important for students to learn. Table 5.1 illustrates the application of the new taxonomy of educational objectives to align a curriculum from the program outcomes, course objectives, learning content and experiences, to related assessments and evaluations.

TABLE 5.1   ALIGNMENT OF A CURRICULUM TO THE NEW TAXONOMY OF EDUCATIONAL OBJECTIVES

RELATED PROGRAM OUTCOME	RELATED COURSE OBJECTIVE	RELATED ACTIVITY LEARNING CONTENT/ ASSIGNMENTS/ LEARNING EXPERIENCES	RELATED ASSESSMENTS OR EVALUATIONS	LEVEL OF PROCESSING							DOMAIN	
				R	C	A	S	M	SS	I	MP	P

A, application; C, comprehension; I, information (declarative knowledge); M, metacognitive; MP, mental procedures (procedural knowledge); P, psychomotor; R, retrieval; S, synthesis; SS, self-system.

A CONTEXTUAL MODEL FOR ALIGNING CURRICULUM AND COURSES

This chapter's author has worked across various levels of nursing education in creating and revising nursing curricula and courses. The dynamic nature in which educational curricula and courses occur prompted her recently to put several concepts she has used over the years to guide both course and curriculum efforts into a model. The Contextual Approach to Navigate Delivery of Outcomes (CANDO) model incorporates selected aspects from general systems, complexity, adult learning, and constructivist theories as well as the backward design process of Wiggins and McTighe (2005). The model offers another way to consider the course or the curriculum within multiple contexts: students, course learning environment, level/program fit, connection to level/program outcomes, clinical workplace, and the larger society. These are identified in Table 5.2.

The model considers that educators continue to learn and they apply that learning to the design and delivery of courses and curriculums. Individual courses and entire curriculums are systems that interface with other systems. The systems are dynamic and are affected by one another. Educators learn and adapt both from previous experiences and from attention to the contexts in which the curriculum and courses operate. Curriculum and courses are aligned to one another by considering the desired end results of learning and working backward in a considered, ongoing process of designing, delivering, and revising curricula and courses. The model is represented by several circles depicting the various external and internal program contexts within which a nursing program and its courses are delivered, and is intended for use at curricular and course levels.

The contexts identified in the CANDO model require educators to ask questions such as: What do I/we need to know and use from this particular context in order to

---

TABLE 5.2 THE CONTEXTUAL APPROACH TO NAVIGATE DELIVERY OF OUTCOMES (CANDO)

GENERAL SYSTEMS THEORY	COMPLEXITY THEORY	ADULT LEARNING THEORY	CONSTRUCTIVIST THEORY	BACKWARD DESIGN
Systems have boundaries but interact with each other (input/ output) and affect one another (feedback)	Systems are connected, open, non-linear, uncertain and unpredictable, complex, and adaptive	Learning incorporates previous experiences, problem-centered, looks to apply knowledge to situations	Integration of prior knowledge with new learning to create new meaning; multiple representations of reality that are complex	Stage 1: Plan course and curriculum starting with determining desired results; Stage 2: determine what constitutes evidence of performance; Stage 3: determine which activities/experiences/ lessons will be used to move learners toward the desired results
(Taplin, 1980)	(Gatrell, 2005; Manson, 2001; What is Complexity Theory?, 2014)	(Merriam, 2001; Kiely, Sandmann & Truluk, 2004)	(Learning Theories/Constructivist Theories, 2014; Terwel, 1990; Brandon, 2010)	(Wiggins & McTighe, 2005)

ensure the delivery of course/curriculum outcomes? Do the outcomes and objectives reflect current and emerging knowledge, skills, attitudes important for practicing nurses? What new content needs to be adapted and what is currently in the curriculum that needs to be revised or removed? What assessments and evaluations are necessary to demonstrate that learners are progressing and meeting objectives and outcomes? and What learning experiences/lessons/assignments will facilitate student's meeting the objectives and outcomes? Although this author used the approach detailed in this model for years, it has not been subject to research. However, in her experience, visualization from this more holistic view has been instrumental in designing and revising courses and curriculums that result in students and graduates who met identified course, level, and program outcomes.

The model is presented here solely as one of many ways to consider how internal program factors and external program factors affect one another and can align in delivering high quality learning outcomes. Research utilizing this model on various types and levels of curriculums would be most welcome. (The CANDO model is complementary to the External and Internal Frame Factors model discussed in Section III of this text for determining the need for curricular revision or for development of new programs.)

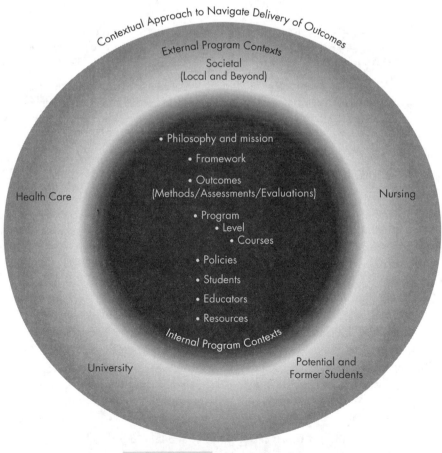

FIGURE 5.1 CANDO model.

CRITICAL THINKING AND TAXONOMY

Nurses practice in fast-paced, complex environments in which chaos and change are often the norm (Goudreau et al., 2009; Rowles & Russo, 2009). Bits of new information bombard us constantly, ensuring that at least some of the content nursing students learn in school today will be obsolete by the time they graduate. These realities require that nurses quickly assess situations (often with only partial information), make rational clinical judgments, follow with sound clinical decision making, and reflect to assess performance and determine continued learning needs. Simpson and Mary Courtney (2002) discussed the urgency for practicing nurses to be able to quickly assess, make decisions, and act in the chaotic and fast-paced environment of health care. This is vital for safe, high-quality care.

Critical thinking requires discernment and a "longing to know—to understand how life works" (hooks, 2010, p. 7). Brookfield (1987) viewed critical thinking through the four components of challenging assumptions, understanding the context of the situation, exploring alternative reasons/causes/influencers, and being a reflective skeptic throughout. Critical thinking is important in nursing and

---

BOX 5.1   DEFINITIONS OF CRITICAL THINKING

Critical thinking is:

- "A purposeful, outcome-directed (results-oriented) thinking . . . [that] requires knowledge, skills, and experience . . . [and helps one] constantly re-evaluate, self correct . . ., and strive to improve" (Alfaro-Lefevre, 1999, p. 9).

- "A rational investigation of ideas, inferences, assumptions, principles, arguments, conclusions, issues, statements, beliefs, and actions that covers scientific reasoning and includes the nursing process, decision making, and reasoning in controversial issues" (Bandman & Bandman, 1995).

- "Reflective and reasonable thinking that is focused on deciding what to do or believe" (Ennis, 1985, p. 45).

- "Purposeful, self-regulatory judgment which results in interpretation, analysis, evaluation, an inference as well as explanation of the evidential, conceptual, methodological, criteriological, or contextual considerations upon which that judgment was based" (Facione, 1990).

- "Those skills (or strategies) that increase the probability of achieving a desirable outcome" (Halpern, 1994. p. 13).

- "An investigation whose purpose is to explore a situation, phenomenon, question, or problem to arrive at a hypothesis or conclusion about it that integrates all available information and that can therefore be convincingly justified" (Kurfiss, 1988, p. 2).

- "The intellectually disciplined process of actively and skillfully conceptualizing, applying, analyzing, synthesizing, and/or evaluating information gathered from, or generated by, observation, experience, reflection, reasoning, or communication, as a guide to belief and action" (National Council for Excellence in Critical Thinking, 1992, p. 201).

- "Thinking about your thinking while you're thinking in order to make you think better" (Paul, 1993, p. 91).

in "everyday life" (Valiga, 2009). A single definition of critical thinking has been elusive, as evidenced by the numerous definitions that have been advanced over the years. A comprehensive definition advanced by Paul (1993) is presented in Box 5.1.

Valiga (2009) conducted an analysis of 17 definitions on critical thinking and found the following aspects in common: (1) a critical thinker is nonbiased, reasoned and truth oriented; (2) critical thinking involves making judgments; (3) thinking can be judged as critical if it holds up to certain evaluative criteria; (4) tied to a belief or action (p. 218).

One of the most articulate scholars on critical thinking is Richard Paul. His 1993 book, *Critical Thinking: How to Prepare Students for a Rapidly Changing World*, challenged educators to fundamentally reconsider how and what content and learning experiences are used in light of developing the thinking skills of students. Paul and Elder published a very informative miniature guide on critical thinking that contains a definition and stages of critical thinking as well as questions and assessment focus areas for determining the development of critical thinking (Paul & Elder, 2007).

Clinical decision making is a term that is becoming more frequently used in nursing programs and in clinical practice. However, critical thinking is foundational to clinical decision making in order to ensure that safe, reasoned actions result. This ability to "think through" various situations is therefore crucial for clarity and discernment among various options (Simpson & Mary Courtney, 2002).

Rowles and Russo (2009) discuss the need for critical thinking in nursing programs. They suggest that educators and students have roles in developing critical thinking. Many educators are moving toward a more facilitative role that incorporates active learning strategies. This approach helps to ensure what and how much is taught is associated with how student thinking develops (Anderson, 2002). It promotes using that knowledge in situations that can then be assessed (Mayer, 2002). Supporting students and acknowledging their accomplishments promote a learning environment that is safe, comfortable, and positive. This atmosphere promotes self-confidence and courage to explore different and creative ways to consider issues and the effects of decisions.

The diversity of previous learning experiences means that students may come from backgrounds in which learning has been passive. Nurse educators see the results of this in students who may come to class unprepared and resist active learning through disengagement or disruption. Critical thinking is complex (Wellman, 2009) and takes time to develop. Nurse educators need to be persistent in engaging students and maintaining expectations for preparation.

Critical thinking is apparent at the higher levels of the taxonomy (Bissell & Lemons, 2006). Friedman et al. (2010) argued that elements of critical thinking exist at every level. Bloom (1994) acknowledged that problem solving associated with critical thinking is based on knowledge and the ability to apply the knowledge "to new situations and problems" (Bloom, 1994, p. 16).

The need for nursing programs to develop and assess critical thinking skills in students was advanced by the National League for Nursing (NLN) in 1991 (Walsh & Seldomridge, 2006). Facione and Facione detailed qualities of critical thinkers and various assessments that can be used to determine if critical thinking is developing in students (Facione & Facione, 1996).

The importance of well-developed critical thinking skills in those about to enter practice is recognized by the National Council of State Boards of Nursing (NCSBN) (Clifton & Schriner, 2010). The main charge of the NCSBN is to protect the safety of the public and the ability to think critically is considered a prerequisite to safe practice. The NCLEX-RN® aims to assess a candidate's ability to think critically by structuring licensure questions at the higher analysis levels of the taxonomy. This is the reason why nearly all questions are written at the application and analysis level (Morrison, Nibert, & Flick, 2006).

ACTIVE LEARNING STRATEGIES

Active learning involves strategies to "engage" versus "explain." Educators place more emphasis on facilitating learning than imparting information. Active learning is more likely to involve students in the use of higher levels of cognition where critical thinking is prominent (McConnell, Steer, & Owens, 2003; Schekel, 2009). Content becomes more relevant as students become more engaged (McConnell et al., 2003). Well-planned active learning strategies enhance motivation and retention of knowledge for use in other settings (Goudreau et al., 2009).

Active learning involves such strategies as inquiry-based learning, problem-based learning, case studies, team-based learning, discussion, questioning that probes thinking, concept mapping, focused reflection, self-assessment, learning portfolios, projects, simulation, and interactive computer modules, and writing assignments (Friedman et al., 2010; Leppa, 2004; Luckowski, 2003; Valiga, 2009). Activities may be individual or occur through collaboration within groups. Collaborative activities promote abilities to learn from one another, work within teams, develop social and communication skills, and develop critical thinking skills through active discourse with one another (DeYoung, 2009).

Developing, implementing, and evaluating active learning strategies take a good deal of thought and time. The activity should correlate with course objectives and connect content to applying and creating new ideas and solutions (Schekel, 2009). Developing active learning strategies that are reflective and authentic or "world focused" can help to motivate learner engagement and critical thinking skills (Halstead in Oermann, 2005; Plack et al., 2007)

Assessments to gauge what students are learning are beneficial in making adjustments in the course such as content emphasis and more application using different situational contexts. The many types of active learning strategies allow for assessment of learning beyond multiple-choice tests (Tomlinson & McTighe, 2006). Nursing programs can reflect the need for ongoing assessment as early as the philosophy statement. It can be realized through the use of outcomes that are subjected to periodic assessment. This can further facilitate success in achieving intended learning outcomes.

SUMMARY

Nurses today are pressed to know, think, and act quickly in health care settings that are increasingly diverse and complex. Nurse educators are challenged to find ways to sift through ever-growing amounts of information and what to include as content, while considering objectives, learning experiences, and assessments. The use of an educational taxonomy provides a framework for developing, executing, and evaluating course, level, and program objectives and outcomes. A particular benefit of the use of taxonomy is attention to the development of critical thinking at all levels. Critical thinking may be facilitated through the use of active learning strategies that both motivate and engage students. Educators' attention to alignment throughout the process of curriculum development and revisions facilitates students' development in their nursing abilities so essential to today's practice.

DISCUSSION QUESTIONS

1. What drove the need for the original Bloom's taxonomy to evolve and what changes resulted?
2. How can taxonomy be used to align student learning to program outcomes?
3. Identify one criticism associated with the use of taxonomy and how it could be overcome.
4. How can the use of an educational taxonomy facilitate the development and evaluation of critical thinking?

LEARNING ACTIVITIES

STUDENT LEARNING ACTIVITIES

1. Write a three-page paper explaining your philosophy of educator and student responsibilities/expectations related to the acquisition of learning outcomes.
2. Select any two, accredited BSN programs that identify program outcomes on their Internet sites. Next, review the most recent literature from the AACN, NLN, ACEN, Commission on Collegiate Nursing Education (CCNE), and Institute of Medicine (IOM). Analyze the outcomes for both programs in light of what abilities are needed (as articulated in the literature you reviewed). Explain the fit of each of the programs to what these professional organizations call for.
3. From the activity above, develop a brief paper showing how the outcomes from the program could be modified to better reflect the abilities needed by nurse graduates for entry into practice.
4. Take one of the program outcomes from the above activity and develop a measurable objective from two of the taxonomy domains (affective, psychomotor, cognitive) for first- or second-semester students in a medical–surgical or professional development course.

NURSE EDUCATOR/FACULTY DEVELOPMENT ACTIVITIES

1. How can a taxonomy table illustrate progression toward learning outcomes at the program, year/semester, and course levels?

2. Using a taxonomy table, plot one of your multiple-choice tests (by item number) into a taxonomy table (cognitive level and knowledge domains). Then exchange your test with a colleague and repeat. Now share the results with your colleague and discuss results. In areas where you differ, review the question and determine whether to revise.
3. Conceptualize your course by aligning it to the program outcomes or end of program objectives. Try using a table or schematic or the CANDO model presented in the chapter to visualize your course in delivering course outcomes.

REFERENCES

Accreditation Commission for Education in Nursing (ACEN). (2014). *Accreditation manual.* Retrieved from http://acenursing.org/accreditation-manual

Airasian, P. W., & Miranda, H. (2002). The role of assessment in the revised taxonomy. *Theory into Practice, 41*(4), 249–254.

Alfaro-LeFevre, R. (1999). *Critical thinking in nursing: A practical approach* (2nd ed., p. 9). Philadelphia, PA: Saunders.

American Association of Colleges of Nursing (AACN). (2014). *The essentials of baccalaureate education for professional nursing practice.* Retrieved from http://www.aacn.nche. edu/publications/order-form/baccalaureate-essentials

Anderson, L. W. (2002). Curricular realignment: A re-examination. *Theory into Practice, 41*(4), 255–260.

Anderson, L. W., & Krathwohl, D. R. (Eds.). (2001). *A taxonomy for learning, teaching, and assessing: A revision of Bloom's taxonomy of educational objectives.* New York, NY: Addison Wesley Longman, Inc.

Asim, A. (2011). Finding acceptance of Bloom's revised cognitive taxonomy on the international stage in Turkey. *Educational Sciences: Theory and Practice, 11*(2), 767–772.

Athanassious, N., McNett, J. M., & Harvey, C. (2003). Critical thinking in the management classroom: Bloom's taxonomy as a learning tool. *Journal of Management Education, 27*(5), 533–555.

Bandman, E. L., & Bandman, B. (1995). *Critical thinking in Nursing* (2nd ed., p. 7). Norwalk, CT: Appleton & Lange.

Biggs, J. (1996). Enhancing teaching though constructive alignment. *Higher Education, 32*, 347–364.

Bissell, A. N., & Lemons, P. P. (2006). A new method for assessing critical thinking in the classroom. *BioScience, 56*, 66–72.

Bloom, B. S. (1956). *Taxonomy of educational objectives, handbook 1: The cognitive domain.* New York, NY: David McKay.

Bloom, B. S. (1994). Reflections on the development and use of the taxonomy. In L. W. Anderson, & L. A. Sosniak (Eds.), *Bloom's taxonomy: A forty-year retrospective* (pp. 1–8). New York, NY: The National Society for the Study of Education.

Booker, M. J. (2008). A roof without walls: Benjamin Bloom's taxonomy and the misdirection of American education. *Academic Questions, 20*(4), 347–355.

Boulton-Lewis, G. M. (1995). The SOLO taxonomy as a means of shaping and assessing learning in higher education. *Higher Education Research and Development, 14*(2), 143–154.

Brabrand, C., & Dahl, B. (2009). Using the SOLO taxonomy to analyze competence progression of university science curricula. *Higher Education, 58*(4), 531–549.

Brandon, A. F., & All, A. C. (2010). Constructivism theory analysis and application to curricula. *Nursing Education Perspectives, 31*(2), 89–92.

Brookfield, S. D. (1987). *Developing critical thinkers.* Milton Keynes, England, UK: Open University Press.

Bumen, N. T. (2007). Effects of the original versus revised Bloom's taxonomy on lesson planning skills: A Turkish study among pre-service teachers. *International Review of Education, 53*(4), 439–455.

Churches, A. (2007). *Educational origami: Bloom's digital taxonomy.* Retrieved from http://edorigami.wikispaces.com/Bloom%27s+Digital+Taxonomy

Churches, A. (2008). *Bloom's taxonomy blooms digitally.* Tech & Learning. Retrieved from www.techlearning.com/artcile/8670

Clifton, S. L., & Schriner, C. L. (2010). Assessing the quality of multiple-choice test items. *Nurse Educator, 33,* 12–16.

Cochran, D., Conklin, J., & Modin, S. (2007). A new Bloom: Transforming learning. *Learning & Leading with Technology, 34*(5), 22–25.

Dave, R. H. (1970). Psychomotor levels. In Armstrong, R. J. (Ed.), *Developing and writing behavioral objectives.* Tucson, AZ: Educational Innovators Press.

DeYoung, S. (2009). *Teaching strategies for nurse educators* (2nd ed.). Upper Saddle River, NJ: Prentice Hall.

Ennis, R., (1985). Critical thinking and the curriculum. *National Forum, 65,* 28–31.

Facione, N. C., & Facione, P. A. (1996). Externalizing the critical thinking in clinical judgment. *Nursing Outlook, 44,* 129–136.

Facione, P. A. (1990). *Critical thinking: A statement of expert consensus for purposes of educational assessment and instruction* (The Delphi Study Report of the American Philosophical Association, p. 3). Millbrae, CA: California Academic Press.

Fink, L. D. (2003). *Creating significant learning experiences: An integrated approach to designing college courses.* San Francisco, CA: Jossey-Bass.

Friedman, D. B., Crews, T. B., Caicedo, J. M., Besley, J. C., Weinberg, J., & Freeman, M. L. (2010). An exploration into inquiry-based learning by a multidisciplinary group of higher education faculty. *Higher Education, 59,* 765–783.

Gatrell, A. C. (2005). Complexity theory and geographies of health: A critical assessment. *Social Science & Medicine, 60,* 2661–2671.

Glennon, C. D. (2006). Reconceptualizing program outcomes. *Journal of Nursing Education, 45*(2), 55–58.

Goudreau, J., Pepin, J., Dubois, S., Boyer, L., Larue, C., & Legault, A. (2009). A second generation of the competency-based approach to nursing education. *International Journal of Nursing Education Scholarship, 6,* 1–15.

Granello, D. H. (2001). Promoting cognitive complexity in graduate written work: Using Bloom's taxonomy as a pedagogical tool to improve literature reviews. *Counselor Education & Supervision, 40,* 292–307.

Hagstrom, F. (2006). Formative learning and assessment. *Communication Disorders Quarterly, 28,* 24–36.

Halawi, L. A., McCarthy, R. V., & Pires, J. (2009). An evaluation of E-learning on the basis of Bloom's taxonomy: An exploratory study. *Journal of Education for Business, 84*(6), 274–380.

Halpern, D. F. (1994). Critical thinking: The 21st century imperative for higher education. *The Long Term View, 2*(3), 13.

Halstead, J. A. (2005). Promoting critical thinking through online discussion. In M. H. Oermann, & K. T. Heinrich (Eds.), *Annual review of nursing education, volume 3, strategies for teaching, assessment, and program planning* (pp. 143–163). New York, NY: Springer Publishing.

Harden, R. M. (2002). Learning outcomes and instructional objectives: Is there a difference? *Medical Teacher, 24*(2), 151–155.

Harrow, A. J. (1972). *A taxonomy of the psychomotor domain.* New York, NY: David McKay Co.

Hauenstein, A. D. (1998). *A conceptual framework for educational objectives: A holistic approach to traditional taxonomies.* New York, NY: University Press of America.

hooks, b. (2010). *Teaching critical thinking: Practical wisdom.* New York, NY: Routledge.

Kiely, R., Sandmann, L. R., & Truluck, J. (2004). Adult learning theory and the pursuit of adult degrees. *New Directions for Adult and Continuing Education, 103,* 17–30.

Krathwohl, D. R. (2002). A revision of Bloom's taxonomy: An overview. *Theory into Practice, 41*(4), 212–218.

Krathwohl, D. R., & Anderson, L. W. (2010). Merlin C. Whitlock and the revision of Bloom's taxonomy. *Educational Psychologist, 45,* 64–65.

Kuhn, M. S. (2008, August). Connecting depth and balance in class. *Learning and Leading with Technology, 36* (1), 18–21.

Kurfiss, J. (1988). *Critical thinking: Theory, research, practice, and possibilities* (ASHE-ERIC Higher Education Report, No 2, p. 2). Washington, DC: Association for the Study of Higher Education.

Learning theories/constructivist theories. (2014). Retrieved from http://en.wikibooks.org/wiki/Learning_Theories/Constructivist_Theories

Leppa, C. J. (2004). Assessing student critical thinking through online discussions. *Nurse Educator, 29*(4), 156–160.

Levine, L. E., Fallahi, C. R., Nicoll-Senft, J. M., Tessier, J. T., Watson, C. L., & Wood, R. M. (2008). Creating significant learning experiences across disciplines. *College Teaching, 56*(4), 247–254.

Luckowski, A. (2003). Concept mapping as a critical thinking tool for nurse educators. *Journal for Nurses in Staff Development, 19*(5), 225–230.

Manson, S. M. (2001). Simplifying complexity: A review of complexity theory. *Geoforum, 32,* 405–414.

Manton, E. J., English, D. E., & Kernek, C. R. (2008). Evaluating knowledge and critical thinking in international marketing courses. *College Student Journal, 42*(4), 1037–1044.

Marzano, R. J. (2013). Targets, objectives, standards: How do they fit? *Educational Leadership, 70*(8), 82–83.

Marzano, R. J., & Kendall, J. S. (2007). *The new taxonomy of educational objectives* (2nd ed.). Thousand Oaks, CA: Corwin Press.

Mayer, R. E. (2002). A taxonomy for computer-based assessment of problem solving. *Computers in Human Behavior, 18,* 623–632.

McConnell, D. A., Steer, D. N., & Owens, K. D. (2003). Assessment and active learning strategies for introductory geology courses. *Journal for Geoscience Education, 51*(2), 205–216.

McNeill, M., Gosper, M., & Hedberg, J. (2011). Academic practice in aligning curriculum and technologies. *International Journal of Computer Information Systems and Industrial Management Applications, 3,* 679–686.

Merriam, S. B. (2001). Andragogy and self-directed learning: Pillars of adult learning theory. *New Directions for Adult and Continuing Education, 89,* 3–13.

Morrison, S., Nibert, A., & Flick, J. (2006). *Critical thinking and test item writing* (2nd ed.). Houston, TX: Health Education Systems, Inc.

National Council for Excellence in Critical Thinking. (1992). *Proceedings of the 12th Annual International Conference on Critical Thinking and Educational Reform* (pp. 197–203, p. 201). Rohnert Park, CA: Center for Critical Thinking and Moral Critique, Sonoma State University.

Noble, T. (2004). Integrating the revised Bloom's taxonomy with multiple intelligence: A planning tool for curriculum differentiation. *The Teachers College Record, 106,* 193–211.

Oermann, M. H. (1990). Psychomotor skill development. *Journal of Continuing Education in Nursing, 21*(50), 202–204.

O'Neill, G. (2010). *Assessment: guide to taxonomies of learning.* Retrieved from www.ucd.ie/teaching

Paul, R. (1993). *Critical thinking: How to prepare students for a rapidly changing world.* Santa Rosa, CA: Foundation for Critical Thinking Press.

Paul, R., & Elder, L. (2007). *The miniature guide to critical thinking concepts and tools.* Tomales, CA: Foundation for Critical Thinking Press.

Pickard, M. J. (2007). The new Bloom's taxonomy: An overview for family and consumer sciences. *Journal of Family and Consumer Sciences Education, 25,* 45–55.

Plack, M. M., Driscoll, M., Marquez, M., Cuppernull, L., Maring, J., & Greenberg, L. (2007). Assessing reflective writing on a pediatric clerkship by using a modified Bloom's taxonomy. *Ambulatory Pediatrics, 7*(4), 285–291.

Prideaux, D. (2000). The emperor's new clothes: From objectives to outcomes. *Medical Education, 34,* 168–169.

Reilly, D. E., & Oermann, M. H. (1990). *Behavioral objectives: Evaluation in nursing.* New York, NY: National League for Nursing.

Roberts, J. L., & Inman, T. F. (2007). *Strategies for differentiating instruction: Best practices for the classroom.* Waco, TX: Prufrock Press, Inc.

Rowles, C. J., & Russo, B. L. (2009). Strategies to promote critical thinking and active listening. In D. M. Billings & J. A. Halstead (Eds), *Teaching in nursing: A guide for faculty* (3rd ed., pp. 238–261). St. Louis, MO: Saunders Elsevier.

Schekel, M. (2009). Selecting learning experiences to achieve curriculum outcomes. In D. M. Billings & J. A. Halstead (Eds), *Teaching in nursing: A guide for faculty* (3rd ed., pp. 154–172). St. Louis, MO: Saunders Elsevier.

Shulman, L. S. (2002). Making differences: A table of learning. *Change, 34*(6), 36–44.

Simpson, B. J. (1966). The classification of educational objectives: Psychomotor domain. *Illinois Journal of Home Economics, 10*(4), 110–144.

Simpson, E., & Mary Courtney, M. (2002). Critical thinking in nursing education: literature review. *International Journal of Nursing Practice, 8,* 89–98.

Sipos, Y., Battisi, B., & Grimm, K. (2008). Achieving transformative sustainability learning: Engaging head, hands and heart. *International Journal of Sustainability in Higher Education, 9,* 68–86.

Sousa, D. A. (2005). *How the brain learns* (3rd ed.). Thousand Oaks, CA: Corwin Press, Inc.

Su, W. M., Osisek, P. J., & Starnes, B. (2004). Applying the revised Bloom's taxonomy to a medical-surgical nursing lesson. *Nurse Educator, 29*(3), 116–120.

Taplin, J. R. (1980). Implications of general systems theory for assessment and intervention. *Professional Psychology, 11*(5), 722–728.

Terwel, J. (1990). Constructivism and its implications for curriculum theory and practice. *Journal of Curriculum Studies, 31*(2), 195–199.

Tomlinson, C. A., & McTighe, J. (2006). *Integrating differentiated instruction: Understanding by design.* Alexandria, VA: Association for Supervision and Curriculum Development.

Tyler, R. W. (1949). *Basic principles of curriculum and instruction.* Chicago, IL: University of Chicago Press.

Valiga, T. (2009). Promoting and assessing critical thinking. In S. DeYoung (Ed), *Teaching strategies for nurse educators* (2nd ed.). Upper Saddle River, NJ: Prentice Hall.

Walsh, C. M., & Seldomridge, L. A. (2006). Measuring critical thinking: One step forward, one step back. *Nurse Educator, 31(4),* 159–162.

Wellman, S. S. (2009). The diverse learning needs of students. In D. M. Billings & J. A. Halstead (Eds), *Teaching in nursing: A guide for faculty* (3rd ed., pp. 18–32). St. Louis, MO: Saunders Elsevier.

What is complexity theory? (2014). Retrieved from http://cw.routledge.com/textbooks/9780415368780/A/ch1doc.asp

Wiggins, G., & McTighe, J. (2005). *Understanding by design (expanded 2nd ed.).* Upper Saddle River, NJ: Pearson.

Wineburg, S., & Schneider, J. (2010). Was Bloom's taxonomy pointed in the wrong direction? *Phi Delta Kappan, 91*(4), 56–61.

Needs Assessment and Financial Support for Curriculum Development

Sarah B. Keating

OVERVIEW

When contemplating a new education program or revising an existing curriculum, a needs assessment is indicated. There are two purposes for conducting an assessment. The first is to validate the currency, academic and professional relevance, and continued need for an existing program. The second is to establish the feasibility for a new nursing program including the demand for it, available resources, academic soundness, and financial liability.

Even though justification for revising a current program usually exists, it is wise to survey constituents and collect information relative to the same factors that are examined in a needs assessment for a new program. This information either reaffirms assumptions about the curriculum on the part of the program planners or identifies gaps or problems that indicate a need for change. It is also useful for accreditation and program review purposes and can serve as the organizing framework for a master plan of evaluation (see Section V). Chapters 6 and 7 discuss the essential components of a needs assessment and offer a model for collecting and analyzing information that is preliminary to new program development or expansion and revision of an existing curriculum. Chapter 8 reviews the need for financial support, and the budgetary planning and management necessary for curriculum development and evaluation.

THE FRAME FACTORS MODEL

Johnson (1977) presented a conceptual model for curriculum development, instructional planning, and evaluation that is similar to the nursing process. Although it is a simple and linear model (P [planning] – I [implementation] – E [evaluation]), Johnson expands it into a complex step-by-step logical process for curriculum development and evaluation. The process includes examining the frame factors or context within which the program exists, setting goals, identifying curriculum content, structuring the curriculum, planning for instruction, and finally, evaluation. Johnson speaks of frame factors as the context in which the curriculum exists. Furthermore, he classifies the context into natural, cultural, organizational, and personal elements (Johnson, 1977, p. 36). This author chose the term of frame factors, external and internal, from Johnson's discussion and adapted it to curriculum development in nursing. It includes the elements that Johnson identified and adds other components that specifically apply to nursing education, health care systems, and the profession.

Frame factors for this text are defined as the external and internal factors that influence, impinge upon, and/or enhance educational programs and curricula. As a conceptual model, it collects, organizes, and analyzes information that is useful for the development and evaluation of curricula. There are two major categories of frame factors, that is, external and internal factors. External frame factors are those that influence curriculum development from the larger environment and outside the parent institution. Internal frame factors are those factors that influence curriculum development and are within the environment of the parent institution and the program itself. Figure III.1 illustrates the frame factors conceptual model.

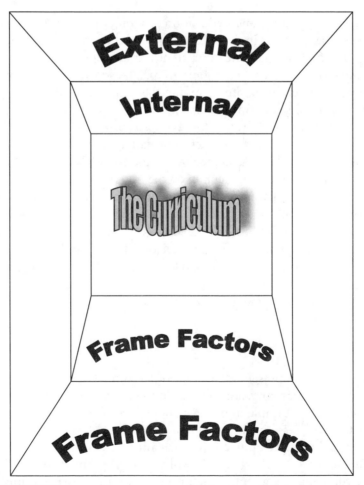

FIGURE III.1   Frame Factors Conceptual model. Adapted from Johnson (1977).

While the principal activities of faculty in curriculum development and evaluation focus on the curriculum plan itself and the need for improvement based on evaluation of its implementation (teaching and learning) and resulting program outcomes, faculty should be involved in the needs assessment. Even if faculty members are not involved in the details of a needs assessment, they need to be cognizant of all of the factors that impact and influence the program. Faculty members sophisticated in the assessment of external and internal frame factors have an advantage for promoting the program through an awareness of the curriculum's financial security, position within the health care system and the profession, and its role in meeting the health care needs of the population. Data from the needs assessment are useful to individual faculty seeking grants and other funding to support research and program development.

It is recommended that nurse educators in both the academic and practice settings use the frame factors model when evaluating education programs, considering revisions of existing programs, or initiating new ones. While administrators take the leadership role in conducting needs assessments, faculty should participate in the decision for what type and how much data to collect and what decisions are made that affect the curriculum.

External Frame Factors

Chapter 6 describes the factors that influence the curriculum from the external environment outside of the parent institution and the nursing education program. They include the community, population demographics, the political climate and body politic, the health care system, the health needs of the population, the characteristics of the academic setting, the need for the (nursing) program, the nursing profession, regulation and accreditation standards, and external financial support. All of these factors influence the curriculum in positive and negative ways and while they may not be in the control of the faculty, they are important to recognize and analyze for their impact on the program. They can "make or break" a program. For example, lack of accreditation for a nursing program can prohibit its graduates from career opportunities and continuing education. Each external factor is discussed in detail and a table provides guidelines for collecting and analyzing data for informed decision making. Chapter 6 initiates a case study that utilizes the conceptual frame factors model and guidelines and it continues in Chapters 7 and 9 to provide a sample needs assessment and the development of a nursing curriculum.

Internal Frame Factors

Chapter 7 discusses the environmental factors within the parent institution and the nursing program that influence the curriculum. The frame factors model identifies the following internal frame factors: description and organizational structure of the parent academic institution; mission, philosophy, and goals of the parent institution; economic situation and its influence on the curriculum; resources within the institution (laboratories, classrooms, library, student services, etc.); potential faculty and student characteristics; and a description of the health care system that supports the curriculum. Similar to the external frame factors, these internal factors influence the curriculum and play a major role in the development, revision, and expansion of programs. As with the external frame factors, faculty uses the information gleaned from an assessment of these factors to arrive at decisions regarding the curriculum. The same data collected for a needs assessment are in fact, related to total quality management of the curriculum and contribute to the evaluation of the program.

RELATIONSHIP OF NEEDS ASSESSMENT TO TOTAL QUALITY MANAGEMENT OF THE CURRICULUM

Establishing a new program is not an exercise that occurs in a vacuum. Preliminary information has an impact on program planners that indicates a possible need for the new program. The same is true for the need to revise a program or expand its offerings; that is, there are trigger mechanisms that initiated the change process. Rather than responding to these external stimuli in a reactive way, faculty and nurse educators should have a master plan of evaluation in place that continuously monitors the program and provides the data needed for planning for changes that are both timely and at the same time, look to the future. Such activities are part of a total quality management process that provides the data for analysis and decisions leading to the continuous improvement and quality of the educational program. The factors discussed in the Frame Factors Conceptual model in this section of the text apply to evaluation strategies as well. Although Section V discusses program and curriculum evaluation at great length, it is useful to incorporate the notion of evaluation as a process when conducting a needs assessment, not only in terms of the present plans for program start-up and changes, but also for planning for the future.

FINANCIAL SUPPORT AND BUDGET MANAGEMENT FOR CURRICULUM DEVELOPMENT AND EVALUATION

An awareness of the financial support and budgeting issues for curriculum development and evaluation is essential for nursing education administrators, managers, and faculty need to ensure the success and continuation of the program. Chapter 8 provides practical guidelines for budget support; seeking funds to develop new programs through grants, endowments, and scholarships; and managing the budget. It discusses the various roles of faculty, administrators, and staff in securing funds and planning and managing budgets for the purposes of curriculum development and evaluation and accreditation activities.

REFERENCE

Johnson, M. (1977). *Intentionality in education.* Albany, NY: Center for Curriculum Research and Services.

External Frame Factors

Sarah B. Keating

OBJECTIVES

Upon completion of Chapter 6, the reader will be able to:

1. Consider the major external frame factors to examine when conducting a needs assessment for the development or revision of a curriculum
2. Analyze external frame factors from the Frame Factors Conceptual model for application to a needs assessment for curriculum development and evaluation
3. Examine a case study that illustrates a needs assessment of external frame factors for a curriculum development project
4. Apply the Guidelines for Assessing External Frame Factors in a simulated or real curriculum development situation

OVERVIEW

Most nurse educators work in an established academic setting or in a health care agency that has a program for staff development and client education. Thus, curriculum development activities usually relate to the revision of the educational program based on feedback from staff, clients, students, faculty, administrators, alumni, and consumers of the program's participants and graduates. It is rather infrequent that new programs are initiated. Whether curriculum development involves a new program or revisions of an existing curriculum, program planners and faculty must evaluate both external and internal frame factors that affect the curriculum, their impact on the current program, and what role they play in forecasting the future.

Chapters 6 and 7 provide detailed information for conducting a needs assessment for the development of a new program and its curriculum or revising an existing curriculum. *A needs assessment for curriculum development* is defined as the process for collecting and analyzing information that contributes to the decision to initiate a new program or revise an existing one.

The first step in curriculum development for faculty and program planners is to examine the environmental and human systems factors that influence the curriculum. These factors can be organized into two major categories: external and internal frame factors (Johnson, 1977). Chapter 6 discusses external frame factors that impact an education program, while Chapter 7 discusses internal frame factors. *External frame factors* are defined as those factors that influence curriculum development in its environment and outside of the parent institution. *Internal frame factors* are those factors that influence curriculum development and are within the parent institution and the program itself. Figure 6.1 depicts the external frame factors that surround the curriculum to consider when conducting a needs assessment.

DISCUSSION

DESCRIPTION OF THE COMMUNITY

The first step in developing or revising a curriculum is to provide a description of the community in which the program exists (or will exist). A needs assessment ensures the relevance of the program to a community need and its eventual financial viability. Existing programs often identify the need for revision of their

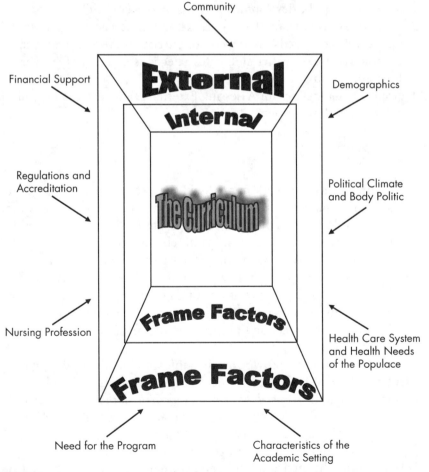

FIGURE 6.1   External frame factors for a needs assessment for curriculum development in nursing. Adapted from Johnson (1977).

curricula based on recommendations from their consumers or an accreditation report. Whether developing a new program or revising an old one, an examination of the external frame factors is essential to assess their impact on the program and its future needs. The program under development or revision is considered in light of its fit to the community that it serves. For the purposes of curriculum development, *community* is defined as a place-oriented process of interrelated actions through which members of a local population express a shared sense of identity while engaging in the common concerns of life (Theordori, 2005, pp. 662–663).

Depending on the nature of the educational program, the community can be as wide as international or as narrow as a small town within a state. Large universities or colleges with research notoriety often attract international scholars, while some state-supported programs attract students who live nearby and intend to spend their professional lives in their home community. *Sectarian* (associated with or supported by a religious organization) or *nonsectarian* (not associated with a religious organization) independent (private) colleges or universities, large or small, face the same challenges when assessing their external environment for curriculum development purposes. Therefore, it is important to identify the community in which the program is situated as urban, suburban, or rural. The location of the community influences factors such as accessibility to students, faculty, learning resources, and financial support.

The major industries and education systems in the community are identified as possible sources for students in the program and for potential partnerships for program support, scholarship, and learning experiences. Industry has resources for scholarship, and financial aid programs and experts in the field who can serve as faculty or adjunct faculty. Health care industries in particular should be participants in the needs assessment and curriculum planning to bring the reality of the practice setting and the community's health care needs into planning. The major religious affiliations, political parties, and systems such as transportation, communications, government, community services, and utilities in the community are additional external frame factors. These factors have an effect on the curriculum as to its relevance to the community and the support it needs to meet its goal. For example, state-supported schools are very dependent upon government funding, while private schools must rely on tuition and endowments.

There are many models in the literature that discuss the major components of a community assessment. Two recent articles discussing the assessment process are Lohmann and Schoelkopf (2009), who discuss the application of a Geographic Information System (GIS) for a community assessment, and Walker, Bezyak, Gilbert, and Trice (2011), who describe the use of a community assessment to develop partnerships to improve the health of the people. The latter article provides examples for collecting and analyzing data.

DEMOGRAPHICS OF THE POPULATION

When considering a new program or revising a curriculum, it is useful to have knowledge of the people who live in the home community of the institution and the broader populace that it will serve. *Demographics* are the data that describe the characteristics of a population, for example, age, gender, socioeconomic status, ethnicity, education levels, and so forth. The demographic information that is vital to program planners includes the age ranges and preponderance of age groups in the population, predicted population changes including immigrant and emigrant statistics, ethnic and cultural groups including major languages, education levels, and socioeconomic groups. This information identifies potential students and their characteristics and to some extent, the needs of the population that the students and graduates will serve.

Educational programs and curricula must be geared toward the needs of the learners. If the student body comes from the region surrounding the institution, the characteristics of the students should be analyzed for special learning needs. For example, if there are nurses seeking to advance their careers, the curriculum needs to focus on adult learning theories and modalities. Younger students about to embark on their first professional degree will need curricula that focus on their developmental needs as young adults as well as the content necessary for gaining nursing knowledge, clinical skills, and socialization into the professional role. Program planners should learn from students coming to the institution from great distances what drew them to the program and if those factors are useful for program planning and recruitment. Faculty should identify potential students with needs for learning resources beyond the usual; for example, a need for tutoring for students whose primary language is not English. It is useful to learn about the financial resources of the potential student body and if there is a need for major financial aid programs. Ethnicity and cultural values in the community and their beliefs about higher education have an impact on recruitment strategies and are especially important in light of the need for increasing the diversity of the nursing workforce.

Another consideration related to demographics is the existence of potential faculty and identification of people who have the credentials to teach. Identifying potential faculty through partnerships with industry and the community is helpful if the program needs to recruit new faculty or seek adjunct faculty and preceptors for clinical experiences. Resources for finding demographic information are plentiful. The U.S. Census Bureau (2013) has national and regional statistical and demographic information that is helpful for assessing the population. Its website is www.census.gov/2010census.

CHARACTERISTICS OF THE ACADEMIC SETTING

Other institutions of higher learning in the nearby community or region have an influence on the program and its curriculum. Identifying other institutions, their levels of higher education (technical schools, associate degree and/or baccalaureate and higher degree), financial base (private or public), and affiliations (sectarian or nonsectarian) gives the assessors an idea of the existing competition for recruiting students, faculty, and staff. Information about the types of programs in nursing that are available from other institutions and their intentions for the future enables developers to understand the gaps in the types of programs and the nature of the competition from other educational programs. For example, if the institution's curriculum offers a nurse practitioner program and two other programs in the region offer similar programs, perhaps the curriculum should be revised to a specialty primary care program such as a pediatric nurse practitioner or geriatric nurse practitioner track, discontinued, or possibly, entered into a joint venture with the other schools. A private institution that is dependent upon tuition and endowments may question whether it should continue to offer a curriculum that is redundant with a state-supported school. Other data to consider are the need for nurses in the area and its surrounds and even though there are multiple programs, the success rates of graduates finding employment in the region.

Benchmarks that the faculty can use to compare its own curriculum against those of its competitors should be identified; for example, the pass rate on the NCLEX-RN®. Other examples include costs of the program, admission, and retention rates, accreditation status, graduate employment rates, reputation in the community, and so forth. It is important to know how the nearby community agencies and health care systems view and hire the graduates of the program. Yet another important factor is the productivity of the faculty members and how their educational credentials, track records in securing grants, publication histories, and research records compare to others.

Suggested resources for collecting data on other academic institutions include the seven regional accrediting associations in the United States. They are:

1. Middle States Association of Colleges and Schools
2. New England Association of Schools and Colleges
3. North Central Association of Colleges and Schools
4. Northwest Commission on Colleges and Universities
5. Southern Association of Colleges and Schools
6. Western Association of Schools and Colleges Accrediting Commission for Community and Junior Colleges
7. Western Association of Schools and Colleges Accrediting Commission for Senior Colleges and Universities

Addresses and contact information for these associations are found in the resources list at the end of the chapter. The accrediting agencies have directories of all of the schools in their regions. The umbrella organization that lists the agencies may be found at the Council for Higher Education Accreditation (CHEA) (2014) website (www.chea.org). National databases may be found at the National Center for Education Statistics (2014) website (http://nces.ed.gov).

Another source for identifying other nursing programs in the region is the list of approved programs provided by the State Board of Nursing. A listing of the state boards and their websites and contact information may be found at the National Council of State Boards of Nursing (2014) (www.ncsbn.org/index.htm).

Once the list of other academic institutions is developed, faculty can find descriptions for each school on their individual websites or in the library. Libraries or admission departments in most institutions of higher learning have current copies of other college and university catalogs; however it is more common and easy to find these descriptions at the institutions' websites.

POLITICAL CLIMATE AND BODY POLITIC

When assessing the community, part of the data describes the public governing structure. For example, if it is urban, it is useful to know if there is a mayor, a chief executive, and a city governing board. Likewise, if it is rural or suburban, vital information to have includes the type of county or subdivision government, who the chief executive is, if the officials are elected or appointed, and what the major political party is.

Equally, if not more, important is information about the *body politic*. A simple definition for the body politic is the people power(s) behind the official government within a community. It is composed of the major political forces and the people who exert influence within the community. The assessors should identify the major players, and their visibility; that is, high profiles or low profiles as the powers behind the scenes. Additional information that reveals the body politic is how those in power influence decisions in the community and how they exert their power by using financial, personal, political, appointed, or elected positions. Specific information that is useful to educators is how the key politicians view the college or university and during elections and other crucial times, if they recognize the power of its people; that is, students, faculty, and staff.

Relative to nursing, the politicians' and the body politic's specific interests in the profession are helpful. For example, if they have family members who are nurses or they have been recipients of nursing care, they are more apt to support nursing education programs. All educational programs need the support of the community and its power structure. Therefore, the information learned from assessing the political climate is vital to planning for the future and seeking assistance when the call comes for additional resources or for political pressure and support to maintain, revise, or increase the program.

THE HEALTH CARE SYSTEM AND HEALTH NEEDS OF THE POPULACE

Providing nurses to care for the health care needs of the populace is of critical interest to the health care system and the consumers of care. It is obvious that information about these two factors is essential to education program planning and curriculum development. Schools of nursing expect that the majority of their graduates will remain in the region. However, nursing is a mobile profession and its members often move to other geographic locations far from their alma maters.

To assess the health care system, it is necessary to identify the major health care providers, types of organizations, and financial bases for the delivery of health care. With the implementation of the Affordable Care Act (ACA), changes in the health care delivery system are occurring rapidly. Thus, it is unwise to discuss at length the U.S. health care delivery system. An overview of the Act is available at www.hhs.gov/healthcare/rights/index.html through the U.S. Department of Health and Human Services (2013). To illustrate the complexity of the impact that the ACA has on the system, Takach (2012) reports that about half of the states in the United States are implementing Patient-Centered Medical Homes for their Medicaid populations. These medical homes integrate primary care, chronic disease, and/or long-term health care as well as behavioral health services. Each participant state or locality responds in different ways to the changes in health care, thus contributing to the confusion about the impact of the changes generated by the ACA on the current system.

A list of major health care organizations and their websites is provided for the readers' convenience in searching for the latest information regarding health care reform. The following is a list of major resources that provide information when conducting an assessment of the health care system for the locality or region that the educational program serves.

- Major health care systems such as Medicare, Medicaid, CHAMPUS, Veterans Affairs (VA), and so on
  - Nonprofit or for-profit health care agencies and eligibility for services
- Sectarian and nonsectarian health-related agencies and eligibility for services
  - City, county, and state public health services
- Services for the underserved or unserved population groups
  - Major primary health care agencies and providers
  - Voluntary health care agencies and their services
- Other community-based health related services staffed by nurses, for example schools, industry, state institutions, forensic facilities, and so on

Information about regional health care systems is available through the following websites, which contain lists of national, regional, and state health care agencies:

- American Health Care Association (2014): www.ahca.org
- American Hospital Association (2014): www.aha.org
- American Public Health Association (2014): www.apha.org
- National Association for Home Care & Hospice (2014): www.nahc.org

Last but not least, the yellow pages of telephone directories or on the web have listings of regional and local health care agencies and facilities.

The assembled list provides an overview of the health care system within which the program is located. It describes the health care resources that are available or not available to the population including the nursing school and institution's populations. It points out the gaps of services in the community and the possibilities for community partnerships including school-based services for the underserved and unserved populations. It identifies trends in health care services and anticipated changes for the future that can influence curriculum development.

It is useful to know if resources within the system, such as health care libraries, are available to students and faculty during clinical experiences or as resources for students enrolled in distance education programs. A review of the list pinpoints existing clinical experience sites and the potential for new ones. Staff of agency personnel department with qualifications as preceptors, mentors, and adjunct faculty are additional resources for possible collaboration opportunities. Scholarship and research opportunities for students and faculty may emerge from the review and can influence curriculum development as well as foster faculty and student development.

An overview of the major health problems in the region contributes to curriculum development as exemplars for health care interventions. The National Center for Health Statistics (2014) website (www.cdc.gov/nchs) provides general information on leading causes of death and morbidity. Vital statistics, health statistics, and objectives for 2020 are located at the Healthy People 2020 (2014) site (www.people.gov/hp2020/comments/default.asp).

THE NEED FOR THE PROGRAM

An examination of the external environment informs the faculty about the increased or continued need for nurses. The following data points act as guides to document the need for the program.

- Characteristics of the nursing workforce and the extent of a nursing shortage, if it exists
  - Predictions for future nursing workforce needs
- Adequate numbers of eligible applicants to the program, currently and in the future
  - Specific areas of nursing practice experiencing a shortage
- Employers' projections for the numbers of nurses needed in the future
  - Employers' views on the types of graduates needed

A brief survey of health care administrators can provide this information, although it is sometimes difficult to expect a good return rate owing to the current pressures on administrators. Another strategy is to conduct focus groups that take no more than 15 minutes in the health agencies. Instructors who use the facilities for students or clinical coordinators are excellent people for collecting the information. There are several resources to identify the national and regional need for nurses. They are the state nurses' associations that can be located through the American Nurses Association (ANA; 2014) (www.nursingworld.org/Functional-MenuCategories/AboutANA/WhoWeAre/CMA.aspx) and the U.S. Department of Health and Human Services (2014) Health Resources and Services Administration (HRSA) Health Professions (http://bhpr.hrsa.gov).

As described previously in the characteristics of the academic setting, knowledge of other nursing programs in the region is useful to avoid curriculum redundancies. The data on the need for the program demonstrate how many of its graduates are currently needed and in the future, the level of education necessary to provide the level of care required, and short- and long-term health care system needs. A current nursing workforce demand indicates the possibility for accelerated programs. Shortages in specialties indicate advanced practice curricula and increased opportunities for registered nurses to continue their education.

THE NURSING PROFESSION

In addition to the need for nurses, it is important to learn about the nursing profession in the region. Professional organizations are rich resources for identifying leaders, mentors, and financial support such as scholarship aid. Curriculum developers should survey faculty and colleagues for a list of the nursing professions in the region. Such organizations include local or regional affiliates of the ANA; the National League for Nursing (NLN); Sigma Theta Tau International; educator organizations such as the American Association of Colleges of Nursing (AACN) and the National Organization of Associate Degree Nursing (NOADN); and the plethora of specialty organizations. Questions to gather information about the profession are: Who are the nurses in the area? Are there professional organizations with which the program can link? What is the level of education for the majority of the nurses in practice? Are there nurses prepared with advanced degrees who could serve as educators or preceptors? Are scholarship and research activities in nursing and health care underway that present opportunities for students and faculty?

REGULATIONS AND ACCREDITATION REQUIREMENTS

Whether the program is new or under revision, state regulations regarding schools of nursing should be reviewed for their requirements and any recent or anticipated changes in them that affect the curriculum. Information on regulations is available through the State Boards of Nursing. For a listing of specific State Boards of Nursing, consult the National Council of State Boards of Nursing (NCSBN) (2014) website (www.ncsbn.org).

National accreditation is not required of schools of nursing; however, it provides the standards for nursing curricula and demonstrates program quality. Sophisticated applicants to the school will look for accreditation. Alumni find it advantageous to graduate from an accredited institution when applying for positions in the job market, future advanced education, and positions in the military. Many scholarships and financial aid programs require that students enroll in accredited institutions. Nursing has two major accrediting agencies and a few specialty-accrediting bodies. The Accrediting Commission for Education in Nursing Inc. (ACEN; 2014a) accredits clinical doctorate, master's/postmaster's certificate, baccalaureate, associate, diploma, and practical nursing programs. Detailed information on its accrediting process and standards may be found at www.acenursing.org. The Commission on Collegiate Nursing Education (CCNE; 2014) accredits baccalaureate and higher degree programs. Information on it may be found at www.aacn.nche.edu/Accreditation/pubsguides.htm.

In addition to accreditation, there are standards and competencies set by professional organizations that serve as guidelines or organizational frameworks for curricula. Several examples for pre-licensure and graduate-level programs are those developed by the AACN for baccalaureate and master's programs and competencies for the clinical nurse leader (CNL) and the doctor of nursing practice (DNP). Access to these documents may be found at the AACN (2013a) website (www.aacn.nche.edu). The ACEN (2014b) lists the standards for all levels of nursing education that they accredit. These standards may be found at www.acenursing.org/resources.

Another external frame factor that influences the nursing curriculum is regional accreditation. The parent institution of a nursing program undergoes periodic review by its regional accrediting body. Members of the nursing faculty are involved in the regional accreditation process and should be mindful of the standards set by that organization as well as those set by the professional accrediting body. For contact information, refer to the Resources list of regional accrediting agencies at the end of the chapter.

Detailed descriptions of accreditation processes and standards for educational programs are described in Section V of this text. It is useful to view them for the standards and limitations they impose during the curriculum development process.

FINANCIAL SUPPORT

An analysis of the finances of the program provides curriculum developers with vital information on the economic health of the program. Indicators of financial health influence how the curriculum will be delivered. Faculty should recognize signs that demonstrate the program's financial viability. If new sources of income for the program are indicated, possible resources need to be identified. The proposed revisions in the curriculum must be realistic in terms of cost. If it is a new program, adequate resources including start-up funds for its implementation must be available. If it is an existing program, faculty and administration should consider whether to continue it at its present level of financial support or increase or decrease support.

Other items of study include how the program is financed and the major sources of revenues such as fees, tuition, state support, private contributions, grants, scholarships, or endowments. Knowing if there are adequate resources to support the program to be self-sufficient is a critical element in the analysis of the financial viability. Although this type of information is the responsibility of administration, curriculum developers must have a basic understanding of the financial support systems that impact curriculum development. Chapter 8 discusses the role of faculty and curriculum planners in procuring funds for support of curriculum development and evaluation and an overview of budgetary planning and management.

SUMMARY

Chapter 6 introduced the first step for conducting a needs assessment in curriculum development and revision. Prior to revising or developing new curricula, an assessment of the factors that influence the education program is necessary. In examining the environment that surrounds the program, curriculum developers look at external frame factors. Table 6.1 serves as a guideline for identifying the external frame factors, collecting the data for an assessment, and analyzing the factors to determine if there is a need for a new program or if changes are necessary for an existing program. Internal frame factors within the parent institution and the nursing program that influence curriculum are considered in Chapter 7.

Analyzing external frame factors in light of proposed new programs or curriculum revisions helps faculty and administrators to determine the type of new program needed or in the case of an existing program, the extent to which changes in the curriculum are indicated. A review of the external frame factors provides a reality check, including the community in which the program is located, the industry for which the program prepares graduates, and the economic viability of the program.

TABLE 6.1   GUIDELINES FOR ASSESSING EXTERNAL FRAME FACTORS

FRAME FACTOR	QUESTIONS FOR DATA COLLECTION	DESIRED OUTCOMES
Description of the Community	Is the community setting conducive to academic programs? What are its major characteristics, such as urban, suburban, or rural?	The institution's campus is located in a safe and supportive environment for its students, faculty, and staff
	What are the major industries and do they financially support the institution as well employ graduates?	Industries are stable and have a history of financial support for the institution and employ its graduates
	What are the major education systems in the community and what is the quality of the programs? How do they feed into the parent institution?	The public and private school systems, kindergarten through 12 provide graduates for the institution and are of high quality. The school counselors have a strong relationship with the institution's admission department
		Community colleges and higher degree institutions collaborate and have articulation agreements for ease of transfer
		Students have easy access at reasonable cost to public transportation to and from home (for commuter students) and to stores and other community services
	What are the community services that provide an infrastructure for the institution, i.e., transportation and communications services?	The community has multiple media communication networks of high quality for marketing, public relations, and education purposes; postal service and other delivery systems are reliable
	What are the community services that provide an infrastructure for the institution, i.e., recreation, housing, utilities, and human and health services?	There are varied and multiple recreation sites for students' leisure activities
		If there are no student health services, the community has quality health and human services for which students are eligible
	What type of government is in place in the community and what are its politics? Is the government supportive of the institution in its midst and does it recognize its contributions to the community?	The government structure is supportive of the parent institution in its community
		Key members of the parent institution serve on advisory boards for the local government

(continued)

TABLE 6.1   GUIDELINES FOR ASSESSING EXTERNAL FRAME FACTORS (*continued*)

FRAME FACTOR	QUESTIONS FOR DATA COLLECTION	DESIRED OUTCOMES
Demographics of the Population	What are the characteristics of the general population?	The population reflects multicultural and ethnic characteristics with a wide range of age groups
	What indications are there that the population supports higher education?	The average income level is at or above the average for the region; poverty levels are low and there are dedicated programs of assistance for the poor
	Within the population, what is the potential for acquiring student, faculty, and staff for the program?	A majority of the population completed high school or higher levels of education and/or there is growing interest in and need for these levels of education
		There is an adequate applicant pool for the program(s); there are potential qualified faculty and staff in the locale
Characteristics of the Academic Setting	Identify other institutions of higher learning in the region. Within those institutions, what types of nursing programs are offered if any?	Other institutions of higher learning in the region have programs not in direct competition with the curriculum and can serve as feeder schools to the program; there are no known future plans that could conflict with the program
	Are there potential or existing competitors?	
Political Climate and Body Politic	Identify the type of government and its structure. Who are the political power brokers in the community?	Key politicians and community leaders support the institution and have working relationships with the people within the educational institution
	What are the relationships of the parent institution to the political power brokers?	
The Health Care System and Health Needs of the Populace	Identify the major types of health care systems and the predominant health care delivery patterns	There are ample spaces currently and for the future for nursing student placements in the various health care systems and settings
	Describe the major health care problems and needs of the populace in the education program's region	The major health care problems and needs match foci in the curriculum
	Describe the role of nursing in the health care system	Nursing, as the largest health care workforce, has a strong representation within the health care system
The Need for the Program	Describe the nursing workforce in the region as well as the state and nation	There is a demonstrated need for nurses in the region, state, and nation currently and in the future
	Describe the numbers and types of nurses needed in the region, state, and the nation for the future	The numbers and types of nurses needed meet the goals and type(s) of preparation available in the education program for the future

(*continued*)

TABLE 6.1	GUIDELINES FOR ASSESSING EXTERNAL FRAME FACTORS (*continued*)	
FRAME FACTOR	QUESTIONS FOR DATA COLLECTION	DESIRED OUTCOMES
The Nursing Profession	List the major professional nursing organizations in the region	There are at least two major nursing organizations in the region that support the program and provide collegial relationships for students and faculty
	Describe the characteristics of nurses in the region	The types of nurses in the region match the potential applicant pool for continued education and/or faculty and mentor positions
Regulations and Accreditation Requirements	Identify the State Board of Nursing regulations for education programs	The nursing education program meets the state board regulations and has or is eligible for approval
	List accreditation agencies that impact the parent institution and the nursing education program	The parent institution is accredited by its regional agency and the nursing program meets the standards of a national professional accrediting body
Financial Support	Analyze the present financial health of the parent institution and the nursing program	The institution and the nursing program are in solid financial condition and there is either guaranteed state support or substantial endowment funds from the local and greater communities for the future
	Develop a list of existing and potential economic resources	There are adequate economic resources for the present and the future of the program
Analysis of the Data and Decision Making	Summarize the findings by generating a list of positive, neutral, and negative external frame factors that influence the curriculum	Make a final decision statement as to the feasibility of the program as it is affected by the external frame factors

CASE STUDY

A case study is presented in this chapter and Chapters 7 and 9 to illustrate a needs assessment and the development of a proposed curriculum. It includes the collection of external and internal frame factors data, their analyses, and a curriculum decision based on the findings.

DESCRIPTION OF THE COMMUNITY

An existing baccalaureate and higher degree nursing program, the home campus of which is located in a suburban town of 20,000 adjacent to the state capital with a population of more than 1,000,000, is about to undertake a needs assessment to determine if the program should expand. The home campus is a private, sectarian, multipurpose higher education institution. It has a long history of liberal arts education and over the past five decades added several professional schools including business, education, engineering, nursing, and the performing arts. All of the professional schools offer baccalaureate and master's degrees in their majors. There are two doctorate programs: one in education (EdD) and the other in business administration (DBA). The undergraduate population numbers 5,000 with 2,000 graduate students. There are a total of 760 faculty members, 300 of those are part time.

Nursing faculty and administrators are aware of the continuing and projected nursing workforce shortage in the nation and in its region, the legislative changes in the health care system and their effect on the nursing workforce, and the trend for preparing advanced practice nurses at the clinical doctorate (DNP) level. They have anecdotal information that employers of nurses prefer baccalaureate or higher degree nurses owing to the complexity of the acute care setting, the shortages of nurses prepared to practice in primary care and community settings, and the Institute of Medicine (IOM) (2010) recommendation on *The Future of Nursing* that recommends the baccalaureate as the threshold for professional nursing.

The nursing program has a basic bachelor of science in nursing (BSN) undergraduate program, (N=200), a registered nurse (RN) to BSN program (N=30), and a master of science in nursing (MSN) program with specialties for family nurse practitioners (FNP), adult/geriatric acute care nurse practitioners, and clinical nurse leaders (N=90). The faculty numbers 30 full-time and 15 part-time members with a dean and two associate deans for the undergraduate and graduate programs. There are five faculty members who have released time to coordinate the five tracks in the program. Three administrative assistants and one information systems and instructional support administrator provide management.

The nursing program is affiliated with a religious-based health care organization of the same denomination as its parent organization. The health care organization is a managed care system and has facilities located throughout the institution's region and the nation. It has been supportive of the nursing program in the past by offering clinical sites for student practice and scholarship or loan forgiveness programs for its staff and students who come to its facilities after graduation. With this information in hand, the dean asks the faculty to conduct a needs assessment for expanding the nursing program by increasing enrollments for entry-level nurses and/or expanding the graduate program to provide additional advanced practice nurses.

Using the Guidelines for Assessing External Frame Factors (see Table 6.1), the faculty initiates a needs assessment. The faculty divides the work into teams of two or three, each to collect information on one of the nine external frame factors. Once the data are collected, they will be presented to the faculty group who will refine the data and analyze them according to the need for the proposed program expansion.

The team assigned to community assessment decides to assess the metropolitan area and its surrounds, which includes six major suburban areas and the adjacent three-county rural area. Of the six suburban areas, half are incorporated as towns or cities. The team conducts a community assessment using portions of the Kazda et al. (2009) framework that uses interviews of key stakeholders and also analyzes GIS data to provide demographic and socioeconomic information according to specific locales. Additionally, the team finds the city, suburban communities, and county websites useful in providing much of the information they seek. The major industries and employers in the area include:

1. The state government
2. Two small but expanding alternative energy manufacturers

3. Several food-processing plants
4. A large inland port
5. A railroad center that serves the region in the transportation of goods and some commuter services
6. An airplane parts manufacturer
7. A rocket engineering and manufacturing plant
8. Retail and recreation/entertainment industry (including two Native American-managed casinos)
9. Primary and secondary education systems
10. Several large health care systems that serve the city, suburbs, and rural neighbors

All of the industries have a long history in the area, are financially stable in spite of the recent recession, and the alternative energy manufacturers plan to expand and employ at least 2,000 additional workers over the next 5 years. The nonhealth-related industries support the business and engineering programs of the parent institution and send many of their workers to the programs for advanced preparation. In the past, two of the manufacturers gave grants to the parent institution for computer engineering scholarships and one manufacturer donated a $25 million grant toward a new business administration building on the home campus.

A state-supported baccalaureate and higher degree program with a nursing program is located in the city. Additionally, there are three state-supported community colleges in or near the city with nursing programs, there is one large university-based medical center with a PhD nursing program to prepare nurse scientists, and the closest private college (without a nursing program) is 300 miles away. The parent institution has existing articulation agreements with all of the community colleges and the state school. There are no DNP programs in the nearby region.

Results from statewide achievement tests reveal that the city's kindergarten through 12th grade system ranked in the 60th percentile. Most of its students prefer to remain in the local area and the majority of those who continue schooling after high school (40%) go to the local community colleges. Students in the three-county area ranked from the 50th percentile (agricultural areas) to the 82nd percentile (suburban areas) on statewide achievement tests. Fifty-five percent of the suburban students continued their education in either community colleges or higher educational institutions; however only 15% of students in rural areas continued their education after high school.

The public transportation system within the city includes buses and a light rail system. The light rail system extends into the three surrounding counties with carpool parking lots available for suburbanites to commute to the city. Three major highways intersect with the city providing easy access for automobile travel. There is a mid-sized airport with commuter planes and major airlines and AMTRAK services are available. Greyhound Bus has a terminal in the city with buses providing interstate transportation. The metropolitan buses and light rail system fares are reasonable and there are discounts for students and senior citizens. There is one major daily paper, several suburban papers, at least 25 radio stations, five major television stations, TV cable service, and telecommunication services for computer access. There are many mailing services in addition to the U.S. Postal Service such as UPS, FedEx, and Pak Mail located throughout the area.

The capital city is located on a major river with three surrounding small lakes and there are several state and city recreation parks for picnicking, swimming, boating, and hiking. The city lies between the ocean and mountains; thus winter, summer, and beach sports are no more than 2 to 3 hours away. Low-rent housing facilities are plentiful owing to the economic recovery owing to more people buying homes. Utilities are fairly reasonable in cost. There are municipal systems for the incorporated cities and county services for delivery of utilities that are for the most part reliable in the delivery of services.

There are four major health care systems that serve their enrolled members. With a projected modest population growth, two of the systems have plans for expansion. Students and/or their parents who are enrolled in these programs are eligible for services. There are public health clinic services for students who do not have health coverage and who are eligible for state-supported health care programs.

The city has an elected city council with a mayor, while the smaller incorporated cities are managed through part-time mayors and city councils with full-time city managers. The counties have elected boards of supervisors and each has a county chief administrator/manager. At the present time, in the urban areas, the Democratic Party has the most representatives in the government. However, the rural areas are more conservative and have elected Republicans to the local governments and representatives to Congress. The three surrounding counties are governed by boards of supervisors with some of the larger suburban communities having local fire department and community services. The three counties have sheriff departments supplemented by state highway patrol services for highway traffic control and serious felonies.

Although the parent institution's board of regents has only one representative in the public government, the president of the college meets periodically with ad hoc committees of the city councils and boards of supervisors to discuss higher education issues that affect their populaces. He has been in the position of president for more than 15 years and is well known and respected throughout the region. This activity on his part contributes to the presence and image of the parent institution in the region.

Preliminary Conclusions

The location and size of the regional community indicate feasibility for expanding the program. The infrastructure of the city and its surrounds and the population base of the region for potential student and health care services support the existing program and could accommodate additional nursing students and graduates. There is only one baccalaureate and higher degree competitor for the nursing program and one university PhD nursing program. However, there are three community colleges with potential applicants to the BSN and RN to BSN programs. These issues will be examined in the Characteristics of the Academic Setting frame factors that follows.

DEMOGRAPHICS OF THE POPULATION

The faculty team assigned to gathering data on the demographics of the region's population seeks information from the websites of the cities and tri-county area. The team learns that the total population of the capital city is a little over 1.4 million.

The racial breakdown by percentage is as follows: White, 45.3; Native American, 1.3; African American/Black, 8.6; Asian, 10.9; Hispanic, 12.6; two or more races, 6.3; and other race, 15.0. The age distribution is as follows: 19 years and younger, 30.2%; 20 to 34, 23.0%; 35 to 44, 15.0%; 45 to 59, 15.9%; 60 to 74, 10%; and 75 and older, 5.9%. The major languages spoken at home are English, 67.4% and languages other than English, 32.6%. (The other major spoken languages are Spanish, Mandarin, or Cantonese.) Forty-two percent of the population has at least one vehicle per household. Of the population, 77.3% hold a high school diploma and 23.7% have a baccalaureate or higher. The major occupations for the working population and their percentage distribution are: management or professional (includes health care), 36.2; services, 16.2; sales or office work, 28.6; fishing, forestry or farming, .4; construction, 7.6; and production, 11.0. The unemployment rate is 9.4 % and steadily decreasing with the improved economic scene. The median household income is $41,200. There are 11.9% of households below the poverty level. Indications are that the population is growing and that the demographics will remain stable.

In contrast, the populations of the three surrounding counties are quite different. The racial breakdown averages over 70% White, 7% African American, 2% Native American, 9% Asian, 12% Hispanic, and 1% other. The average median income is $51,000 and less than 5% households were below poverty level. The average age distribution in the counties reveals a somewhat older population than the city with 11% ages 0 to 9 years, 7% 10 to 19, 9% 20 to 29, 11% 30 to 39, 22% 40 to 49, 15% 50 to 59, 12% 60 to 69, 8% 70 to 79, and 4% 80+. About 23% of the counties' residents hold a high school diploma, 17% hold baccalaureates, and 31% had some college education but no degree.

Preliminary Conclusions

Overall, this population is growing and compared to other parts of the state and nation, is economically stable. Its diverse ethnic population meets the program's goal to increase cultural diversity in its student population, while at the same time, there may be need for programs to assist students whose primary language is not English. There is a large percentage of individuals who are educated beyond high school and who are potential faculty and staff for the program and might be interested in second-career opportunities. Age breakdowns in the population indicate a large percentage of potential college students between the ages of 18 to 44.

CHARACTERISTICS OF THE ACADEMIC SETTING

The team assigned to identify other institutions of higher learning goes to the regional accrediting body. They find a listing of accredited colleges and universities in the region. They decide to identify those institutions within the selected city and 75 miles outside the radius of the city line. They also look at the city's website that lists all of the institutions. Once all schools are identified and they learn which schools have nursing programs, they divide the work among themselves to gather data from the programs' websites and interview the administrators of the schools of nursing. The information they seek includes the types of nursing programs and tracks offered, the applicant pool, admission date(s), the enrollments, graduation rates, licensure examination (NCLEX) pass rates, where the majority of graduates work, and the impressions of the administrators for the need for an additional program or expansion of existing programs in the area. The purpose for the interviews is twofold, such as, it gives basic information about other nursing programs in the region, and it also informs them of the potential for another program or expansion. The faculty is aware that the interviews must be handled delicately with sincere reassurance to the administrators that the proposed program is meant to complement existing programs. This sets the pathway for continued collaborative relationships and in the future should the program begin.

The academic setting team learns that the three community colleges offer associate degree in nursing (ADN) programs and the state-supported school offers a generic BSN program as well as an accelerated RN to BSN program. It has four master's specialty tracks, one in education, one in nursing administration, one in community health nursing, and a FNP program. Additionally, the faculty learns that the program recently developed an online RN to BSN track that is proving to be very popular. They also note that there is one statewide online RN to BSN program and multiple nationwide programs for RNs to earn their baccalaureates.

The three community colleges are about equal in size and their administrators report that their total enrollments approximate 150 with 50 graduates each year. Their qualified applicant pool numbers 350 each, although they believe they may be drawing from the same applicant pool. Their admission rates to fill slots averages 93% to 95% leaving a waiting list each year of about 50 qualified applicants. There are no plans to increase enrollments in the near future owing to the lack of state support for program expansion. The administrators report pass rates on NCLEX ranging from 82% to 100%. The vast majority of their graduates remains in the local area to practice and are either in acute care, nursing home, or home health agencies.

The state-supported BSN and higher degree school administrator reports that they have a total enrollment of 300 students in the basic BSN program, 100 RNs in the RN to BSN program, and 150 in the graduate programs. The MSN nurse practitioner program is the most popular with the community health nursing and education tracks each enrolling approximately 20 students each year. About 75% of the basic BSN students transfer in from the community college, having completed their nursing prerequisites. The remainder enters as freshmen. The basic BSN program graduates approximately 65 each year with an average NCLEX pass rate of 87% for the past 5 years. About 80% of its graduates remain in the area to practice. The qualified applicant pool for the basic BSN program is 350 and again, the administrator believes some of the applicants may be in the same pool as the ADN programs. Owing to constraints on state-supported funds, there are no plans to expand enrollments in the near future.

The RN students come from regional health care agencies and based on the response to the online version of the program, the school may discontinue its traditional RN to BSN program. Most master's students come from the region as well and are seeking additional education for career mobility purposes. Although the MSN applicant pool is small compared to the capacity of the program (200 for 150 slots), the program remains viable. The administrator notes that there have been requests recently from those who have baccalaureates or higher degrees for a master's or second-degree program. Upon further investigation with the ADN administrators, the faculty learns that they too have experienced these requests, and in fact, have students enrolled in their programs that have bachelor's or higher degrees other than nursing.

The university medical center currently has medical, dental, pharmacy, and nursing programs. It is a research extensive health sciences center and therefore offers a PhD research–focused degree in nursing. Graduates of the program hold positions as researchers in medical centers and as faculty in schools of nursing. In a discussion with the university's dean of nursing, the assessment team learns that the university-based program has no immediate plans to expand the program owing to the nature of the health sciences institution and research focus. It has about 36 students enrolled in the program in various stages of doctoral study, graduates about 10 students each year, and admits approximately 8 to 10 students per year. Although the program is not a direct competitor for nursing students and programs in the region, it provide potential faculty for schools of nursing.

Preliminary Conclusions

In addition to its own program, the region has five nursing programs, three ADN, one baccalaureate and master's degree, and one PhD in nursing program. There appears to be an adequate qualified applicant pool for these programs and there are waiting lists for the generic programs (ADN and BSN). The RN to BSN pool seems satisfied with the new online program offered by the state-supported school and there are multiple other options for them to complete a baccalaureate in nursing. All of the clinical specialties at the master's level are viable. One tantalizing fact is the interest on the part of college graduates in becoming nurses. There are no fast-track baccalaureate or entry-level master's programs in the region. The faculty team recommends collection of additional data about this possibility.

POLITICAL CLIMATE AND BODY POLITIC

The initial description of the community identified the city's government as consisting of a city council and a mayor. At the present, the Democrats are the political party in control. The adjacent counties have mayoral and council governments for the smaller cities and boards of supervisors for the county government. The counties are predominantly Republican although recently there have been some elected posts captured by Democrats. The team assigned to investigate the political climate and body politic decides to attend a board of supervisors meeting in each county and a city council meeting. They also read the local newspapers' metro sections and the editorial pages. They interview faculty and staff who live in the region and the director of extended education to seek opinions on the political climate in the city and counties as they relate to the parent institution and the health care system. They ask people who live in the three counties to attend a board of supervisors meeting and/or city council meetings to learn about the major political issues in the region.

The meeting of the city council of the major city, which the team attended, happened to have health care issues on its agenda. Citizens were concerned about the pending proposal to close two of the city's public health clinics owing to a shortfall in the state budget and a trickling down effect of less public funds for the clinics. The faculty noted several political action groups in attendance who were vocal in their protests about the closures. It being an election year, the mayor and council members listened carefully to their pleas and by the end of the meeting, assured them that the clinics would remain open. The team observed that the mayor was a strong leader with little dissension among the council members on the various issues.

The survey team was quite interested in learning that the mayor was an RN and knowledgeable about health care issues. They decided to seek an interview with the mayor and were successful in meeting with her for a half-hour. At the meeting, they gained the mayor's support for the possible expansion of the program as long as the other nursing programs in the area supported it. She was well aware of the nursing shortage and the need for preparing additional nurses as well as those for advanced practice related to the changes in the health care system from the ACA (2014).

Faculty and staff who attended county board of supervisors meetings heard many of the smaller issues facing county governments such as the downturn in residential and business development, the need for additional public safety services, and what services to cut when planning for the next fiscal-year budget. Health and nursing-related issues did not come up in the meetings but the people who attended introduced themselves to the board members and identified where they worked. The purpose was to begin to establish a recognition of the role of the college and its contributions to the community.

The city's newspaper had several articles on the closure of the public health clinics and the editorial opinion page had a glowing account of the mayor's support for the groups who opposed the closures. The articles discussed the nursing shortage as well; thus, it was concluded that information about the increasing need for nurses was reaching the public. The assessment team scanned local newspapers and decided to continue to do so in order to keep abreast of the news in the region and also to have contact sites if there was a need to publicize the program.

The director of extended education felt that most of the city's and counties' populations were aware of the parent institution from the college's media campaign. The School of Extended Education runs spot announcements on the radio and even gained some free public service announcements on television, as one of its students is the manager of one of the major stations. The director runs advertisements in the local newspaper, usually a month before the semesters start. The director described his role on the ad-hoc committee on higher education for the city council. This role gives him the opportunity to meet other key educators and helps raise the visibility of the institution in the community. It was his overall impression that the reputation of the institution and its quality were gaining in the community.

Preliminary Conclusions

The faculty team concluded that although the parent institution's educational programs are relatively new in the community, key members of the body politic and the public recognize the institution. They felt they had the initial support of the mayor who is a leader in the community, but felt that the nursing program will need to nurture a relationship with her to gain further support. In addition, there is a need to publicize the program in the three-county area and to continue to build relationships with the political leaders. Depending on other findings in the needs assessment, the team felt that there would be, at the very least, no opposition to the program and, at the most, moderate support. One caution was issued and that was the need to work with the administrators and faculty of the existing nursing programs as colleagues. It would be advantageous to develop a program that would complement existing programs and not create a threat to them.

THE HEALTH CARE SYSTEM AND HEALTH NEEDS OF THE POPULACE

As identified in the community assessment, there are four major health care systems serving the city and surrounding region. The team assigned to assess this frame factor gathers data through the website of the American Hospital Association and the National Association for Home Care as well as looking in the yellow pages of the telephone directory. They check the Morbidity and Mortality Weekly Reports (MMWR, 2014; www.cdc.gov/mmwr, the state health department's health statistics), and GIS Inventory (2014) maps (http://gisinventory.net/index.php?page_id=624_) for comparisons of the tri-county area's and the capital city's health indicators with the national and statewide data.

One health care system is a nonprofit large health maintenance organization that has a nationwide network. There are two nonprofit regional health care systems providing enrollees with a wide array of services. One is sponsored by the same religious-based organization as that of the nursing program's parent institution. The other is a federation of former independent nonprofit community hospitals that merged to share resources for cost savings. There is no public hospital except for the state-supported university medical center; however there are public health clinics that provide primary care for the medically indigent. The medically indigent receive Medicaid services through the existing health care systems and the Medicaid program (federal and state/county) reimburses the agencies for the services provided.

The VA has a large medical center with acute care with all specialties except maternity and pediatrics, which it subcontracts with the other regional hospitals, outpatient services, a nursing home wing, and a rehabilitation center. It prefers RNs with baccalaureates for staffing and employs master's- and DNP-prepared clinical nurse leaders, clinical specialists, acute care and primary nurse practitioners, managers and administrators. It provides clinical practice sites for both undergraduate and graduate students for all of the nursing schools in the region and encourages its staff to continue its education with released time and educational stipends as incentives. It is especially supportive of the CNL program and uses many of the school's graduates. It is interested in collaboration with the school on a DNP program as it uses the graduates in advanced practice roles and as administrators.

There are three for-profit agencies that in addition to patient care services supply medical equipment. There is one nonprofit visiting nurse association and that agency is under contract with several of the heath care systems for home and hospice care. Most school districts have one school nurse, there is a nurse practitioner with four RNs assigned to the city jail, and three of the major industries have occupational health nurses.

The major health care problems of the populace match those of the morbidity and mortality statistics of the state and the nation. The population is aging and thus the need for health services for seniors and chronic diseases is expected to rise. The systems appear to meet the acute care needs of the populace. For those enrolled in health maintenance organizations, health promotion services seem adequate; however additional nurse practitioners are indicated in the near future to staff primary care services owing to the increased numbers of insured clients. The local Women, Infants, and Children (WIC) programs have public health nurses who provide health education and follow-up home visits but the public health department does not have a system-wide health education program, providing only immunizations and primary care services in their clinics. With the increase in insured individuals from the effects of the ACA, the need for more advanced practice nurses, public health nurses, and staff nurses is indicated.

The team interviewed either the chief administrator of nursing or the associate administrator in the major health care systems. The team members learned that the majority of staff nurses are associate degree graduates. All of the large health care systems employ clinical specialists or acute care nurse practitioners and those with primary care services employ nurse practitioners. A few have staff educators, although those nurses also serve as risk managers. The university-based medical center has an all RN staff and employs more clinical specialists and acute care nurse practitioners than the other systems. The public health clinics use public health nurses prepared at the baccalaureate level for follow-up visits and nurse practitioners staff the few primary care clinics. Since the two clinics at risk for closure will remain open in response to public pressure, additional public health nurses and nurse practitioners will be needed. The visiting nurse organization uses both public health nurses and RNs for home visiting and hospice services. It indicated the need for additional advanced practice nurses. All of the organizations use licensed practical nurses (LPNs) and the administrators report that they would like to encourage these nurses to continue with their education since they prefer RNs.

The administrators reported that they welcome nursing students and have existing clinical placement agreements with the regional nursing schools. The team decided to collect additional information in their interviews to share with the faculty team assigned to the "The Need for the Program" frame factor. The administrators said they could accommodate additional students for learning experiences, particularly if the program were to hold experiences on evening shifts or weekends. The religious-based system was especially open to having additional students in their agencies and indicated that the program's students would receive priority placements. All nursing specialties were represented in the agencies, although some had larger specialty units than others. A list was made of the agencies, their specialty units, and numbers of potential advanced practice and experienced nurses who could serve as preceptors, mentors, clinical instructors, or faculty.

Preliminary Conclusions

The faculty concluded that there is a wide variety of health care agencies with a plethora of potential clinical experiences available for students in an expanded program. Nursing administrators welcomed the idea of an expanded program to increase the numbers of baccalaureate and higher degree nurses in the region. This information would be passed on to the team investigating "The Need for the Program." The health care problems and needs of the populace are not unique and match the existing content of the curriculum. There is a need for health promotion activities and increased primary care services, especially for the poor and the aging population, which present opportunities for faculty and student practice.

THE NEED FOR THE PROGRAM

The faculty assigned to the frame factor that describes the need for the program go to the state's board of nursing website and the state nurses' association for information on the nursing workforce in the region. They learn that there are 1,450 RNs of whom 1,250 are employed. The four major health care systems report a vacancy rate of 10% and the schools, public health clinics, and home care agency report a total of 50 vacant positions. The team did not include skilled nursing facilities in the survey; however, they learned from a few directors of nursing that they too are experiencing shortages of nurses with a rapid turnover of staff who move to acute care facilities. Calculating the needs for nurses in numbers of vacant positions, the team estimated that there are at least 200-plus available positions. They note that the existing nursing programs plan to only graduate 125 entry-level nurses. The number of vacancies does not account for the numbers of nurses in the workforce who plan to retire within the next 5 years, especially in light of the fact that the average age of the nurse in the region is 48.5 years.

In addition to entry-level positions, 100% of the administrators of the nursing services programs told the team that they anticipated increasing their staff owing to the growing demand and complexity of health care. They reported shortages in staff nurses and those in advanced practice, especially acute care clinical specialists and nurse practitioners. The administrators indicated a preference for baccalaureate prepared nurses and when informed about entry-level master's, fast-track RN to master's programs, and DNP programs, their interest increased, especially if the programs are accelerated. They voiced a sense of urgency related to the increased need for nurses prepared at higher levels of education. The team's review of state and national trends demonstrated a similar need for nurses and an ever-increasing shortage of nurses over the next decade.

Preliminary Conclusions

There is a documented need for entry-level nurses in the capital city, the region, state, and nation. In addition, nursing administrators report an increased need for baccalaureate prepared graduates and advanced practice nurses. The needs thus far match the types of options in the nursing program, such as basic BSN, RN to MSN, and advanced practice roles.

THE NURSING PROFESSION

The team assigned to analyze the nursing profession in the nation and region goes to the websites of the major nursing organizations in the nation. Nationally, nursing is responding to the IOM (2010) recommendations and to the effects of the ACA (2013) calling for advanced practice nurses, particularly in primary care. According to the AACN (2013b), the numbers of baccalaureate and higher degree programs across the United States are increasing. BSN to DNP programs are increasing and there are well over 180 DNP programs with additional programs poised to become accredited. The trend is for advanced practice education to occur at the doctoral level, replacing master's level programs.

The team discovers that the state-supported baccalaureate and higher degree program sponsors a local Sigma Theta Tau chapter as does the home school of nursing, the state nurses association has a regional affiliate, and there is a coalition of specialty organizations in the city. The nurse executive group meets periodically and is loosely affiliated with the American Organization of Nurse Executives. The administrators of the nursing schools belong to this group and their faculty clinical coordinators have a group of educators who meet twice a year with staff educators in the four major health care systems. There is one health care providers union and that union represents nurses in two of the health care systems.

About 60% of the employed nurses work in acute care; the remainder are in community-based agencies. About 71% of the working nurses have an ADN or diploma, 22% have a BSN, 6% have a master's, and less than 1% have a doctorate. It was difficult to match the educational preparation of the nurses to the type of position they held, although anecdotal information demonstrated that the majority of master's-prepared nurses were top administrators (vice presidents), clinical specialists, clinical nurse leaders, or nurse practitioners. The BSN nurses were employed in public health, schools, home care, or as case managers or administrators. Only eight nurses with doctorates were found in practice: two were researchers at the university-based medical center; one was a researcher at the VA, another was the staff development/patient education director for the VA, and two were DNPs in advanced practice at the VA; the remaining two were researchers in the large health care system. The faculty did not survey faculty of schools of nursing; however, it was acknowledged that there are additional master's and doctorate-prepared nurses in the community, some of who were faculty in other schools of nursing.

Preliminary Conclusions

There are several nursing organizations whose members can serve as preceptors and mentors. There are eight known doctorate-prepared nurses who could serve as research mentor, preceptors for advanced practice students, and perhaps, faculty. There are master's prepared nurse practitioners, clinical nurse leaders, educators, administrators, and clinical specialists who are potential students, clinical faculty, preceptors, or mentors.

There is a shortage of nurses in the region, state, and nation. The existing workforce does not meet the preferred need for baccalaureate and advanced practice prepared nurses. The existing schools of nursing cannot meet the current regional demand for nurses and employers of nurses forecast an increasing need in the future. There is a need for programs to increase the numbers of nurses with BSNs and for advanced practice roles.

REGULATIONS AND ACCREDITATION REQUIREMENTS

The dean of the nursing program and the associate deans of the undergraduate and graduate programs act as the team to investigate regulations and accreditation requirements. The program is due for a Commission for Collegiate Nursing Education (CCNE) re-accreditation visit in 2 years. The nursing program has approval of the State Board of Nursing. A phone call to the executive director of the State Board by the dean verifies that the Board must approve any expansions of the program that affect any of the licensure or state certification requirements. A proposal for changes in the program must be presented to the Board at least 6 months in advance of initiation of the revised program. The Board has guidelines for the proposal and will send it to the administrator of the program. Guidelines include a list of qualified faculty, adequate student services, including library facilities, approved clinical facilities, and adequate classroom and learning laboratories. Approval comes through the Education Committee of the Board and can be reviewed within 3 months of receipt of the proposal.

The parent institution has regional accreditation. A call to that agency and a review of its standards indicate that new degree programs must be preapproved by the agency at least 6 months prior to the enrollment of the first class. The criteria for approval are much the same as the State Board of Nursing. In addition to the requirements of the State Board of Nursing, the regional agency looks for evidence of infrastructure feasibility and educational effectiveness. The usual turn-around time for a response to a proposal is 2 months.

The nursing program has national accreditation through the CCNE. A call to a consultant at that agency finds that education programs must submit a substantive change report no earlier than 90 days prior to implementation or no later than 90 days after its implementation.

Preliminary Conclusions

If the faculty and administrators of the nursing program revise or develop new tracks in the program, the proposal for the changes must be completed and submitted to the Board of Nursing and the regional accrediting agency at least 6 months prior to start-up of the program. A description of the program should be submitted to the CCNE 90 days prior to its initiation.

FINANCIAL SUPPORT

The dean and associate deans of the undergraduate and graduate nursing programs prepare a report and business case on the financial resources of the parent institution and the nursing program. They consult with the comptroller of the institution as well as the director of Human Resources. The parent institution has an endowment fund of over $120 million. It has an active alumni association and raises at least $2 million each year for scholarships. Its capital operating costs match that of the tuition and fees income each year. It has several million-dollar grants from private and federal sources for research in science and for program development in education. The nursing program has one federal grant ($300,000) for the nurse practitioner program, $10,000 from the federal advanced education nursing traineeships, one health care system grant for $50,000 for preparing RNs to MSNs, and several scholarship funds totaling $10 million in endowments. The financial-aid programs include a statewide tuition assistance program for needy students, the federally sponsored work–study programs and traineeships, PELL grants, nursing loan programs, and a forgivable loan program from a health care agency for students who agree to work for that agency for 2 years upon graduation. In addition, there are numerous private scholarships that are available to nursing students from external sources.

The comptroller assures the team that the institution will provide a business plan for the nursing program to calculate start-up costs and the economic feasibility of an expanded program. If the program appears to be economically sound, the parent institution will provide the start-up costs. In addition to an analysis of the financial health of the institution, the team examines possible income sources for the expanded program. They contact the nursing administrators of the four major health care systems to discuss possible program development support, physical sites for student classrooms and laboratories, and scholarships or loans for nursing students. The religious-based system has some labs that students could use for clinical skills practice and they are quite interested in scholarship programs or forgivable loans for students who commit to a 2-year contract with that agency upon graduation.

Preliminary Conclusions

The parent institution and the nursing program are financially stable. There is the promise of start-up funds and professional consultation for a business plan if the decision to expand the program is realized. In addition to the traditional economic resources, there are potential sources of income and support from the health care system. See Table 6.2 for a summary of the findings and conclusions of the external frame factors needs assessment.

TABLE 6.2 ANALYSIS OF THE EXTERNAL FRAME FACTORS NEEDS ASSESSMENT DATA AND DECISION MAKING

FRAME FACTOR	FINDINGS			CONCLUSIONS
	POSITIVE	NEGATIVE	NEUTRAL	
Community Description	Size, location, and infrastructure of the region support the needs of the college Industry and services are variable but steady		Politics vary according to location	*Positive* The community location and support systems can accommodate an expansion of the program The political systems support the institution
Demographics	Diverse About 30% with higher degrees Adequate potential applicant pool	Possible language barriers	Middle-income predominates	*Positive* Potential applicant pools for entry-level and higher degree are adequate; population is diverse *Neutral* Socioeconomic variables indicate ability to enroll in private education with some financial aid support *Negative* Some students whose primary language is not English may need support
Academic Settings	Adequate applicant pool for all five schools. There are three ADN and one BSN Program whose graduates are potential applicants for the graduate program Clinical specialties are viable with FNP popular Interest in accelerated second baccalaureate or entry-level MSN and DNPs. RNs like online format	The FNP track may be redundant to owing to the state-supported FNP program	Five existing nursing programs in the region	*Positive* There is interest in online format and accelerated or entry-level master's programs There are no DNP programs in the region The existing PhD program may provide future faculty *Neutral* While there is an adequate applicant pool and there is interest in entry-level programs including the entry-level graduate programs, there are five existing nursing programs *Negative* FNP track may be in direct competition with state school

(*continued*)

TABLE 6.2 ANALYSIS OF THE EXTERNAL FRAME FACTORS NEEDS ASSESSMENT DATA AND
DECISION MAKING (*continued*)

FRAME FACTOR	FINDINGS			CONCLUSIONS
	POSITIVE	NEGATIVE	NEUTRAL	
Political Climate	The parent institution is recognized in the community The mayor of the capital city is an RN, a strong leader and supports the program	Need to work with existing nursing programs to avoid conflict and redundancies	No opposition to expanded program The faculty and staff are in the process of developing relationships with community leaders to increase awareness of the program	*Neutral* The expanded program has a strong potential of success if it works with existing nursing programs and builds positive relationships with the body politic
Health Care System and Health Needs of the Population	There is a wide variety of health care agencies for learning experiences Nursing administrators favor and support BSN or higher degree programs Health care needs match curriculum content		There are possible opportunities for student and faculty practice in health promotion and primary care activities	*Positive* The health care system is supportive and offers many learning opportunities for students Health care needs match curriculum content There is need for increased health promotion and primary care services
Need for Program	There is a need for additional entry-level nurses in light of current and future shortages There is a demand for BSN-prepared nurses Existing program offerings match the demand			*Positive* An expanded program could meet the regional demand for additional nurses at the entry-level and advanced practice at the DNP level

(*continued*)

TABLE 6.2 ANALYSIS OF THE EXTERNAL FRAME FACTORS NEEDS ASSESSMENT DATA AND DECISION MAKING (*continued*)

FRAME FACTOR	FINDINGS			CONCLUSIONS
	POSITIVE	NEGATIVE	NEUTRAL	
Nursing Profession	There are several nursing organizations with nurse leaders that support the program The majority of nurses are ADN prepared		There are eight doctorate-prepared nurses as potential mentors or faculty Master's-prepared nurses are in advanced roles	*Positive* Professional nursing organizations and their members are potential supporters, mentors, and faculty for the program The potential applicant pool for baccalaureate and higher degrees is promising
Regulations and Accreditation			A proposal for a new degree program must be submitted to the regional accrediting body and the State Board of Nursing A report should be sent to CCNE 90 days prior to its start	*Neutral* Proposals must be submitted to the accrediting and regulating bodies in advance of initiation if the assessment of external and internal frame factors is favorable toward an expanded program
Financial Support	Financial reports indicate economic health and stability The parent institution will provide start-up funds; at least one health care system offered financial assistance		There are other potential financial resources	*Positive* The financial picture is excellent There are future potential resources that need to be explored further
Overall Decision				20 positive conclusions 10 neutral conclusions 3 negative conclusions

CONCLUSION

A needs assessment of nine external frame factors revealed a positive external environment for an expanded program when compared to the desired outcomes of the "Guidelines for Assessing External Frame Factors." The faculty recommend that the program continue to study the potential for the program by conducting a needs assessment of the internal frame factors impacting the curriculum. Thus far, findings indicate a demonstrated need to increase the numbers of nurses in the region at the entry level and advanced practice levels. Nursing administrators in the region are supportive, the community body politic is supportive in the capital city, there are possibilities for support in the surrounding counties, and there is strong support from one of the key health care systems. The parent institution indicates support by offering to develop a business case and start-up funds should the faculty recommend an expanded program. Several recommendations were made based on the needs assessment thus far:

1. Consider an entry-level graduate program, increase enrollments in the BSN program, accelerate the RN to BSN to MSN program, assess the MSN tracks for their need in the community to determine if any should be discontinued, remain at present levels, or new ones developed, consider online formats, and possibly develop a DNP program for master's-prepared nurses in the region or as an entry-level program from the BSN
2. Conduct focus groups of potential entry level and advanced practice students to determine community interest in the proposed programs
3. Plan meetings with existing nursing education program administrators, health care system administrators, county politicians, and the mayor to nurture relationships
4. As the work continues, keep records that can eventually be the basis of a proposal, both as an internal document and as a report to regulating and accrediting bodies

DISCUSSION QUESTIONS

1. Conducting a needs assessment is time consuming. Debate the value of conducting the assessment by paid consultants rather than faculty.
2. How does the process of a needs assessment apply to both curriculum development and curriculum evaluation?

LEARNING ACTIVITIES

STUDENT LEARNING ACTIVITY

As a student group, examine the community around you for its potential for a nursing program. Use Table 6.1, "Guidelines for Assessing External Frame Factors," to collect data on the external frame factors that you need to consider. After you collect the data, summarize your findings and compare them to the desired outcomes listed in the table. Based on the findings, justify why or why not a new nursing program is needed.

NURSE EDUCATOR/FACULTY DEVELOPMENT ACTIVITY

Using Table 6.1, "Guidelines for Assessing External Frame Factors," assess your nursing curriculum. Collect data for each external frame factor as it applies to the curriculum. Summarize your findings and compare them to the desired outcomes listed in the table. In light of your summary, is a curriculum revision indicated? Explain your reasons for the decision to revise or not to revise.

REFERENCES

Accreditation Commission for Education in Nursing. (2014a). Retrieved from http://www .acenursing.org/about#numaccred

Accreditation Commission for Education in Nursing. (2014b). *Resources. Accreditation manual.* Retrieved from http://www.acenursing.org/resources

Affordable Care Act. (2014). *Health and human services.* Retrieved from http://www .hhs.gov/healthcare/rights/index.html

American Association of Colleges of Nursing. (2013a). Retrieved from http://www.aacn .nche.edu

American Association of Colleges of Nursing. (2013b). *Annual report.* Retrieved from https://www.aacn.nche.edu/aacn-publications/annual-reports/AnnualReport12.pdf

American Nurses Association (2014). Retrieved from http://www.nursingworld.org/ FunctionalMenuCategories/AboutANA/WhoWeAre/CMA.aspx

American Public Health Association. (2014). Retrieved from http://www.apha.org

Commission on Collegiate Nursing Education. (2014). Retrieved from http://www.aacn .nche.edu/Accreditation/pubsguides.htm

Council for Higher Education Accreditation (CHEA). (2014). Retrieved from http://www .chea.org

GIS Inventory. (2014). *The National States Geographic Information Council (NSGIC).* Retrieved from http://gisinventory.net/index.php?page_id=624

Institute of Medicine. (2010). *The future of nursing: Leading change, advancing health.* Washington, DC: National Academies Press.

Johnson, M. (1977). *Intentionality in education.* (Distributed by the Center for Curriculum Research and Services, Albany, NY.). Troy, NY: Walter Snyder, Printer, Inc.

Kazda, M., Beel, E., Villegas, D., Martinez, J., Patel, N., & Migala, W. (2009). Methodological complexities and the use of GIS in conducting a community needs assessment of a large U.S. municipality. *Journal of Community Health, 34*(3), 210–215. Retrieved from CINAHL database.

Lohmann, A., & Schoelkopf, L. (2009). GIS—A useful tool for community assessment. *Journal of Prevention & Intervention in the Community, 37*(1), 1–4.

Morbidity and Mortality Weekly Reports (MMWR). (2014). Retrieved from http://www .edc.gov/mmwr and http://www.cdc.gov/mmwr/international/relres.html

Takach, M. (2012). About half of the states are implementing patient-centered medical homes for their Medicaid populations. *Health Affairs, 31*(11), 2432–2440.

Theordori, G. L. (2005). Community and community development in resource-based areas: Operational definitions R=rooted in an interactional perspective. *Society and Natural Resources, 18*(7), 661–669.

U.S. Department of Health and Human Services. (2013). *About the law.* Retrieved from http://www.hhs.gov/healthcare/rights/index.html

Walker, A., Bezyak, J., Gilbert, E., & Trice, A. (2011). A needs assessment to develop community partnerships: Initial steps working with a major agricultural community. *American Journal of Health Education, 4*(5), 270–275.

RESOURCES

American Health Care Association. Retrieved from http://www.ahca.org

American Hospital Association. Retrieved from http://www.aha.org

Healthy People 2020. Retrieved from http://www.healthypeople.gov/hp2020/Comments/default.asp

Middle States Association of Colleges and Schools
Middle State Commission of Higher Education (MSCHE)
3624 Market St. 2nd Floor Annex
Philadelphia, Pennsylvania 19104-2680
Phone 267-284-5000 Fax 215-662-5501
E-mail: info@msche.org
www.msche.org.

National Association for Home Care & Hospice. Retrieved from http://www.nahc.org

National Center for Education Statistics. Retrieved from http://nces.ed.gov

National Center for Health Statistics. Retrieved from http://www.cdc.gov/nchs

National Council of State Boards of Nursing. Retrieved from http://www.ncsbn.org

New England Association of Schools and Colleges
Commission on Institutions of Higher Education (NEASC-CIHE)
209 Burlington Road
Bedford, Massachusetts 01730
Phone 781-271-0022 Fax 781-271-0950
E-mail: CIHE@neasc.org
www.neasc.org

North Central Association of Colleges and Schools
The Higher Learning Commission (NCA-HLC)
30 North LaSalle Street, Suite 2400
Chicago, Illinois 60602
Phone: 312-263-0456 Fax: 312-263-7462
E-mail: info@hlcommission.org
www.ncahigherlearningcommission.org

Northwest Commission of Colleges and Universities (NWCCU)
8060 165th Avenue, NE, Suite 100
Redmond, Washington 98052
Phone: 425-558-4224 Fax: 425-376-0596
E-mail: selman@nwccu.org
www.nwccu.org

Southern Association of Colleges and Schools (SACS)
Commission on Colleges
1866 Southern Lane
Decatur, Georgia 30033
Phone: 404-679-4500 Fax: 404-679-4528
E-mail: bwheelan@sacscoc.org
www.sacscoc.org

U. S. Census Bureau. *United States census 2010*. Retrieved from http://www.census .gov/2010census

U.S. Department of Health and Human Services. *HRSA health professions*. Retrieved from http://bhpr.hrsa.gov

Western Association of Schools and Colleges Accrediting Commission for Community and Junior Colleges (WASC-ACCJC)
10 Commercial Boulevard, Suite 204
Novato, California 94949
Phone: 415-506-0234 Fax: 415-506-0238
E-mail: accjc@accjc.org
www.accjc.org

WASC Senior College and University Commission
985 Atlantic Avenue, Suite 100
Alameda, California 94501
Phone: 510-748-9001 Fax: 510-748-9797
E-mail: wascsr@wascsenior.org
www.wascweb.org

Internal Frame Factors

Sarah B. Keating

OBJECTIVES

Upon completion of Chapter 7, the reader will be able to:

1. Evaluate the internal frame factors that affect a nursing education program for the need to either develop a new program or revise an existing one
2. Compile resources for the collection of data related to internal frame factors for comparing the data to desired outcomes for program development
3. Analyze a case study that illustrates a needs assessment of internal frame factors for a curriculum development project
4. Apply the guidelines for assessing internal frame factors in a simulated or real curriculum development situation

OVERVIEW

Section III introduced the reader to the Frame Factors model and Chapter 6 discussed the external frame factors that nurse educators should review when conducting a needs assessment for program planning and curriculum development purposes. The data collected from a review of the external frame factors provide information related to the external environment of the educational program and feed into the decision-making process for developing new programs or revising existing ones. These factors can have a major impact on the program's existence and decisions regarding changes. Chapter 6 initiated a case study as an example of a needs assessment, using the Frame Factors model that is continued in Chapter 7 with the internal frame factors to consider. See Figure 7.1 for a conceptual model of the internal frame factors that impact the curriculum (Johnson, 1977). This chapter discusses the components of the curriculum and continues the case study with recommended revisions of the current program and a proposal for a new doctor of nursing practice (DNP) program based on the needs assessment.

Faculty continues to be responsible for curriculum development and evaluation and is part of the process for collecting information about the internal frame factors that impact the educational program. The internal frame factors include a description and organizational structure of the parent academic institution; mission and purpose, philosophy, and goals; internal economic situation and its influence on the curriculum; resources within the institution (laboratories, classrooms, library, academic services, instructional technology support, student services, etc.);

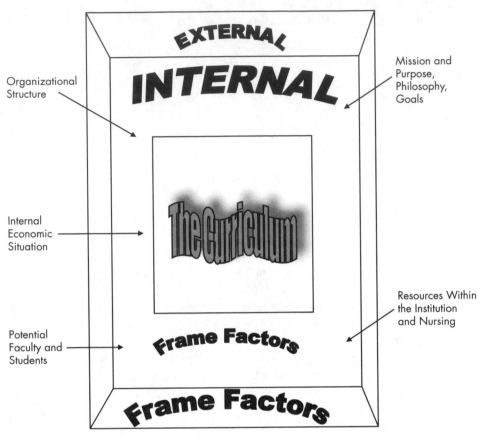

FIGURE 7.1   Internal frame factors for a needs assessment for curriculum development.
Adapted from Johnson (1977).

and potential faculty and student characteristics. The information related to these factors is analyzed for its relevance to the program and the findings are weighed as to their importance to the quality of the program, its existence, and possible changes.

Chapter 7 provides detailed information about each of these internal frame factors and there is a table with guidelines for collecting information about the factors and assessing the need according to the desired outcomes. The chapter ends by continuing the case study of a fictional nursing school that is conducting a needs assessment for revising and expanding the program.

DISCUSSION

DESCRIPTION AND ORGANIZATIONAL STRUCTURE OF THE PARENT ACADEMIC INSTITUTION

When looking at the environment that surrounds a nursing education program, the parent institution in which it resides is examined in light of the scenario it sets for the program. The physical campus and its buildings create the milieu in which the program exists with the nursing program a reflection of its place within the institution. The nature of the institution influences the structure of the campus and for nursing education programs, can be located in health care agencies, academic medical centers, liberal arts colleges, large research universities, land grant universities, multipurpose state-supported or private universities, or community colleges. The history of the institution is important to know such as its growth or change over the years and the role the nursing program had in its political fortunes or misfortunes. In small private institutions, the school of nursing can be one of the largest and most influential constituents, while in statewide university systems, nursing can be a small department within a health-related college that is within the greater university.

All educational institutions and health care agencies have organizational structures, usually of a hierarchal nature. Faculty should analyze the structure of the parent institution as well as that of the nursing program to describe the hierarchal and formal lines of communication that guide the faculty in developing and revising programs. For example, as described in Chapters 2 and 3, curriculum proposals and changes must be approved first on the local level (the nursing curriculum committee and faculty), moved to the next level of organization such as a college curriculum committee and dean, and finally, to an all-college or university-wide curriculum committee with its recommendations going to the faculty senate (or its like) for final approval. There can be administrative approval along the way from department heads, deans, and perhaps academic vice presidents or provosts; especially in regard to economic and administrative feasibility. Nevertheless, the major approval bodies are those that are composed of faculty and within faculty governance prerogatives.

At the same time, it is useful to include the major players within the faculty and administrative structures in order to discuss with them the plans and rationale for proposed new programs or curriculum revisions. Prior consultation with these key people can help to smooth the way when the proposals are ready to enter the formal arena and they can give advice related to changes that might enhance approval or advice on the best presentation formats that facilitate an understanding of the proposal. These contacts can be of a formal or informal nature; however, a word of caution: to avoid disastrous results, never blindside an administrator or decision maker. It is wise to keep them informed of new proposals or possible changes to place them in the advocate role as the approval process wends its way through the system.

MISSION AND PURPOSE, PHILOSOPHY, AND GOALS OF THE PARENT INSTITUTION

The mission/vision and purpose, philosophy, and goals of the parent institution determine the character of the nursing program. Most institutions of higher education focus their missions and philosophies on three endeavors: education, service, and scholarship/research. Nursing must examine the mission and philosophy of its parent institution to determine its place within these three basic activities. For example, a state-supported university may have as part of its mission and philosophy the education of the people of the state for professional, leadership, and service roles. Thus, the nursing program could focus its mission and philosophy on the preparation of nurses for leadership roles and provision of health care services to the people of the state. If the statewide system is the predominant preparer of nurses within the state as compared to independent colleges, then the additional mission or purpose might be to provide an adequate nursing workforce for the state.

In contrast, independent or private colleges and universities may have missions and philosophies that have a sectarian flavor such as preparing individuals with strong liberal arts foundations for public service or roles in the helping professions. Again, a nursing program's mission is usually compatible with this mission. Academic medical centers are yet another example of nursing's match to health disciplines that are housed in one institution and whose mission is to prepare individuals for the health professions. Community college or junior college missions usually focus on technical education or on prerequisite preparation for entering into upper division level colleges and universities. Although the debate still rages about the role of nursing programs in these institutions, there is no question that they fit the mission of the 2-year college as most expect that their graduates will function as registered nurses (RNs) and continue with their education at the baccalaureate and higher degree levels. Rosa (2009) surveyed associate degree in nursing (ADN) faculty members to identify the factors that contributed to their advising students to continue their education and earn a baccalaureate. She found that faculty members felt a moral commitment to advise students as professional colleagues to continue their education. Another factor influencing their advisement was the extent to which the ADN school was affiliated with baccalaureate completion programs.

INTERNAL ECONOMIC SITUATION AND INFLUENCE ON THE CURRICULUM

As stated in Chapter 6, the economic health of the institution has a significant impact on the nursing program and curriculum. How much of the share of resources, income, and expenditures that the nursing program has can affect program stability and room for expansion. For example, nurse-managed clinics must be self-supporting or economic recessions can cause their demise. For state-sponsored programs, the parent institution is subject to the state economy during periods of recession and prosperity. Independent colleges, unless heavily endowed, depend on tuition, student fees, or other income-generating operations.

All institutions depend upon endowments, financial aid programs for students including scholarships, loans, and grants. Nursing programs are eligible for many federal grants and have a history of securing other types of grants from private foundations, state-supported programs, and private contributions including those from alumni associations. These income-generating programs illustrate to the parent institution that the nursing program is viable and at the same time, the institution's reputation and ability to garner external financial resources help the nursing program to secure funding.

Institutions usually have support systems for assisting faculty to write grants and to seek outside financial support. Nursing programs should have close relationships with these support systems and have a plan in place for securing additional funds. Faculty plays a major role in writing grants with the perks related to them, if funded, of released time for program development and scholarship and research activities. Two sources for funding to support program development on the national level are the Health Resources and Services Administration (http://bhpr.hrsa.gov/nursing) and the National Institutes of Health (http://www.ninr.nih.gov). The latter focuses on clinical research; however, it is possible that faculty may wish to conduct curriculum and educational program research. A list of private foundations with funding opportunities for program development is located at www.research.ucla.edu/ocga/sr2/Private.htm (University of California-Los Angeles, 2014).

Assessment of the economic status of the parent institution and the nursing program provides a realistic picture of the potential for program expansion and curriculum revision. When developing curriculum, the first demand for financial support comes with the need for resources to conduct a needs assessment such as the costs of released time for those who are conducting the assessment, review of the literature, and surveys of key stakeholders. A cost analysis for revising a curriculum or mounting a new one requires a business case to justify the costs and to forecast its financial viability. Unless there is a nursing program financial officer, the nursing program administrator and faculty should work closely with the parent institution's business office or chief financial officer in developing the business case.

RESOURCES WITHIN THE INSTITUTION AND NURSING PROGRAM

An analysis of the existing resources within the institution and the nursing program supplies information related to possible program expansion and curriculum revisions. First, there should be adequate classrooms, learning laboratories, library staff and resources, computer facilities, clinical practice simulations, instructional technology support, and distance education resources for the current program. When planning for revisions of the curriculum or for new programs, the need for expansion of these facilities and additional staffing should be identified. If expansion is not possible, then creative approaches to scheduling for the maximum use of these facilities can be examined, for example, evening classes, weekend learning experiences, and online delivery of courses.

Academic support services such as the library, academic advisement, teaching-learning resources, and instructional technology contribute to the maintenance of a quality education program and are internal frame factors that should be assessed when developing new programs or revising existing ones. If there are to be new programs or expansion of current curricula, the library resources must be adequate. Library resources include not only those resources on campus but also services for off-campus programs and students. There should be Internet and web-based library access for students and faculty and this is especially true when the campus has a large commuter student population, distance education programs, or proposes new programs. Library and instructional technology support staffing must be large enough and knowledgeable about nursing education needs. Thus, faculty should have strong relationships with librarians and the instructional technology staff in order to build the resources needed to revise the curriculum or develop new programs.

Academic advisement services play an important role in program planning as new programs can require additional staffing. If the curriculum is revised, updates for academic advising are necessary so that the faculty and its support staff who provide the services have current information to impart to the students. Teaching–learning resources need to be available to keep faculty current in instructional strategies, particularly if the revisions to the curriculum have an effect on instructional design. For example, a baccalaureate program may decide to convert its RN program to a web-based delivery system. In this case, faculty needs training in preparing and implementing web-based courses.

Instructional support systems are part of planning as well since the nature of the proposed program or the revised curriculum may call for additional resources. These resources include programmed instruction units, audio–visual aids, hardware and software, computer technologies, high-fidelity and low-fidelity mannequins for simulated clinical situations, and so forth. They can generate large costs to the program and should be calculated into the business case and the costs associated with their maintenance and replacement expenses over time. Some instructional support systems include monthly or annual students fees as well. For new programs or revisions, these costs are often included in requests for additional student lab fees or external funding. If the updating or creation of new laboratory/simulation practice labs are one-time costs, external funding through donations, grants, or endowments are possibilities.

Student support services are equally important to nursing education programs and are an integral part of the curriculum development process. Major student services include enrollment (recruitment, admissions, registrar activities, and graduation records), maintenance of student records, advising and counseling, disciplinary matters, remediation and study skills, work study programs, career counseling, job placement, and financial aid. Depending upon the size of the university or college, these services can be congregated into one department or subdivided into several. Their role in curriculum development is important, as expanding or changing educational programs requires student services support. For example, if a new program is proposed, then the recruitment and admissions staff will need to be apprised of the program to best serve the needs of the new program in recruitment and admission activities.

Financial aid programs are crucial to the recruitment, admission, and retention of students and if the proposal brings in new revenues through grants or other financial support structures, the financial aid staff must be cognizant of the proposal. They can provide useful information to program planners and thus a partnership between the student services staff and the nursing program staff is beneficial.

Work–study programs and job placement information can supplement the curriculum, if these programs are in concert with the educational plan and not in conflict with the program of study. An example of a conflict is a revised curriculum that calls for accelerated study and clinical experiences that disallow student employment and therefore prohibits enrollment in the work–study program. Another aspect is the potential influence of students' part-time employment on the curriculum and its role in intended and unintended outcomes on the educational experience. With the preponderance of adult learners in nursing programs, the reality of their outside employment while enrolled in studies must be taken in to account.

The informal curriculum often takes place through the planned activities of the student services department. Again, partnerships between them and nursing faculty increase the effectiveness of the formal curriculum. Students who could benefit from remediation or learning skills workshops should be referred to student services. Faculty work with student services staff to identify the learning needs of nursing students and this is especially relevant when curriculum changes are taking place. Additionally, student services staff work with faculty concerning the special needs of students with learning disabilities and the accommodations they require without imperiling the student's individual needs or the safety of the clients for whom the students provide care. Brock (2010) describes essential student support services for at-risk groups and their success in improving graduation rates. Nursing students who are at risk for failure should be identified early in the program and referred to student support staff to facilitate their success in the program.

POTENTIAL FACULTY AND STUDENT CHARACTERISTICS

When proposing new educational programs or revising existing curricula, thought needs to go into the characteristics of the existing faculty and the student body who will participate in the educational program. If a new program is proposed, the faculty composition is reviewed. There should be adequate numbers of faculty members who represent diversity in gender and ethnic backgrounds and to reach the desired faculty to student ratio. Depending upon the nature of the program, clinical supervision of students requires a low student to faculty ratio but can differ according to program. For example, master's and doctoral students are usually RNs and therefore may not need the close supervision required for entry-level students. However, for some advanced practice roles, there is a need for close faculty supervision. However, in these latter cases, preceptorships or internships are the usual format and a faculty member can supervise more students in collaboration with the clinical preceptors. In entry-level programs, the student to faculty ratio is usually 8 to 10; however, in the senior year, it is possible to have preceptorships with approximately 12 to 15 students, depending on the nature of the clinical experiences. While lectures can accommodate many students, seminars and learning laboratories demand fewer numbers of students and therefore additional faculty. Enrollment in online courses can vary with as few as 10 to 12 at the graduate level and seminar-type courses to didactic online courses that accommodate as many as 30 or more students. In the case of the latter, the format for the course is modified to adjust to the larger number of students and the resultant teaching load for the instructor. These are practical issues that must be addressed owing to the quality perspectives and cost factors that they present when developing curricula.

Yet another consideration related to faculty is the match of knowledge to the subject matter, clinical expertise, and pedagogical skills. Information on the numbers and types of faculty needed, their required educational levels, and scholarship and research history feed into decisions about curriculum development since faculty knowledge and expertise are critical to the delivery of the curriculum. As with faculty considerations, the characteristics of the student body and the types of students the faculty hopes to attract to the new program or the revised curriculum are important. If it is a new program, the potential applicant pool should be identified according to interest, numbers, availability, and competition with other nursing programs. If a new program is contemplated, its type dictates the kind of applicant pool that the program and the admission department need to target. If it is a curriculum revision to update the program and plan for future demands, the applicant pool might be the same as the current one.

The characteristics of the students in the program help to tailor the curriculum according to their learning needs. For example, if it is an entry-level associate degree or baccalaureate program, the applicants may be a mix of new high school graduates, transfer students with some college preparation, and adult learners with some work experience. The curriculum is then planned to meet a diversity of learning needs from traditional pedagogical learning theories to adult learning theories. Diversity of racial, ethnic, and cultural characteristics are other factors to consider and the educational program must plan to be culturally responsive as well as preparing professionals with cultural competence.

SUMMARY

Chapter 7 reviewed the internal frame factors to consider when conducting a needs assessment for developing new educational programs or revising curricula. These factors follow the assessment of external frame factors that influence the educational program and are equally important to the decision for changing a curriculum or developing a new program. While the external frame factors examined the macro-environment surrounding the program, the internal frame factors looked at those factors that are closer to the program and include the parent institution as well as the nursing program itself.

Factors that were examined include the characteristics of the parent institution and its organizational structure. How the nursing program fits into this structure can determine the economic, political, and resource support for program changes. It sets the stage for the processes that the nursing faculty must undergo to gain approval for the proposed changes. The mission and purpose, philosophy and goals of the parent institution influence the nature of the nursing program and to ensure success, the nursing program must be congruent with those of the parent institution. The internal economic status and the available resources of both the parent institution and the nursing program are assessed for the financial viability as well as the necessary additional resources and support services for proposed revisions to the curriculum or proposed new programs. Finally, the characteristics of the faculty and the potential student body are reviewed to determine their match to the proposed change. See Table 7.1 for guidelines to assess the internal frame factors when conducting a needs assessment for curriculum revision or new program proposals.

TABLE 7.1	GUIDELINES FOR ASSESSING INTERNAL FRAME FACTORS	
FRAME FACTOR	QUESTIONS FOR DATA COLLECTION	DESIRED OUTCOMES
Description and Organizational Structure of the Parent Academic Institution	In what type of educational institution is the nursing program located? What is the milieu of the parent institution in regard to the nursing program? What is the organizational structure of the parent institution? What place in the institution does the nursing program hold? What influence does it have? In what order must a program go through the approval process? Who are the major players in the various levels of approval processes? What are the layers of approval processes for program approval and curriculum revisions?	The nursing program is recognized in the institution for its place in education, scholarship, and service to the community There is a supportive organizational system for program planning and curriculum revision A fair and comprehensive review process that results in economically sound and high quality educational programs exists The approval process benefits the nursing program through the education of other entities by nursing about the program, which results in their support for it
Mission and Purpose, Philosophy, and Goals of the Parent Institution	What are the mission, philosophy, and goals of the parent institution? Are they congruent and supportive of the nursing program?	The mission and purpose, philosophy, and goals of the parent institution are congruent with and supportive of the nursing program
Internal Economic Situation and its Influence on the Curriculum	What is the operating budget of the nursing program? Is it adequate for the support of the existing program? Are there resources for program or curriculum development activities? Does the program have a financial officer or administrative assistant who can develop a business plan for the proposed program or curriculum revision? If not, are there resources available from the parent institution for this activity?	The nursing program has adequate resources for supporting its educational program from the parent institution The nursing program has the resources for program or curriculum development activities The nursing program has a business plan, the resources, and administrative support for mounting a new program or revising the existing curriculum

(continued)

TABLE 7.1	GUIDELINES FOR ASSESSING INTERNAL FRAME FACTORS (*continued*)	
FRAME FACTOR	QUESTIONS FOR DATA COLLECTION	DESIRED OUTCOMES
Resources Within the Institution and Nursing Program	How many classrooms, clinical practice, simulation, and computer laboratories does the nursing program have and are they under the control of the nursing program? Can they accommodate additional students or newer technologies in the proposed program or curriculum revisions? Are the plans for these facilities included in the proposal and are their costs calculated in the business plan?	The current physical facilities such as classrooms, offices, clinical practice and simulation laboratories, and computer facilities are adequate and can accommodate curriculum revisions or new programs *or* there are plans for expansion in place that are part of the business plan and have the support of the financial bodies of the institution
	What are the available resources for program planning and curriculum revision? Is there released time available for those involved? Is there staff support available? Are there teaching-learning continuing education programs available to faculty?	There are teaching and learning support systems for faculty that facilitate program planning and curriculum revisions
	What instructional and technology support systems and staff are in place in the institution and the nursing program? Are they adequate and up to date? Are there plans for increasing and updating the systems and staff according to the revised or new program needs?	There are adequate instructional and technology support systems and staff available for the current program and for proposed future programs
	How many texts and journal holdings as well as electronic databases does the library have and will they meet the needs of students and faculty in the future, especially if new programs are developed or major revision are planned?	The current and proposed library and electronic holdings are adequate to meet the needs of the nursing program and proposed curricular revisions
	Is there adequate librarian and technical support?	There are reasonable hours/days and staff support for students and faculty to access the library and other electronic communications
	What are the available hours/days and staff support for students and faculty to access the library and other electronic communications?	

(*continued*)

TABLE 7.1	GUIDELINES FOR ASSESSING INTERNAL FRAME FACTORS (*continued*)	
FRAME FACTOR	QUESTIONS FOR DATA COLLECTION	DESIRED OUTCOMES
	Is the current academic advising system working to students' and faculty's satisfaction?	The academic advising system can accommodate appropriate faculty-student ratios and there are support systems within in it to ensure the quality of advisement
	Are there appropriate faculty-to-student ratios for academic advising? Will a revised curriculum or new program require additional faculty or staff for academic advising purposes?	The student services system (recruitment, enrollment, registrar, financial aid, remediation, student counseling, and other services) works in partnership with nursing faculty to enhance the informal and formal curricula
	What are the current relationships of the nursing program's administration, faculty, and staff with those of student services? Is the student services department aware of the proposed revisions or proposed new programs and have they been consulted regarding future students services needs that may be impacted by the changes?	The parent institution and the nursing program can currently, and in the future, support the curriculum with adequate facilities and services
	What are the current facilities and services related to classrooms, laboratories, computer facilities, clinical experience laboratories, the library, instructional support systems, teaching-learning support, academic advising, and student services? Are they adequate for the current program and for future program planning and/or curriculum revisions?	
Potential Faculty and Student Characteristics	Describe the characteristics of the current student body and the history of the applicant pool to the nursing program. Has the program been able to meet its enrollment targets in the past 5 years? If not, what strategies have taken place to meet the target?	The parent institution and the nursing program have the resources to recruit, educate, and graduate the type of student body that the new program or curriculum revision requires
	What are the characteristics of the student body for the proposed program or revised curriculum? Is there an adequate applicant pool to fulfill enrollment targets? Has the nursing program a partnership and plans with the admissions department for recruiting and retaining students?	

(*continued*)

TABLE 7.1	GUIDELINES FOR ASSESSING INTERNAL FRAME FACTORS *(continued)*	
FRAME FACTOR	QUESTIONS FOR DATA COLLECTION	DESIRED OUTCOMES
	Describe the characteristics of the current faculty	
	Are the numbers of faculty sufficient? Do they meet program requirements, educational level, clinical expertise, scholarship/ research, and teaching experience qualifications? Do they represent diversity? Are there plans to recruit additional faculty if indicated?	There is a sufficient number of qualified faculty that represent diversity and meet faculty to student ratio standards
Analysis of the data and decision making	Summarize the conclusions by generating a list of positive, negative, and neutral findings that can influence the curriculum and program planning	Develop a final decision statement as to the feasibility for developing a new program or revising the curriculum based on the needs assessment of the external and internal frame factors

CASE STUDY

The case study initiated in Chapter 6 presented a fictional baccalaureate and higher degree school of nursing seeking to expand its offerings in order to meet the region's increasing nursing shortage and need for additional advanced practice nurses. The faculty was divided into teams and each team gathered data related to the external frame factors that influence program and curriculum development. Thus far, the information they gathered indicate a positive milieu for expanding the program for either entry-level baccalaureate or higher degree students, an accelerated track for RN to master of science in nursing (MSN) students, and the possibility for a bachelor of science in nursing (BSN) to DNP with a postmaster's DNP program for advanced practice nurses. The next step is to assess the internal frame factors that can further impact the decision for revising the existing programs and/or developing new ones.

DESCRIPTION AND ORGANIZATIONAL STRUCTURE OF THE PARENT ACADEMIC INSTITUTION

The school of nursing dean and the associate deans of the undergraduate and graduate programs put together a description of the parent institution (college) and the school of nursing. The most recent accreditation reports for the Commission on Collegiate Nursing Education (CCNE) and the State Board of Nursing provide the description including the organizational structure for both the college and school.

With a few minor edits of the documents to update them, they have the report ready to analyze for information related to the proposed expansion.

The home campus of the college is located on the outskirts of a large metropolitan area with the campus a self-contained unit in a pleasant pastoral setting. The school of nursing shares offices, classrooms, and several laboratories with the science department. In addition, it has one clinical skills lab and one low-fidelity simulation lab that are under its control. There is easy access to public transportation to travel into the metropolitan area where many learning and leisure time experiences for the students take place.

The school of nursing represents about 6% (230 undergraduates and 90 master's) of the student body and was founded within the 100-year-old institution almost 60 years ago, becoming the first professional school in the college. The institution averages an enrollment of 4,500 undergraduate students each year with the graduate school enrollment at 500. It has six schools including arts and sciences (46% of the enrollment), business administration and economics (26% of the enrollment), computer science (6% of the enrollment), education (8% of the enrollment), extended education (8% of the enrollment), and nursing. All but the arts and sciences school have graduate programs and education is a graduate-only school. The highest degree that the institution awards is the doctoral degree (EdD and DBA) and it awards the bachelor of arts, bachelor of science, and master of science degrees. It has an excellent reputation in the community for its dedication to community service and high-quality programs, all of which hold regional and national accreditation.

Although the original purpose of the college had strong liberal arts and religious foci, the institution became multipurpose with the addition of the professional schools including business, education, and nursing, with computer sciences a relatively young school, having started 10 years ago. The school of extended education offers distance education programs in business administration, computer sciences, and education from the home campus and works collaboratively with nursing on the RN to BSN program. Extended education is currently under study for a needs assessment to determine if some programs should be cut or additional programs added. Each school has a dean and the school of nursing dean has been in his position for 12 years and therefore has a strong voice in the council of deans owing to his history within the college. There is an academic provost to whom the deans report. The president, who is an ordained minister within the religious sect that sponsors the college, is its chief executive officer. There is a comptroller, a dean of student affairs, a dean of enrollment services, director of human resources, and a director of the library, information services, and instructional support.

The faculty full-time equivalents total about 210 with an additional 100 or more part-time lecturers. There is an academic senate composed of two representatives from each school's faculty, three members-at-large, undergraduate, and graduate student representatives, a presidential appointee, and the academic provost. There are three major committees of the senate: the curriculum, graduate, and faculty affairs committees. The faculty elects the chair of the senate, chair-elect, and secretary. The faculty votes for members of the three committees from the senate membership. The committee members elect committee chairs to their positions. There is one nursing faculty member on the graduate committee, one nurse is chair of the faculty affairs committee, and another is a member-at-large of the senate.

The school of nursing faculty and the senate curriculum committee must approve new academic programs and curriculum revisions. If the proposals emanate from graduate programs, the graduate committee recommends approval after review and sends them to the senate with recommendations.

The school of nursing faculty has 30 full-time tenured/tenure-track faculty and 15 part-time clinical faculty, not including the dean and three administrative support staff. One member of the administrative staff serves as the instructional support and informational systems support person for the school. A part-time clinical instructor serves as the clinical placement coordinator. There are two associate deans, one each for the graduate program and the undergraduate program. They have 30% released time for coordination duties. The five tracks in the nursing program (BSN, RN to BSN, family nurse practitioner [FNP], adult /geriatric acute care nurse practitioner [ACNP], clinical nurse leader [CNL]) have coordinators who have 20% released time for these functions. The part-time faculty's teaching role occurs primarily in supervising students during their clinical experiences. The faculty members teach in both undergraduate and graduate programs, although some are predominantly assigned to one or the other depending upon their clinical expertise and academic preparation. Seventy-five percent of the full-time tenure track faculty members have doctorates and there are currently three enrolled in doctoral programs. The school of nursing faculty meets once a month during the academic year and there are four major committees, that is, curriculum, graduate, peer evaluation, and student affairs. All program and curriculum revisions must be approved through the appropriate nursing committee structure and then approved by the faculty as a whole with final administrative review and approval by the dean. Approved proposals are forwarded to the appropriate senate committee who makes recommendations to the senate who vote for approval or disapproval. On approval of the senate, the provost completes a final review and makes recommendations to the president.

Preliminary Conclusions

The college has a strong reputation for high-quality liberal arts and professional education programs within the region and the school of nursing has a significant role within the college. The dean of nursing is an active and respected member of the college's administrative structure with a sense of the history of the college and school of nursing.

There are clear hierarchal lines of communication for administrative decisions and for gaining curriculum and program approval. The school had three senators with two on senate committees, but none on the curriculum or graduate committee. Thus, some political maneuvering will be necessary to educate the senate about proposed changes to solicit their support. The president, provost, and comptroller have been aware of the needs assessment and potential program changes and are supportive owing to their awareness of the community's demand to prepare more nurses for the health care system.

MISSION AND PURPOSE, PHILOSOPHY, AND GOALS OF THE PARENT INSTITUTION

Because of the institution's religious base, nursing's mission is congruent with the institution's mission and goals that focus on the preparation of compassionate and responsible citizens for society and professionals who provide services to the community. Although the school of nursing sometimes finds itself in conflict with the large school of arts and sciences that emphasizes strong liberal arts and science foundations for all undergraduate students, nursing often allies itself with the other professional schools and thus can forestall additional prerequisites by arts and sciences that can overburden the student prerequisite load for the undergraduate degree in nursing.

Preliminary Conclusions

The school of nursing's mission and purpose, philosophy, and goals are in congruence with those of the college. It recognizes the need to educate key individuals from the other schools about the nursing shortage and the need to increase enrollments. At the same time, it must collaborate with them in regard to the impact a new or revised program might have on the other schools.

INTERNAL ECONOMIC SITUATION AND ITS INFLUENCE ON THE CURRICULUM

The same team who examined the organizational structure of the college meets with the comptroller of the college to discuss some additional issues related to the economic situation and its effect on the proposed expanded or revised program. When conducting the assessment of the external frame factors, faculty found that both the college and school of nursing are financially stable, the comptroller is willing to help develop a business case for a proposed program and there are potential external funding resources for a new program should it start up. Recently, the nursing faculty identified several state and federal programs that might fund a new program; especially if it included strategies to reduce the current nursing shortage and increase educational levels of professional nurses. However, this requires released time for faculty to write the grants. It is calculated that two faculty members each need 5% released time for the next semester to write these grants. The comptroller refers the dean and faculty to the provost who may have some faculty development funds that could cover the costs for this released time. The provost agrees to provide a total of $5,000 as released time for the next semester for faculty to write grant proposals for program development.

Thus far, there has been no financial support for the needs assessment and as it progresses, the dean and faculty feel the need for some support to continue to develop the proposal. Of special concern is the need to provide released time for curriculum development when and if expansion is approved. This would involve at least three faculty members and would take about 5% of their workload in assigned time activities to develop or revise the existing curriculum. This released time needs to be built into the next year's budget for the school of nursing. The comptroller suggests that the dean of nursing place this on the agenda when the council of deans and the provost develop next year's proposed budgets. The dean discussed this with the provost who is willing to place the item into next year's budget request.

Preliminary Conclusions

The college and the school of nursing are economically stable. The college administration indicated support for developing a business case for an expanded and/or revised *program. The business plan will calculate estimated start-up costs and program main-tenance funds for 3 years when the program becomes self-sufficient. The provost will provide $5,000 next semester for faculty-released time to write grants for program development funds. The dean will include the cost for faculty-released time for curriculum development into next year's budget with the approval of the provost.*

RESOURCES WITHIN THE INSTITUTION AND NURSING PROGRAM

A team of faculty composed of representatives from the laboratories, the clinical coordinator, the library, informational systems and instructional support liaison, the school's curriculum committee chair, and the undergraduate and graduate associate deans assess the resources within the college and the school of nursing. Since the proposed change or new programs must match the resources of the existing program, and meet the needs of students who may be at a distance from the school, the team assesses resources needed for possible distance outreach.

The on-campus classrooms, learning laboratories, and computer classrooms, although not under the school's control, are adequate in size and number for the present on-campus student enrollment. However, even if enrollments expand, there is a need to upgrade the clinical practice laboratory and add at least one additional simulation lab with high- and low-fidelity mannequins. These upgrades imply an additional room to house the simulation with an adjacent control and observation room. The library has one of the largest holdings in the region for nursing journals and texts as well as for other disciplines. Recently, the library upgraded its off-campus access through Elton B. Stephens Company Information Services databases with full text journal articles. The instructional support services department and the school of extended education have distance education programs including videoconferencing with a dedicated broadcasting suite and there is a contract with a web-based delivery system for computer-based courses. These facilities were developed for the schools of business administration and education graduate programs as well as the RN to BSN program. The director of the library, information systems, and instructional support services meets with the team and indicates that nursing has access to these technologies, although videoconferencing services dictate scheduling of classes to avoid conflict with the school of extended education programs. She indicates that monthly in-service workshops by library staff are held for faculty to improve teaching effectiveness as well as to learn new technologies such as developing web-based courses and designing videoconference classes. Many nursing faculty attend these workshops and are always welcome as new programs and technologies are developed. While staff seems adequate at this point, new programs or new delivery systems will require additional staffing.

As for off-campus facilities, the team knows from the assessment of the external frame factors that the dean of extended education indicated that the classrooms he rents in the proposed off-campus outreach program site are available for rental by the nursing program as well. These rooms include office space for faculty, one office for the coordinator of the program, a traditional classroom, and a dedicated high technology computer and videoconferencing room that can be shared with other extended education students. Special clinical learning laboratories near the site are available to the program, rent free, from the religious-based health maintenance organization.

The academic advisement system in the school of nursing requires that each faculty member carries an average of 20 advisees. Advisees are matched to faculty members' expertise and interests. In the graduate program, advisors are usually the students' thesis or research project chairs and therefore advisors have fewer student advisees.

The team assesses student services needs for a possible expanded program. They meet with the director of enrollment services and discuss recruitment, student records, counseling services, financial aid programs, and work–study options for nursing students. The proposed program calls for at least one additional staff member in enrollment services for all of the services mentioned above, although it is possible that such a person could work with the extended education program staff located in its off-campus site should the program decide to offer classes off-site. This needs to be included in the business plan and is duly noted for bringing to the attention of the comptroller.

Preliminary Conclusions

Current facilities and services for the school of nursing are adequate for the on-campus program. However the following is a list of the needs if the program expands or an outreach web-based program are decided on. Areas that indicate additional costs to fill the needs include:

- *Classrooms and office space: Rooms shared with extended education include a rental fee.*
- *Computer and videoconferencing classroom: One room shared with extended education. There is a rental fee*
- *Clinical practice and simulation facilities: At least one room with equipment; possible donations by the health care system*
- *Library and instructional support systems: Current facilities are adequate and accessible; there may be need for additional staff depending on type of program and upgrading of web-based platforms*
- *Academic counseling: Additional faculty and staff*
- *Student services: Services are in place; however additional staff may be necessary*

POTENTIAL FACULTY AND STUDENT CHARACTERISTICS

Four faculty members representing the undergraduate and graduate programs are charged with identifying potential faculty and student characteristics and the need for an expanded program. They agree that a full-time coordinator for a new program is necessary during the planning stages as well as for managing the program when it commences. At that time, depending upon the size of the student enrollment, that person could assume some teaching responsibilities in addition to coordinating the program. Faculty characteristics and needs must match those of the current faculty with tenure track and clinical positions available to the program. Educational levels, clinical expertise, scholarship and research, and teaching experience qualifications of new faculty must be matched to the needs of new programs and/or revision of existing ones. The size of the faculty will be determined by the choice of program, specialty, if it is or is not a pre-licensure program, and the delivery mode of the program. For example, some lecture courses might be developed and delivered through videoconferencing or web-based courses that are already part of the on-campus program and the faculty's repertoire, while new faculty will be needed for clinical supervision of students and some theory and learning laboratory courses if the existing program expands or a new program is instituted. Although precise numbers of teachers cannot be calculated until the final decision is made to offer the program and what kind of program it will be, a plan for additional tenure track faculty for teaching didactic material and clinical supervision of students as well as part-time clinical faculty is essential.

Like the faculty, the characteristics and size of the student body depends upon the decision to expand or to offer new programs and the types of program. Based on the needs assessment of the external frame factors, the decision appears to be going toward an expansion of the RN to BSN program to an MSN program, a possible entry-level MSN program for college graduates with the development of a BSN to DNP and postmaster's DNP program. If an expansion of the undergraduate program such as a fast track baccalaureate is initiated for college graduates, the numbers of students are likely to be larger than for an entry-level master's program. However, since either program is a prelicensure program, the faculty to student ratio for clinical supervision must be calculated into the costs for mounting the program. A calculation is necessary for the critical mass of number of students needed to meet the cost of mounting the program. The same prerequisites and other admission criteria for students on the home campus program must be applied to a potential outreach program.

With these factors in mind, the faculty team members look at the enrollment and retention patterns of the school of nursing's home campus. In spite of the competition with the lower cost, state-supported nursing programs, the undergraduate program enrollments have been stable for the past 5 years; however the applicant pool decreased in the past 4 years by 8% with a slight increase this past year. The team attributed the slight increase in the applicant pool to the lay public's increasing awareness of the nursing shortage. Although enrollment targets were met for the past 5 years, the result was that students that were admitted to the program had lower overall high school GPAs and scores on the SAT. Although they met the prerequisites and admission criteria, the average overall GPA and SAT scores fell by 3% points. Thus, the students required more academic counseling and remediation programs than in the past for retention purposes and the attrition rate increased slightly from 6% to 8%. The NCLEX passing score for first-time takers averaged around 85% over the past 5 years.

Faculty informally survey entry-level MSN programs across the county and learn that the NCLEX pass rates exceed 90% and graduates are gainfully employed in nursing positions. Although formal studies were not conducted, anecdotal information indicates high satisfaction with the entry-level MSN graduates on the part of faculty, the graduates' employers and the graduates. The majority of faculty members reported that they enjoyed working with these students and found them challenging owing to their adult-learner needs, previous work experience, and new perspectives on nursing as a profession.

The nursing faculty learns from the admissions department that there are many college graduates in the nursing applicant pool based on the news of the nursing shortage in the public media. Based on their experiences, the admissions staff believes that recruitment for both types of students into the undergraduate or graduate programs should be fairly easy; although owing to the other existing nursing programs, the entry-level master's program is more attractive as there is no competition for those types of students. They report that they have many inquiries for a DNP program and estimate they receive about 10 calls per week. The inquiries come from nurses who are in advanced practice roles. However, establishing a DNP program will require meetings of the staff with regional college and university advising centers' staff, public media advertisements and spot announcements, and on-site information meetings. These activities would have to be included in the business case.

Preliminary Conclusions

Although the current overall nursing faculty to student ratio is 1 to 13, which is lower than the other schools in the college, any new programs will require a coordinator, additional faculty, and staff. A full-time coordinator for any new programs is necessary to build relationships within the college and the community, and to help admissions staff recruit students. Eventually, the coordinator role could include some teaching activities. Current faculty may be able to deliver their lectures and theory-type courses to larger audiences; however, expanded supervised skills labs, simulation labs, and clinical experiences will require part-time clinical faculty services at the very least.

The coordinator and faculty will need to work closely with enrollment services in the recruitment of students into the program. A marketing and recruitment plan including a timetable needs to be developed. See Table 7.2 for a summary of the findings and conclusions of the needs assessment based on the internal frame factors.

TABLE 7.2   ANALYSIS OF THE INTERNAL FRAME FACTORS

FRAME FACTOR	FINDINGS	NEGATIVE	NEUTRAL	POSITIVE	CONCLUSIONS
Description and Organizational Structure of the Parent Academic Institution	The college and school of nursing have positive reputations. Organization and hierarchal communication lines are clear for program and curriculum development processes and approvals. The dean has influence in the college. The college administrators are aware of the proposed program and supportive thus far.	There are no nursing senators on the senate curriculum or graduate committees		The school has three senators on the academic senate Organization lines are clear There is administrative support The dean has influence The school has a positive reputation	*Positive* The college organizational structure and administrators are supportive The dean has influence *Neutral* There is a need to educate key members of the senate about the program

(continued)

TABLE 7.2	ANALYSIS OF THE INTERNAL FRAME FACTORS (*continued*)				
FRAME FACTOR	FINDINGS	NEGATIVE	NEUTRAL	POSITIVE	CONCLUSIONS
Mission and Purpose, Philosophy, and Goals of the Parent Institution	The school of nursing's mission, purpose, etc., match the college mission, purpose, philosophy, and goals It has good relationships with the professional schools	A few of the other schools may present roadblocks to the development of an expanded program if it impacts their programs		Mission is congruent Relationships with professional schools are good	*Positive* Nursing's mission congruent with the college mission. Nursing has the support of the professional schools. *Neutral* A campus-wide education effort about the nursing shortage and need for advanced practice nurses is indicated
Internal Economic Situation and its Influence on the Curriculum	The college and nursing are financially secure. The college administrators favor the proposed program and will develop a business case for it. There is $5,000 released time for faculty to write grants.	There is no support for the needs assessment and program or curriculum development		The college and nursing are financially secure The costs for released time to develop the curriculum will be included in next year's proposed budget	*Positive* The college and nursing are financially secure. The comptroller will develop a business case for the proposal. There is money for faculty to write grants. *Negative* Plans for released time for curriculum development must be included in next year's budget
Resources Within the Institution and Nursing Program	The current on-campus program has adequate resources and services. The costs for some facilities may be offset by donated space.	An outreach on-ground program will require rental fees for classroom, labs, offices, a coordinator, support staff, and faculty		Some support staff and instructional support services can be covered by existing services	*Positive* The college and school have adequate resources for the on-campus program, some of which can be shared with the outreach program. The RN to BSN online program is successful.

(*continued*)

TABLE 7.2	ANALYSIS OF THE INTERNAL FRAME FACTORS (*continued*)				
FRAME FACTOR	FINDINGS	NEGATIVE	NEUTRAL	POSITIVE	CONCLUSIONS
		A new simulation lab and furnishings is indicated		Current resources on campus are adequate for on-campus programs	*Negative* The business case must include increased costs for coordinators, faculty and support staff, and physical facilities
		Additional staff for the library, instructional technology, and labs may be indicated			
		Student services may need to increase staff for marketing and recruitment			
	The current faculty is well qualified	A coordinator for new programs and support staff for start-up is necessary		Faculty is qualified	*Positive* Faculty is well qualified
	Inquiries from college graduates are increasing			The applicant pool to the baccalaureate had a slight increase in the past year	An increased interest in entry-level master's program
	Entry-level master's graduates and employers are satisfied	Part-time faculty at the very least will be necessary for learning lab and clinical supervision purposes		There have been increased inquiries from college graduates and from advanced practice nurses for a DNP	Entry-level MSN have high NCLEX pass rates with employer satisfaction
	NCLEX pass rates are excellent	Recently, the quality of the undergraduate applicant pool decreased		Entry-level MSN programs are successful	Increased interest and need for DNP prepared advanced practice nurses
		Additional marketing and recruitment services are indicated for recruiting students			*Negative* Need to select new coordinators for new programs
Overall Decision					15 positive conclusions 11 negative conclusions 0 neutral conclusions

CONCLUSION

The needs assessment of the internal frame factors clarified some of the issues raised by the assessment of the external frame factors. Overall, the college and school of nursing has the experience and knowledge to expand its programs. Other schools in the college, particularly the professional schools and extended education are supportive of nursing. The nursing faculty is well prepared and the library, technology, and instructional support systems of the college can facilitate the development of new programs within certain financial limitations. The library and instructional and technology support services will work with nursing to ensure adequate resources and staffing for faculty and student support. Released time for faculty ($5,000) to write grants for external funding for program development is available. However released time for program planning and curriculum development is of highest priority. The dean, provost, and comptroller plan to develop a business case and request support for these activities into next year's budget. Student services works closely with the school and with a small increase in staffing can provide marketing and recruitment support.

Applications and enrollment patterns have been stable for the school of nursing, although the RN to BSN and master's programs have been more stable than the undergraduate program. Specific items for the business case have been iterated. The recommendations from the needs assessment of the external factors and the conclusions reached from the assessment of the internal factors led to the decision to decrease the basic baccalaureate enrollments by 10 new admissions each year and expand the RN to BSN program into an accelerated master's program with the majority of the courses online, as there is no other program in the region that accelerates RNs to the MSN. Interest from college graduates supports the initiation of an entry-level master's program that provides college graduates with the equivalent of a baccalaureate in nursing to move into the master's program. In addition, a DNP program will be initiated to accommodate master's prepared advanced practice nurses and to provide a pathway for graduates of the BSN and entry-level master's, the RN to MSN, and MSN graduates to continue into the doctoral program. Since the state-supported school prepares nurse practitioners, it was decided that the FNP program limit its enrollment to 20 per year in light of the other program in the region. The acute care nurse practitioner (adult/geriatric) and the clinical nurse leader tracks will remain steady at 20 per year. The plans call for a decrease of 30 students in the MSN specialty track to accommodate 30 new entry-level students and 10 RN students. However as the curricula are revised and new ones developed, it is anticipated that enrollments will grow each year except for the basic undergraduate program, which will decrease slightly. Eventually, graduates of the BSN program can move into the DNP program, while the MSN programs are phased out. The program thus follows the national trend to offer advanced practice education at the doctoral level.

It was determined by the faculty and administrators that there is an adequate applicant pool for the programs, there are no other programs like them in the region, and the school meets the demand for preparing additional nurses prepared at the baccalaureate and higher degree levels for the workforce. The first order of business is to identify program coordinators for the DNP and entry-level MSN to lead curriculum development, marketing of the programs, and recruitment of students. (The existing RN to BSN coordinator can continue with the RN to MSN program.) A new coordinator will be appointed for the entry-level MSN and the FNP coordinator will assume coordination of the DNP program. The following are the recommendations for initiation of the program and plans for their follow-up.

1. Develop an entry-level MSN curriculum to meet the needs of college graduates (baccalaureates or higher *not* in nursing)
   a. Appoint a coordinator for the program and support staff
   b. Work with the associate deans and coordinators of the MSN programs to develop the curriculum for the entry-level MSN that is congruent with upper-division-level BSN courses and provides a segue into the existing MSN tracks
   c. Investigate and prepare reports on the development of the program for eventual accreditation and program evaluation requirements
   d. Initiate information meetings about the program for the college community and the public
2. Expand the RN to BSN program into an accelerated RN to MSN program
   a. Work with the associate deans, coordinator of the RN to BSN program, and the coordinators of the MSN tracks to expand the curriculum
   b. Appoint faculty to revise the existing RN to BSN curriculum to accelerate students into the MSN program
   c. Investigate and prepare reports on the development of the program for eventual accreditation and program evaluation requirements
   d. Work with faculty to revise the format of courses to an online delivery
3. Work with the undergraduate and graduate associate deans and the coordinators of the MSN tracks to develop a postmaster's DNP program
   a. Appoint a task force to develop the curriculum for the DNP
   b. Investigate and prepare reports on the development of the program for eventual accreditation and program evaluation requirements
   c. Initiate information meetings about the program for the college community and the public
4. Establish an infrastructure for program development, planning, and implementation, for the expanded RN program and the initiation of the entry-level MSN and DNP programs
   a. Develop a business case for the proposed plans in collaboration with the comptroller for presentation to the college community
   b. Work with the comptroller to develop a business plan for a start-up year and implementation of the program for the following 3 years leading to self-sufficiency
   c. Identify all costs for management and planning for the program, support staff, faculty, facilities, resources, and services
   d. Balance the costs with income from start-up grants, tuition, and fees

5. Initiate start-up activities for the program including the following plans
   a. Meet with key stakeholders about the program, for example, the provost, body politic, other nursing program directors and faculty, focus groups of potential students, health care facilities administrators and educators, potential funding agencies, and feeder educational institutions
   b. Hold information and planning meetings with the dean and other deans of schools within the college, the provost and the president, the director of the library, information system, and instructional support services, the dean of enrollment services, nursing faculty, the nursing graduate committee, current enrolled entry-level master's students and graduates of that program, and members of the senate
6. Begin a written record for the program to incorporate into grant proposals, accreditation reports, and proposals for approval by the school of nursing and the academic senate
   a. Complete the Program Evaluation Review Technique chart
   b. Develop an evaluation plan for each program that is congruent with the nursing master plan of evaluation
   c. Develop reports to meet regional and national accreditation criteria and standards and State Board of Nursing regulations

REFERENCES

Brock, T. (2010). Young adults and higher education: Barriers and breakthroughs to success. *Future of Children, 20*(1), 109–132.

Health Resources and Services Administration. (2013). *Health professions. Nursing grant programs.* Retrieved from http://bhpr.hrsa.gov/nursing

Johnson, M. (1977). *Intentionality in education.* (Distributed by the Center for Curriculum Research and Services, Albany). Troy, NY: Walter Snyder, Printer, Inc.

National Institutes of Health. National Institute of Nursing Research. (2014). *Building the scientific foundation for clinical practice.* Retrieved from http://www.ninr.nih.gov

Rosa, J. M. (2009). Factors that influence the advisement of nursing students regarding baccalaureate completion: Associate degree nursing faculty *perspectives. Teaching and Learning in Nursing, 4*(4), 128–132.

University of California-Los Angeles. Office of Contract and Grant Administration. (2014). *Private foundations and organizations.* Retrieved from http://www.research.ucla.edu/sr2/Private.htm

CHAPTER 8

Financial Support and Budget Planning for Curriculum Development or Revision

Sarah B. Keating

OBJECTIVES

Upon completion of Chapter 8, the reader will be able to:

1. Analyze the influence that financial costs and budgetary management have on curriculum development or revision
2. Itemize the costs associated with curriculum development or revision
3. Identify resources for financial support for curriculum development and revision activities
4. Analyze the roles of faculty, administrators, and staff in budgetary planning, management, and the procurement of funds for curriculum development and revision

OVERVIEW

Activities associated with curriculum development for new programs or revision of existing ones require financial support for the time spent by personnel on the project and its associated costs. The costs may be minor or major depending upon the extent of the changes or new program development. For example, if it is a revision, it may not call for additional faculty, but perhaps renovation of the physical facilities and other instructional support needs are indicated. These costs apply to new programs but also could indicate the need for additional faculty and staff. New programs usually require start-up costs associated with their initiation such as the time spent on developing the program prior to student admission, approval from accreditation agencies and regulating bodies, and increased recruitment activities for students and new faculty. Chapter 8 discusses the types of costs that occur; their impact on the proposed program or revision, budget planning, and management; and possible resources for funding. The roles of administrators, faculty, and staff are described.

FINANCIAL COSTS AND BUDGETARY PLANNING

Financial Costs

The process for evaluating an existing program for possible revision and conducting a needs assessment for possible changes or creating a new program involves administrative, faculty, and staff. Depending upon the extent of the change or development, the time spent may be part of the usual role of these personnel. For example, faculty curriculum committee members review recommendations for change in the curriculum as part of committee activities, which in turn are part of the service role expectations for faculty. Another example is when planning and managing the budget, the administrator may find that one of the tracks in the overall program is losing money owing to low student enrollments, while another track is turning away applicants. Analyzing the problem and bringing it to the attention of the faculty is the next step to address the problem and is considered a usual administrative responsibility.

Although activities associated with program changes normally take place in faculty curriculum committees and the time spent on these activities is considered a part of the faculty service role, faculty time over and above the usual service activities may be necessary. The costs associated with the additional time occur in the form of released time or a stipend for individual faculty members, or a consultant may be hired to coordinate the project. Staff support for the activities such as taking and recording minutes for meetings held, coordination of participants' schedules for meeting times, collecting data for assessment, and so on must be included in the costs.

When calculating the costs associated with curriculum development, both direct and indirect costs must be considered. Direct costs are those that can be attributed to new costs and includes additional personnel; physical facilities such as offices, labs, classrooms, and furnishings; staff and instructional support equipment; computers and their hardware and software; office supplies, and so on. Indirect costs are those associated with the use of existing staff, physical facilities such as offices and meeting rooms, utilities, furnishings, and supplies that the institution provides from its resources. These indirect costs are usually estimated on a percentage basis of the total and can range from approximately 3% to 40% of the total costs. Personnel costs represent the largest expenditure for supporting curriculum change or development. However, there are a few other associated direct costs such as fees associated with data collection when conducting a needs assessment, office supplies, new computer hardware and software, and travel for data collection or consultation purposes.

Costs of Nursing Programs in Academe

Although the literature on the costs of program development is sparse, two articles were identified that related to the cost of nursing programs in comparison to other disciplines and how to estimate the costs and benefits for a new program. The reader may find them useful when involved in curriculum development and planning. A summary of the articles follows.

Nursing programs must often defend themselves from other disciplines that assume that nursing education is an expensive proposition. Certainly, the nursing faculty to student ratio required for clinical supervision in health care agencies is costly. However, large theory classes where lecture prevails as the modality for entry-level programs and the use of simulation help to counterbalance the expense. Also, clinical instructors are often part time or serve as adjunct faculty who cost less than tenured or tenure-track faculty who are full time. Booker and Hilgenberg (2010) conducted a study in a small private university and developed a model for comparing the costs of nursing in comparison to other academic programs The model examined the quality (Q), potential (P), and cost (C) (QPC) of programs to compare disciplines from a cost-benefit perspective. In using the model, the authors demonstrated that while nursing fell into the costly category, it also rated as a high-quality discipline with a moderate potential index, especially for the RN to bachelor of science in nursing (BSN) program. Based on the results from the use of the model, and the decrease in applications to the basic program, the decision was made to increase enrollments for the RN to BSN program and modestly cut back on enrollments in the baccalaureate program. The QPC model described in the article provides details for measuring the quality, potential, and cost of an educational program that can be useful to other programs in the process of curriculum development or revision. It provides details for analyzing the costs and the potential benefits from a program and contributes to the decision-making process within a sound financial environment.

Fagerlund and Germano (2009) describe a cost and benefit analysis model for development of a nurse-midwifery educational program that is useful in identifying not only the costs for starting a program but also the potential benefits to the public, home institution, the health care system, clinical sites, and students. Costs that apply to an academic institution fall into three categories: (1) direct costs, such as faculty and staff salary and benefits; (2) indirect costs, such as library and student services; and (3) capital costs, such as building additions, improvement, or replacement. Universities tend to have complex financial and accounting structures and, while it is possible to list each indirect cost, for the purposes of the cost-benefit model described by the authors, indirect costs were allocated on a percentage basis. For this study, a 40% indirect cost rate was applied. The 40% indirect cost rate was used because, according to the authors, it is a typical rate used by academic institutions for estimating indirect costs for federal grants. The prototype used in this model provides a persuasive argument for the establishment of a program and is a useful model for other institutions planning new programs.

Budgetary Planning and Management

The chief nursing officer (CNO; dean, director, or chair) of the educational program is responsible for managing the budget. Administrative support staff assists in the management of the budget allocation, although in some smaller nursing programs, these responsibilities may be included in the expectations for the CNO. Planning for the future, both annually and long term, is part of the CNO role. Schools of nursing and their parent institutions have strategic goals and plans for the future, usually within a 5-year framework. In addition, most schools have a master plan of evaluation. These plans, with their goals and objectives, provide guidelines for projected curriculum revisions, new program proposals, and program and accreditation activities. Thus, a section in the budget for curriculum development and evaluation should be part of the planning process. When planning annual budgets in association with the development of short- and long-term goals, administrators should involve faculty and staff to assist in the identification of current and potential needs for curriculum revision and the development of new programs and their related costs.

Specific items in budgets that relate to curriculum planning include faculty released time to identify possible revisions or new programs; released time for conducting a needs assessment; consultant fees if indicated for major revisions or new program development; and additional staff support, office supplies, and communications and technology support. According to the program's long-range goals or strategic plan, these costs may be for 1 year or several depending upon the extent of the changes. As the planning process develops, indications for change or new programs require further planning for the future based on the costs for developing new programs and, perhaps, discontinuing programs that no longer meet the goals of the program. Table 8.1 lists the elements to consider in planning annual budgets as they apply to curriculum revision or development of new programs.

Costello (2011) discusses a planning process for annual budgeting that ties program costs, including maintenance of the program and anticipated needs, to the overall program goals. He offers a budget balanced scorecard model that lists items and their costs and assigns values to them and their contribution to the program goals. He recommends limiting the number of items so that they are achieved within the year rather than having numerous unachieved goals. Costello describes the process of planning as "gathering correct information, having clear goals, understanding the risk, and outlining an approach that's more like a path than a tightrope" (p. 64).

A description for building a business plan for a small grant and its management serves as a model for planning budgets (Sakraida, D'Amico, & Thibault, 2010). The authors expand on Sahlman's (1997) formula for critical factors to consider when budget planning (people, opportunity, context, risks, and rewards). Included in their expanded considerations are the personnel involved and their tasks, communication systems, and the establishment of networks of key people for support. They recommend that people who manage the grant have training in preparing budgets, working with administrators who oversee the project, knowledge of institutional policies, conducting monthly reviews of expenses according to allowable costs, and ensuring that expenditures tie to the goals of the project.

Several articles from the literature discuss the financial aspects for new program planning. Stuart, Erkel, and Shull (2010) report on the planning process in a school of nursing that considered the development of a new doctoral program that would not add to the costs of the existing nursing program. The authors present a model for analysis of the costs for existing tracks in a program that lead to decisions for cutting programs that are no longer financially viable. Items for analysis

TABLE 8.1	BUDGET ELEMENTS FOR CURRICULUM ASSESSMENT AND PLANNING			
ITEM	ASSOCIATED COSTS	POTENTIAL BENEFITS	RISKS	TOTAL COST
Faculty Released Time	% of released time necessary (salary)	Faculty development in curriculum planning and assessment; faculty ownership of the curriculum	Time away from teaching activities; development of barriers and resistance to curriculum change	$
Consultant	Fees, travel, lodging	Expert assistance for identifying needs, redundancies, and nonproductive programs	Insufficient or inadequate product compared to expense	$
Staff	% of released time necessary (salary) or new temporary position	Experienced program management perspectives or 100% of time devoted to the activity	Time away from usual activities; temporary positions are difficult to fill	$ (salary and benefits)
Office Supplies	Flash drives, paper, desk supplies, etc.	Support for the process	None	$
Needs Assessment	Access to data-bases, travel to agencies, mailing costs, telephone charges, etc.	Documents needs; develops potential partnerships with outside agencies	Time consuming; can be slanted; missing data	$
Reports	Time of personnel office supplies	Record for documentation and planning purposes	Time consuming	$
Total				$

of costs and revenues for each track included faculty resources, faculty to student ratios, student enrollments, faculty salaries and benefits, and revenues from tuition and fees. While not addressing the costs of the time spent on the analysis and for planning a new program, the model provides ideas for managing nursing education budgets and planning for change.

Gantt (2010) describes how to use the strategic planning model SWOT (strengths, weaknesses, opportunities, threats), for building a business case to add a simulation lab for a nursing program. Gantt points out that the plan provides for annual review to measure the success or failure of the program as to its match to the program's overall strategic plans and thus justifies its existence.

Poirrier and Oberleitner (2011) describe in detail an entry-level accelerated BSN program designed for nonnurse college graduates. The school of nursing collaborated with four large medical centers to secure funding for a 5-year project to prepare the college graduates for nursing. Five other smaller hospitals participated in the project by providing additional clinical sites for student practice. More than $1 million were donated to the school from the health care agencies and the university contributed funds from students' tuition and fees as additional funds to manage the program. The article describes in detail budget items that were included to fund the program and is useful for budget planning purposes. As mentioned previously, financial environments can influence the development and maintenance of educational programs and in this instance, the program was phased out after the 5-year period owing to changes in the financial and employment climates.

If a program decides to offer a new program based on the findings from a needs assessment, planning for a budget to start the program and maintain it is a crucial step. Costs to develop the curriculum, recruit students, and add faculty, staff, and physical facilities and supplies must be part of the cost side of the budget, along with the revenue side of the budget for its source of financial support. See Table 8.2 for a listing of the items to include in a budget when planning for a new program.

SOURCES FOR FINANCIAL SUPPORT

There are three major sources of funding for curriculum development and planning other than the home institution's support in its regular budget. Depending on the nature of the home institution, the majority of funds for the budget come from the general funds (if state-supported), tuition and fees, endowments, grants, and donations. When considering funds for curriculum development, the three major resources for funds are grants (private and public), philanthropy (donations and endowments), and partnerships with the community. Each of these sources is discussed with ideas from the literature for procurement of funds.

Grants

The major resource for program development and student and faculty support at the federal level comes from the Health Resources and Services Administration (HRSA), Division of Nursing (2014). Included in the program of grants are traineeships for advanced practice students, faculty loans, support for nurse managed health care services, and program development. The program development funds, for the most part, focus on starting up new programs and a large part of the funds support curriculum development. It is not permanent funding and is intended as an incentive to increase the advanced practice nursing workforce and to support other types of advanced nursing education programs, for example, education and public health. For detailed information on this major resource, go to the HRSA website (http://bhpr.hrsa.gov/nursing/index.html).

In addition to federal grants, there are major private foundations and organizations interested in supporting nursing education programs. They include the Bill

TABLE 8.2 ELEMENTS FOR BUDGET PLANNING FOR NEW PROGRAMS

ITEM	YEAR 1	YEAR 2	YEAR 3	YEAR 4	YEAR 5
COSTS					
Salaries and benefits of existing faculty, administrators, and staff for curriculum development					
Salary and benefits for coordinator of program					
Salary and benefits for program faculty					
Consultant fees and costs					
Salary and benefits for support staff					
Recruitment of personnel					
Recruitment of students					
Capital improvements/ additions					
Supplies, services, technology, and information services and staff					
Library additions and staff					
INCOME					
Student enrollments/tuition (include admissions, anticipated attrition rate, and graduations) (part time full time if applicable)					

(continued)

TABLE 8.2   ELEMENTS FOR BUDGET PLANNING FOR NEW PROGRAMS *(continued)*

ITEM	YEAR 1	YEAR 2	YEAR 3	YEAR 4	YEAR 5
INCOME					
Student fees					
Grants, endowments, donations, other					
Totals					

Note: Five-year budget planning recommended with annual review for adjustments.

and Melinda Gates Foundation (2014), Robert Wood Johnson Foundation (2014), the W. K. Kellogg Foundation (2014), the Josiah Macy Jr. Foundation (2014), the Gordon and Betty Moore Foundation (2014), and many others. A listing of other private resources can be found at the UCLA Office of Contract and Grant Administration (2014; www.research.ucla.edu/ocga/sr2/Private.htm).

Many universities and colleges offer courses in grant writing and there are a few that are online. One online site from the General Services Administration (2014) offers ideas for *Developing and Writing Grant Proposals* (www.nmfs.noaa.gov/trade/howtodogrants.htm).

Partnerships

There is a long history of partnerships between nursing education programs and health care agencies. The purpose for these partnerships is not only to provide clinical experiences for students, but also to support schools of nursing in preparing professionals for the workforce. These partnerships take many forms, including work–study or internship experiences for students who may earn a modest salary and at the same time earn academic credits, contribution of nursing clinicians to the school as instructors, use of facilities for laboratory and simulation experiences, continuing education and research opportunities for both faculty and staff, and scholarship or loan programs for students in exchange for contracts to work for the agency upon graduation. The numbers and amount of financial support available from agencies seem to ebb and flow according to nursing workforce demands and the financial climate at the time.

A model for partnerships between health care systems and educational institutions is the Veterans Affairs (VA) Nursing Academy project, which supplied $60 million to establish partnerships with the VA and baccalaureate schools of nursing. It funds faculty positions using expert clinicians from the VA system (or the community if there is a lack), provides clinical practice experiences for students, and recruits new graduates into the VA system. There are four established regions including the western, midwest, south, and northeast regions of the United States. Benefits for the schools and the VA include current updates on clinical practice and an increase in the faculty workforce as well as the nursing workforce. This model serves as an example for other health care systems wishing to increase the nursing workforce and, at the same time, participate in updating nursing curricula and addressing the nursing faculty shortage (Bowman et al., 2011).

Bentley and Seaback (2011) describe a collaborative program among 12 nursing programs and two clinical agency partners to provide faculty development workshops on clinical simulation strategies. Its purpose was to increase student enrollments and enhance their clinical experiences and skills. It was funded by a grant from the Texas Team and the Texas Workforce Commission. Thirty percent of the nursing programs were able to increase enrollments owing to faculty's increased use of simulation in place of clinical experiences.

Budgeting schemata for forging partnerships between health care agencies and nursing education programs are discussed by De Geest et al. (2010). The University of Pennsylvania and the University of Bezel in Switzerland developed academic and service partnership models that provide guidelines for developing partnerships between health care agencies and nursing education programs. The models are useful tools on how to balance agreements between the two institutions and include specific budgetary items for planning and management of the financial support system. Of special interest is the appointment of a full-time coordinator to manage the agreement when the arrangements become complex and involve many personnel, students, and resources from both institutions.

Philanthropy

Philanthropic funds come from donations to the nursing programs. A large majority of these donations are earmarked for scholarships for students. However, there are times when programs receive donations for program development. For example, Andrews et al. (2011) describe a partnership established between several schools of nursing and the Transcultural Nursing Society to prepare nursing faculty and students in cultural competence. The project was funded by a federal grant; however, the society had a major role in helping to develop the program and serves as an example of how professional organizations can contribute to nursing curricula development.

Peeples (2010) presents recommendations for universities and colleges, especially Historically Black Colleges and Universities, which apply to nursing educators for securing funding for curriculum development. She recommends three major strategies to obtain donations from philanthropic individuals and organizations. These are (1) identify funders who connect to your institutional mission and vision (p. 258), (2) infuse creativity and collaboration into your strategy (p. 256), and (3) engage alumni in giving (p. 259).

Alumni organizations are a good resource for nursing programs and schools should encourage the support of alumni organizations through special functions such as reunions at the time of graduation, research events, and guest lecturers. Fostering alumni participation can begin early in the professional socialization process through the nursing student association with faculty mentoring and support. An editorial describing the importance of alumni building contains useful material for schools of nursing to gain support from alumni associations (Cleary, Jackson, Vehviläinen-Julkunen, Lim, & Chan, 2012).

ROLE OF ADMINISTRATORS, STAFF, AND FACULTY IN FINANCIAL SUPPORT FOR CURRICULUM DEVELOPMENT ACTIVITIES

Administrators and Staff

When a curriculum revision is indicated or a new program is in the offing, additional administrator and faculty time is expected and usually it is over and above the normal job expectations. Therefore, released time and related costs are expected and must be planned for in the budget. Administrators, with faculty input, should include a line item for program planning in the budget to cover these anticipated costs. While indirect funds from a grant can provide for the released time spent on program planning, they usually are not available until after the fact, that is, the grant is approved and funded after initial activities took place. Depending on the institution's policies regarding indirect funds, administrators may have the discretion to use funds for program development generated from other grants. Otherwise, funds for program planning should be part of the regular budgeting process.

If administrative staff has responsibility for the management of the school budget, records of expenditures for curriculum revision or new program development should be kept. They are especially useful to illustrate the purpose for the funding and its tie to the grant/project goals. If the administrator manages the budget, the same processes apply and provide documentation for accounting purposes. Each year, during the budget review and projections for the future, administrators, staff, and faculty should identify continuing funding needs for program development. Needs vary according to the amount of curricular revision or new program development indicated. A discussion on the costs of program review, evaluation, and accreditation can be found in Section V, "Program Evaluation and Accreditation."

Faculty

Curriculum development and evaluation is an ongoing process built into the educational program activities. Nurse educators in the process of delivering the curriculum through instructional activities such as classroom lectures, seminars, conferences, laboratory practice, simulation activities, and clinical supervision gather information on how well the curriculum is delivered. This ongoing assessment of teaching effectiveness and student learning outcomes is part of the role of teaching. It is a job expectation and, therefore, as part of the usual responsibilities, is supported through faculty salaries. Yet another aspect of faculty work is the participation in work groups such as course and level and curriculum committee meetings. These activities are considered part of the service role for faculty and from a budgetary point of view are a part of the salary paid to faculty and the expected responsibilities of the role. If major curriculum revisions or a new program are indicated, conducting a needs assessment and developing the curriculum can require faculty time over and above the usual expectations. In that case, the administrator and faculty in the program need to identify sources of funds to support the released time for these activities and to plan for them in the budget.

SUMMARY

Chapter 8 discusses the importance of financial support for curriculum revision and program development. It reviews the costs, benefits, and budget planning and management activities associated with curriculum development and revision. Resources for funding these activities are offered and the roles of administrators, staff, and faculty in seeking funding, planning, and managing the budget are described.

DISCUSSION QUESTIONS

1. What influence do you believe finances have on developing and maintaining a vibrant curriculum?
2. What individual or group do you believe has the responsibility for procuring funds for program development and curricular revision? Provide a rationale.

LEARNING ACTIVITIES

STUDENT LEARNING ACTIVITIES

1. Interview a member or chair of the curriculum committee for her or his perspectives on financial support for program development and curriculum revision. Interview questions you might consider asking are:
   a. How much time do you spend on curriculum activities?
   b. Are you compensated in any way for this time or is it an expectation of your role? Do you believe faculty should have released time for curriculum development activities? Why or why not? How would you pay for overtime?
   c. When was the last curriculum revision? Do you expect a revision in the near future? Are there plans for review and revision of the curriculum in the school strategic plan?
   d. Do you participate in planning for future curriculum committee activities and development and are budgetary issues involved in the planning?
   e. Are you aware of any resources to support curriculum change or new program development? If yes, what are these sources?

NURSE EDUCATOR/FACULTY DEVELOPMENT ACTIVITIES

1. Survey your community/region for existing partnerships between nursing education programs and clinical agencies. Other than providing clinical experiences for students, are there any other financial support programs related to curriculum revision or new program development in the partnership?
2. Identify needs for and possible partnerships to support nursing education in your region. Indicate your strategies for developing the partnership and its maintenance over time

REFERENCES

Andrews, M. M., Cervanitez Thompson, T. L., Wehbe-Alamah, H., McFarland, M. R., Hanson, P. A., Hasenau, S. M., . . . Vint, P. A. (2011). Developing a culturally competent workforce through collaborative partnerships. *Journal of Transcultural Nursing, 22,* 300.

Bentley, R., & Seaback, C. (2011). A faculty development collaborative in interprofessional simulation. *Journal of Professional Nursing, 27,* e1–e7.

Booker, K., & Hilgenberger, C. (2010). Analysis of academic programs: Comparing nursing and other university majors in the application of a quality, potential, and cost model. *Professional Nursing, 26,* 201–206.

Bowman, C. C., Johnson, L., Cox, M., Rick, C., Dougherty, M., Alt-White, A. C., . . . Dobalian, A. (2011). The department of veterans affairs nursing academy: Forging strategic alliances with schools of nursing to address nursing's workforce needs. *Nursing Outlook, 59,* 299–307.

Cleary, M., Jackson, D., Vehviläinen-Julkunen, K., Lim, J., & Chan, S. (2012). Editorial: Nursing alumni building a strong voice for the future. *Journal of Clinical Nursing, 21*(9/10), 1197–1198.

Costello, T. (2011). Better budget planning. *TI Professional, 13*(5), 64, 62–63.

De Geest, S., Sullivan Marx, E. M., Rich, V., Spichiger, E. Schwendimann, R., Spirig, R., & Van Malderen, G. (2010). Developing a financial framework for academic service partnerships: Models of the United States and Europe. *Journal of Professional Scholarship, 42*(3), 295–304.

Fagerlund, K., & Germano, E. (2009). The costs and benefits of nurse-midwifery education: Model and application. *Journal of Midwifery and Women's Health, 54*(5), 341–350.

Gantt, L. T. (2010). Strategic planning for skills and simulation labs in colleges of nursing. *Nursing Economics, 28*(5), 308.

General Services Administration. (2014). *Developing and writing grant proposals.* Retrieved from http://www.nmfs.noaa.gov/trade/howtodogrants.htm

Peeples, Y. T. (2010). Philanthropy and the curriculum: The role of philanthropy in the development of curriculum at Spelman College. *International Journal of educational Advancement, 10*(3), 245–260.

Poirrier, G. P., & Oberleitner, M. G. (2011). Funding an accelerated baccalaureate nursing track for non-nursing college graduates. *Nursing Economics, 29*(3), 118–126.

Sahlman, W. (1997). How to write a great business plan. *Harvard Business Review, 75*(4), 98–108.

Sakraida, T. J., D'Amico, J. D., & Thibault, E. (2010). Small grant management in health and behavioral sciences: Lesson learned. *Applied Nursing Research, 23,* 171–177.

Stuart, G. W., Erkel, E. A., & Shull, L. H. (2010). Allocating resources in a data-driven college of nursing. *Nursing Outlook, 50*(4), 200–206.

RESOURCES

Bill and Melinda Gates Foundation. (2014). Retrieved from http://www.gatesfoundation.org

Gordon and Betty Moore Foundation. (2014). Retrieved from http://www.moore.org

Health Resources and Services Administration. Division of Nursing. (2014). *Nursing grant programs.* Retrieved from http://bhpr.hrsa.gov/nursing/index.html

Josiah Macy Jr. Foundation. (2014). Retrieved from http://www.macyfoundation.org

Robert Wood Johnson Foundation. (2014). Retrieved from http://www.rwjf.org

UCLA, Office of Contract and Grant Administration. (2014). Retrieved from http://www.research.ucla.edu/ocga/sr2/Private.htm

W. K. Kellogg Foundation. (2014). Retrieved from http://www.wkkf.org

Curriculum Development Applied to Nursing Education and the Practice Setting

Sarah B. Keating

OVERVIEW

Prior to discussing curriculum development, it is useful to review the definition of curriculum. According to this text, a curriculum is the formal plan of study that provides the philosophical underpinnings, goals, and guidelines for the delivery of a specific educational program. Chapter 9 introduces the components of the curriculum and the process for its development followed by specific chapters on associate, baccalaureate, master's, advanced practice doctorates, and research-focused doctoral degrees. The last chapter in this section discusses application of the components of the curriculum to the development of education programs in the practice setting.

Experienced educators will testify to the fact that as a curriculum ages, changes occur that were unintended in the original curriculum plan. These changes occur in response to feedback from students, faculty, and consumers; faculty's individual interpretations of the course content; changes in faculty personnel who are not familiar with the curriculum; changes in the practice setting; and the expansion of nursing knowledge. Unless there is continuous evaluation of the curriculum, the plan will eventually become so corrupted that it is barely recognizable.

Section V describes in detail the value of evaluation activities as they apply to approval, review, and accreditation of nursing programs. However, it is wise in this section on curriculum development to recognize the need for continually monitoring the program, at least annually, to ensure that it is meeting the original mission, framework, goals, and objectives of the curriculum. The data collected from evaluation reviews and the recommendations issuing from them indicate to faculty the need for revising the curriculum, discontinuing certain programs within it, or initiating new tracks. If this exercise is conducted every year, maintaining the integrity of the curriculum becomes easy and there are fewer hoops to go through in seeking approval for major or minor changes. Annual review and minor revisions contribute to a curriculum that is current and is a living, vibrant organism that prepares nursing professionals for current and future markets.

PURPOSE OF CURRICULUM DEVELOPMENT

The overall purpose of curriculum development is to meet the learners' needs by ensuring that it meets educational and professional standards and that it is responsive to the current and future demands of the health care system. To accomplish this long-term goal, the curriculum serves as the template for faculty to express its vision, mission, philosophy, framework, goals, and objectives of the nursing program. While curriculum development is the prerogative of the faculty, consumers of the program need to be involved in the process. Consumers include the students, their families, the health care system that utilizes its graduates, nurse educators, staff in the practice setting and, last but not least, the patients that receive nursing care from students and graduates.

COMPONENTS OF CURRICULUM DEVELOPMENT

The classic components of a school of nursing curriculum include (1) the mission and vision (for the future) of the program; (2) the philosophy of the faculty that usually contains beliefs about teaching and learning processes; critical thinking, scholarship, research, and evidence-based practice; and other selected concepts, theories, essentials, and standards that define the specific nursing education program; (3) the purpose or overall goal of the program; (4) a framework by which to organize the curriculum plan; (5) the end-of-program objectives or student learning outcomes (SLOs); and (6) an overall implementation plan (program of study). The components should be congruent with the parent institution's mission and philosophy. Chapter 9 discusses the components in detail and the pros and cons of frameworks to organize the curriculum plan including the use of nursing and other disciplines' theories and concepts and professionally defined standards or essentials of education.

LEVELS OF NURSING EDUCATION

Chapters 10 through 14 apply the components of the curriculum to the various levels of nursing education including the associate degree, the baccalaureate, master's, doctor of nursing practice (DNP), and research-based doctorates, for example, the PhD and doctor of nursing science (DNS). Each chapter provides a summary of the role that each level of education plays in the mission, philosophy, organizational framework, goals, and end-of-program objectives for its parent institution. Issues that apply to each such as entry into practice, opportunities for further education, advanced practice, contributions to nursing education and the profession, evidence-based practice, and research are discussed.

CURRICULUM DEVELOPMENT APPLIED TO THE PRACTICE SETTING

Chapter 15 assists staff developers in adapting the information in the text to their arena of nursing practice. Although the major focus of the text is on curriculum development and evaluation in schools of nursing, many of the same components and activities for curriculum planning apply to staff development even though the target audience differs. The processes for conducting a needs assessment, and setting the mission/vision, philosophy, purpose, and goals for an education program in the practice setting must be in line with the health agency's mission, vision, and purpose. This applies to all types of staff development programs including orientation, specialty and cross training, maintenance of skills competency, and continuing education. The current role of educators in nursing practice settings, their qualifications, and desired educational levels are discussed. Issues and trends that apply to staff development are reviewed.

The Components of the Curriculum

Sarah B. Keating

OBJECTIVES

Upon completion of Chapter 9, the reader will be able to:

1. Compare curriculum development activities among various types of educational institutions and levels of nursing education
2. Distinguish the formal curriculum from the informal curriculum
3. Analyze the components of curriculum development according to their role in producing a curriculum plan
4. Analyze a case study that illustrates the revision of an existing program and development of a new program
5. Assess an existing curriculum or educational program by using the "Guidelines for Assessing the Key Components of a Curriculum or Educational Program" (Table 9.1)

OVERVIEW

Chapter 9 provides an overview of types of educational institutions in higher education and how the various levels of nursing education fit into them. It continues with a discussion about the classic components of the curriculum, which include:

- Mission/vision
- Philosophy
  - Beliefs about teaching and learning processes
  - Critical thinking and its application to nursing
  - Liberal education and the sciences
  - Health care system, organization, policy, finance, and regulation
  - Clinical prevention and population health/cultural competence
  - Interprofessional communication and collaboration
  - Professionalism, professional values, and nursing practice
  - Social justice and advocacy
  - Scholarship, research, translational science, and evidence-based practice
  - Information systems and patient care technology
  - Quality health care and patient safety

- Organizational framework and concept mapping
- Overall program goal and purpose
- Implementation plan
  - SLOs (student learning outcomes; end-of-program objectives)
  - Level objectives
  - Course objectives
- Course prerequisites
- Course descriptions
- Content outlines
- Course schedule
- Learning activities
- Evaluation methods
  - Program of study

This chapter provides a sample nursing curriculum developed from the fictional case study in Chapters 6 and 7, the needs assessment. Table 9.1 provides guidelines for assessing the key components of a curriculum or educational program. Chapters 10 through 15 discuss in detail levels of nursing education from the associate degree through the PhD with Chapter 14 applying the components of the curriculum to staff development and health education. Chapter 20 responds to the issues that arise from the myriad levels the nursing education for entry into practice and proposes a plan that promotes a unified approach to nursing education for the readers' consideration and debate.

TYPES OF INSTITUTIONS

Types of higher educational institutions are classified as *private* and *public*, and undergraduate or graduate. The types of nursing education programs addressed in this text range from the associate degree to the doctorate level. Many nursing curricula include step-in and step-out educational programs that provide career ladder opportunities for nurses. Most institutions of higher education identify themselves according to classifications found in the Carnegie Foundation for Advancement of Teaching Classification (2014). The Carnegie classification was first published in 1970 with the most recent classification occurring in 2010. The 2010 designations are according to what institutions teach (undergraduate and graduate programs), whom they teach (student profiles), and the size and setting of the institution. The basic classifications include:

- Undergraduate Instructional Program Classification
- Graduate Instructional Program Classification
- Enrollment Profile Classification
- Undergraduate Profile Classification
- Size and Setting Classification (Carnegie Foundation for Advancement of Teaching, 2014)

A listing with a detailed description of each type of classification is available at http://classifications.carnegiefoundation.org/descriptions/index.php.

For the purposes of this text, the discussion about types of higher education institutions includes private (nonprofit and for-profit) and public institutions (federal, state, or regionally supported) as well as community colleges, small liberal arts colleges, large multipurpose or comprehensive colleges and universities, research-focused universities, and academic health science/medical centers.

Sectarian and *nonsectarian institutions* are yet another classification with sectarian institutions reflecting a religious affiliation, for example, Catholic University, Southwest Baptist University, Brigham Young, and so on. While curriculum development activities are quite the same across types of institutions, the differences arise when examining the overall purpose of the institution and the financial and human resources that are available for revising or initiating new programs.

LEVELS OF NURSING EDUCATION

The levels of nursing education discussed in this text include associate degree programs that are usually housed in community colleges. These colleges are regional, public-supported institutions; however, there are some privately funded 2-year colleges that include nursing programs. Baccalaureate, master's, and doctorate nursing programs are found in both state-supported and privately funded institutions. There are a few "single-purpose," nursing-only schools. Many of these schools are or were former diploma, hospital-based programs with the latter converting to associate degree or baccalaureates in nursing. There are relatively few diploma program left owing to the financial constraints they face as well as the need for providings the liberal education and basic sciences that undergird nursing programs. Most hospital-based diploma programs are affiliated with higher degree programs, for example, community colleges and baccalaureate and higher degree programs. According to the American Association of Colleges of Nursing (AACN) Nursing Fact Sheet (2014d), diploma programs account for roughly 10% of all nursing programs in the United States. VickyRN (2014) reports that most of the remaining diploma schools are located in the east and midwest United States.

For all types of programs, administrators and faculty should plan in advance for financial support of curriculum development and evaluation activities and investigate possible external resources for support such as grants for curriculum changes and program development activities. A program that has been available over the years for nursing program development or expansion is the Health Resources and Service Administration's (HRSA) division of nursing programs that include Advanced Education Nursing Traineeship (AENT), Advanced Nursing Education (ANE), Advanced Nursing Education Expansion (ANEE), Innovative Nurse Education Technologies (INET), Nurse Anesthetist Traineeship (NAT), Nurse Education, Practice, Quality, and Retention (NEPQR), Nurse Faculty Loan Program (NFLP), Nurse Managed Health Clinics (NMHC), Nursing Assistant and Home Health Aide (NAHHA), Nursing Workforce Diversity (NWD), and Personal Home Care Aide State Training (PHCAST) (U.S. Department of Health and Human Services, Health Resources and Services Administration, Health Professions, 2014). See Chapter 8 for a discussion on financial support for curriculum development.

THE FORMAL AND INFORMAL CURRICULA

The *formal curriculum* is the planned program of studies for an academic degree or discipline. It includes the components of the curriculum that are discussed in this chapter and the curriculum plan is visible to the public through its publication in catalogs, recruitment materials, and on websites. The *informal curriculum* is sometimes termed the hidden curriculum, or co-curriculum, or is composed of extracurricular activities. These planned and unplanned influences on students' learning should be kept in mind as faculty assesses and develops the curriculum. Examples include special convocations with invited speakers, student organization activities that parallel course work, and outside-of-class meetings with students and faculty to enrich learning experiences. The co-curriculum incorporates planned activities such as collaboration with other academic units, student affairs meetings (information meetings, orientation, counseling sessions, etc.), field trips, work–study programs, service learning, and planned volunteer services in the community. Examples of extracurricular activities are athletics, social gatherings, and student organization events.

Some examples of the informal curriculum's influence in nursing are student services activities and counseling, special convocations, graduations, honor society meetings, study groups, student nursing association meetings, student invited attendance at faculty meetings, participation in academic committees, and so on. Many schools of nursing schedule informal student–faculty meetings, holiday parties, and special events such as pinning ceremonies, honors convocation, and so on. These activities provide opportunities for student–faculty interchanges to enrich and supplement the formal classroom setting as well as facilitate leadership opportunities for the students.

Effects of Student–Faculty Interactions on the Curriculum

Student–faculty relationships are important factors to consider and influence the unplanned curriculum. Micari and Pazos (2012) studied student and faculty interactions in organic chemistry classes and the influence that the interactions had on students' performance and perceptions about the course. They found that students' grades and confidence in the courses were positively correlated with their interactions with faculty. They offer useful suggestions for faculty on how to connect to students to foster a positive learning experience.

THE CAMPUS ENVIRONMENT

The physical environment for the delivery of the educational program is important to the image of the home institution and plays a major role in building a sense of belonging for students and alumni alike. Broussard (2009) talks about the influence of the architecture and landscape of the home campus that creates lasting relationships among students, alumni, faculty, staff, and the community. He talks about "transformational places" on campus where the college community has time to congregate and share ideas and experiences. He makes a point about commuter students and the need for campuses to build into the landscape places where they too can experience a feeling of community.

Elkins, Forrester, and Scott (2011) conducted a study of students' perceptions of the college campus sense of community according to how they were involved in campus activities other than those associated with formal learning. Using factors identified in the literature and adjusting them to their campus, they found that the sense of community differed according to the types and extent of students' extra-curricular activities. Additionally, they found that the more students were involved, the more they gained knowledge of the history and traditions of the institution and this gained sense of community contributed positively to student learning.

Fuggazato (2009) describes the close ties of the institution's mission to its physical facilities. The mission can serve to structure buildings and rooms to enact its mission, for example, a student activities center that provides opportunities for student governance and participatory citizenship. He describes how institutions can evaluate their effectiveness by examining the mission and how physical structures on campus serve to realize elements of the mission.

While the physical environment plays a small role in programs that are delivered in cyberspace, some colleges and universities require periodic on-campus academic program meetings or residencies and special events for distance education students to experience the on-site campus. Another strategy is to provide program information materials that include pictures of the campus and campus life. This helps students to identify with the physical location and landscape to form images unique to the home campus. Other strategies for delivering the informal curriculum and an academic environment online include virtual faculty office hours and student and faculty meeting rooms.

Greener (2010) conducted a qualitative study (detailed grounded analysis of interviews of faculty) to discover their perceptions about the virtual learning environment (VLE) for courses taught online. The author introduces the notion of plasticity in the online learning environment, for example, adapting to the learning styles of students and learning activities according to the subject and different student needs. This is in contrast to the in-person, structured classroom environment. The VLE offers challenges for teachers to develop learning strategies and the opportunity to become more interactive with the student in order to meet learner needs. Building in activities that connect the online learner to the physical campus contributes to the students' sense of belonging and community. On-campus orientation meetings, defense of scholarly works, and graduation activities can serve to connect the online learner to the campus.

COMPONENTS OF THE CURRICULUM

The following discussion examines each of the major components of the curriculum from the vision or mission statements to the philosophy statement that embraces faculty beliefs and values about teaching and learning; critical thinking; liberal education and the sciences; the health care system, organization, policy, finance, and regulation; clinical prevention and population health; interprofessional collaboration; professionalism, professional values, and nursing practice; social justice and advocacy; scholarship, research, translational science, and evidence-based practice; information systems and technology; and quality health care and patient safety. A description follows on how the organizational framework, overall goal or purpose, SLOs (end-of-program objectives), and level objectives constitute the implementation plan that flows from the mission and philosophy statements.

THE MISSION OR VISION STATEMENT

[handwritten margin notes: 3 elements in a mission — teaching/learning, svc, scholarship/research OR VISION STATEMENT, outlook oriented institution future plans dreams]

Traditionally, higher education institutions in the United States have three major elements included in their mission, that is, teaching/learning, service, and scholarship/research. The mission statement for each institution depends upon the nature of the institution and the three major elements are often divided into separate permutations. In more recent times, some organizations either replace or supplement the mission statement with a vision statement. For the purposes of this discussion, the *mission statement* is the institution's beliefs about its role and responsibilities for the preparation of its graduates (outcomes). It may discuss the classic teaching/learning, service, and scholarship functions as they relate to the purpose of the institution. A *vision statement* is outlook oriented and reflects the institution's plans and dreams about its direction for the future. It is usually short, visionary, and inspirational.

Meacham (2008) conducted an analysis of mission statements in higher education. He studied over 300 missions of universities identified by *The Princeton Review* (2001) as the 331 best colleges across the United States. Findings were similar to those of Morphew and Hartley (2006) with most missions emphasizing liberal arts, service, and social responsibility. Meacham discusses the utility of mission statements for orientation of new faculty and administrators to the history and purpose of the institution, assessment of the program and its relevance to current goals, utilization for campus-wide discussions on current issues confronting the institution, and visualization of the future direction of the university/college.

Colder (2011) surveyed Canadian higher education institutions' website mission and vision statements. He found that 81% (n = 65) of the institutions went through a planning process to develop the statements. He states that while a mission should focus on the outcomes or purpose of the institution in order to provide direction for its members, many spoke of learning processes and the means to achieve the outcomes rather than the outcome. Regarding vision statements, Colder found that many institutions described their current state, rather than the future and many were lengthy rather than the brief, short, to-the-point visions for the future.

Chief administrators (presidents) of institutions of higher learning assume much of the responsibility for assuring that the mission and vision are current and reflect the purpose of the college or university. They provide the leadership and resources for administrators, staff, faculty, and students to implement the mission and vision, to maintain its relevancy in the community, and to meet future education needs. Developing or revising mission and vision statements are usually a part of a strategic planning process that involves all of the constituents within the institution.

The purpose/mission of the institution is examined and a vision statement is developed that looks into the future for the next decade or two. These activities foster creativity and a movement toward the future that provide the framework for planning. After consensus is reached, the mission and vision statements serve as the guiding documents for developing long-range goals and implementing them. Another consideration related to the mission is the congruence of the statement with its actual implementation. Measures to determine if the mission is realized throughout the educational process and according to the expectations of graduates' performance in the real world, give feedback as to how well the mission is met. For example, if the mission has a strong research emphasis, there should be adequate support and funding for faculty to write grants to sponsor research, and released time and facilities to conduct their studies.

Another aspect to the implementation of the mission is a cost analysis of the budget to relate the amount of monies allocated to the various functions of the program that support the mission. Academic and infrastructure support systems are analyzed for congruency with the mission. An example from nursing is an institution's support and commitment to a nurse-managed primary care clinic that serves the underserved and unserved populations of the community in which the institution is located. In this example, the clinic meets the institution's mission to serve the community.

Unless the school or department of nursing is a stand-alone academic entity, the mission of the major academic division, for example, college or school, in which it resides, is examined in addition to that of the parent institution. Both the missions of the parent institution and its academic subdivision should be congruent with each other and provide guidelines for the mission statement of the nursing program. These statements depend upon the nature of the institution and the nursing program. Smaller institutions may focus on liberal arts as a basis for all disciplines and professional programs to meet societal needs, while large research-oriented universities or academic health sciences centers might espouse new knowledge breakthroughs by its faculty's and graduate students' research. In the case of the former, nursing's mission statement would reflect the graduation of well-prepared nurses to meet current and future health care demands; the latter would have an emphasis on nursing research and leadership in the profession.

As with the presidents of universities and colleges, deans and directors of nursing education programs have a leadership role in developing program missions and visions that are not only congruent with the parent institutions, but look to the future. Additionally, the mission needs to be examined frequently for its relevance to the rapidly changing health care system and the needs of society.

PHILOSOPHY

A definition for *philosophy* is listed in Merriam-Webster (2014) as a "critical examination of the rational grounds of our most fundamental beliefs and logical analysis of the basic concepts employed in the expression of such beliefs." The philosophy for a curriculum should flow from the mission and vision. It gives faculty members the opportunity to discuss their beliefs, values, and attitudes about nursing and an education that imparts a body of knowledge and skills for the next generation of care providers. Faculty members discuss their beliefs about their specific school of nursing and its role in preparing nurses for the future, including statements on teaching and learning theories, the development of critical thinking, and beliefs about the essentials of nursing education including liberal education and the sciences; the health care system, organization, policy, finance, and regulation; clinical prevention and population health; diversity; interprofessional collaboration; professionalism, professional values, and nursing practice; social justice and advocacy; scholarship, research, translational science, and evidence-based practice; information systems and patient care technology; and quality health care and patient safety. Each individual member holds his or her own personal philosophy of education and nursing and thus the development of a philosophical statement can become an arduous task to agree on. Nevertheless, the resulting statement reflects the faculty's (as an entity) rationale for the school of nursing's existence and it serves to flavor the remainder of the curriculum components, their implementation, and their outcomes.

The first task in the development of a philosophy statement is to look at those of the parent institution and the subdivision of the parent in which nursing is housed. The ideal nursing philosophy incorporates all of the components of the other two philosophies, although at times there are mismatches to some of the specific components. In those instances, a rationale as to why that incongruence exists and how the nursing program meets other components of the philosophy should be discussed. Eventually, this rationale is documented so that members of the school and external reviewers understand the fit of the nursing program within its parent institution and subdivision.

Some examples of incongruence of a nursing program's philosophy with its parent institution's philosophy occur when the program is within a traditional, liberal arts college that has no other professional programs. In this case, the nursing program's philosophy speaks to the importance of a strong liberal arts foundation for its graduates and the role of the nursing program to produce graduates who provide health care for the community. Another example is a nursing program housed within a school of engineering, along with several other professional programs such as computer science and journalism. In this case, nursing emphasizes the professional education aspects and preparation of professionals who serve the community.

The majority of nursing education programs' philosophies include basic theories, concepts, beliefs, and values of faculty. The statement can be brief and succinct or lengthy; however, it should offer guiding principles for the remainder of the curriculum and should be evident in the organizational framework(s), goals, objectives, and implementation plan. The following discussion reviews many of the concepts found in nursing education program philosophies and is offered as a way for faculty to share ideas and beliefs and find consensus for developing or revising the program's philosophy.

BELIEFS ABOUT TEACHING AND LEARNING PROCESSES

Beliefs about teaching and learning form the premise for the delivery of the nursing curriculum. In the past, courses were traditionally delivered through classroom lecture, clinical laboratory sessions, and clinical experiences in the reality setting. The emphasis was on teaching and the curriculum reflected that modality. In the more recent past, with the focus on program outcomes and the advent of technology, the emphasis changed to learner-centered education. The role of the teacher, instead of transmitter of knowledge, became a role of expert, mentor, and coach. Teaching strategies fostered student participation in learning activities instead of acting as passive receivers of knowledge. With the change in focus to the learner, theories and principles of teaching and learning served as guides for assessing the characteristics of the learners and adapting those theories and principles to the needs of the learner. Chapter 4 of this text reviews learning theories applicable to nursing education.

Cox, McIntosh, Reason, and Terenzini (2011) investigated what factors influence a "culture of teaching" in institutions of higher learning. They surveyed 45 colleges and universities representing liberal arts, comprehensive, and research institutions with 5,512 usable faculty members' responses. They found that the major influence on faculty's perceptions of the institution's "culture of teaching" focus was dependent upon the type of institution and not its policies. The public and academe continue to value research institutions and place faculty's research productivity above teaching activities. The authors conclude that in spite of the findings that academic policies have little influence on building a learner-centered environment, there remains a need to develop a culture and environment in all institutions that place emphases on learner-centered teaching and SLOs.

CRITICAL THINKING AND ITS APPLICATION TO NURSING

Chapter 5 of this text discusses educational taxonomies and strategies for developing critical thinking that give faculty members ideas on how these theories and concepts apply to their specific nursing program. The resultant sharing and discussions are summarized and become part of the philosophy statement. Development of critical thinking is essential to the preparation of nurses for clinical decision making and judgment. Most philosophies for nursing curricula contain some mention of it and thus it is useful for faculty to discuss its place in the curriculum and how it applies to its specific nursing program. Chan (2013) conducted a review of the international literature on critical thinking in nursing and identified themes related to the definition of critical thinking as it applies to nursing. From the review, she identified the characteristics of critical thinkers as "(i) gathering and seeking information, (ii) questioning and investigating, (iii) analysis, evaluation, and inference, and (iv) problem solving and application of theory" (p. 237). Four major influences on the development of critical thinking include the student, teacher, educational system, and the environment. In addition, some of the articles described strategies for developing critical thinking but as the author points out, further study is indicated to assess the efficacy of these strategies.

LIBERAL EDUCATION AND THE SCIENCES

One of the essential skills taken from the liberal arts and integrated into nursing education is the ability to write effectively. Troxler, Vann, and Oermann (2011) conducted a review of the literature related to the development of writing skills in undergraduate nursing programs. The purpose of the study was to identify various strategies for developing writing skills that are essential to nurses' communication skills in their relationships with patients and in the written word. Among the strategies identified in the review were key writing assignments across the curriculum, intensive nursing writing courses, ombudsman programs, and online writing tutorials.

Pavil (2011) reviews the connections between the arts and nursing education and practice. She reviews the literature that identifies instructional strategies for fostering creativity in nursing through artistic expression such as poetry, painting, music, sculpture, and so on. To integrate the liberal arts with nursing, and use creativity, students write a scholarly paper on a case study of a clinical experience with a patient and create a presentation to their peers that depicts the experience, such as role playing, reciting a poem, painting, music, and so on. Students, although reluctant about the assignment at first, expressed their enthusiasm about the experience and the opportunity to blend the arts with nursing.

Lapum et al. (2012) describe the integration of the social sciences into nursing education with experiences for students to investigate social justice issues and begin to assume the role of advocate for the oppressed. The authors describe how the teacher presented a poem applied to an oppressive experience in which she was involved and had the students write notes on their reactions to the story. The notes were assembled into a continuing poem and provided the teacher and students the opportunity not only to explore social justice issues and experience the negative feelings associated with them, but also to enter a threshold for developing solutions to the problems. The article illustrated the integration of the social sciences into education and practice and it demonstrated a strategy for participative student learning.

The integration of the liberal arts into nursing practice was studied by DeBrew (2010) when comparing the perceptions of RN to bachelor of science in nursing (BSN) and prelicensure BSN graduates. DeBrew describes AACN's (2014c) *Essentials for Baccalaureate Nursing* and the application of the liberal arts to nursing. The author surveyed RN to BSN and entry-level BSN graduates (n = 92) and found that the RN to BSN and entry-level BSN graduates were quite similar in their responses to the value of the liberal arts. The graduates reported that the liberal arts helped them communicate with patients, contributed to cultural competence, provided an academic background to grow professionally, and caused them to think globally and critically, which supported clinical decision making.

As a capstone experience in undergraduate work, Beuttler's (2012) persuasive essay argues for a return to a senior level moral philosophy course to integrate knowledge from the liberal arts. He reviews how American education moved away from the liberal arts and became more discipline specific. He argues that if institutions say in their missions, visions, and philosophies that they prepare graduates with moral character, good citizenship, leadership qualities, self-reliance, and worldviews, there should be a senior level course to integrate the liberal arts knowledge gained. Professional education, such as nursing, usually has senior-level capstone courses for the purpose of integration of knowledge gained through the previous years. However, as Beuttler points out, there needs to be a similar course that integrates the liberal arts to ensure the preparation of graduates who have strong moral characteristics.

To demonstrate the critical contribution that science has to nursing, Wolkowitz and Kelley (2010) surveyed 149 directors of associate degree, baccalaureate, diploma, and practical nurse nursing programs who utilized the Test of Essential Academic Skills (TEAS). TEAS assesses entrance into academe. They also utilized the Assessment Technology Institute (ATI) results to assess students' knowledge of the fundamentals of nursing. Multiple regressions compared science, mathematics, reading, and English TEAS scores to successful completion of student scores on the ATI fundamentals. They found that *science* was the major factor contributing to success in the fundamentals of nursing.

Along with the traditional requisite sciences of anatomy, chemistry, microbiology, nutrition, and physiology for nursing, genetics is now included in most programs as a separate course or integrated throughout the curriculum. The AACN *Essentials* documents (2014b) include genetics as part of the essentials. The continual breakthroughs of knowledge from the National Human Genome Project (HGP) illustrate the important contributions genetics have on the health of individuals. The latest information from the HGP may be found at www .genome.gov/10001772 (2014). Several articles on the integration of genetics into the curriculum that may be helpful to nurse educators as they plan a curriculum include DeSavo (2010); Lea, Skirton, Read, and Williams (2011); and Tonkin, Calzone, Jenkins, Lea, and Prows (2010).

THE HEALTH CARE SYSTEM, ORGANIZATION, POLICY, FINANCE, AND REGULATION

Knowledge of how the health care system is organized, financed, and regulated is essential for nurses to understand how it functions and nursing's role in it. Nurses must be prepared to provide leadership in the management of health care services and to address policy issues. The current organizational system of health care in the United States is in a state of flux owing to the enactment and implementation of the Affordable Care Act of 2010 with its legality subsequently upheld by the Supreme Court in 2012. Pulcini (2013) provides an update on its implications for patients and nursing including health insurance coverage in a competitive market, expansion of Medicaid benefits, availability of prescription medications, and the impact on advanced practice nurses' services and reimbursement. The federal government provides the full text of the Act and updates related to it at www.hhs .gov/healthcare/rights/law/index.html (U.S. Department of Health and Human Services [HHS], 2014).

Nurses are first in a Gallup poll as being the most ethical of professions (Nurses earn . . . 2014) and, in the same article, the American Nurses Association (ANA) encourages policy makers to involve nurses in key health care groups such as advisory and governing boards and working with coalitions of consumers, politicians, and professionals. How to prepare nurses for leadership in the health care arena should be part of the discussion by faculty when developing the philosophy for the curriculum. Faculty's beliefs about the health care system's organization, regulations, and financing are reviewed and the profession's responsibility in shaping public policy should be part of the educational program.

The extent of the education and experiences for students on these issues will vary according to the level of education, that is, entry-level or advanced nursing. Logan, Pauling, and Franzen (2011) present the Grand View Critical Analysis model as a tool for baccalaureate nursing students to examine and analyze a health care issue, focus on the issue, form colleagueships to address the issues, analyze evidence-based practice related to the issue, and develop a proposal related to the issue with an action plan to carry it out. This type of activity builds leadership skills for nurses in the policy-making arena.

On the graduate level, Aduddell and Gorman (2010) present an example of how their nursing program for advanced practice nurses integrated concepts on health care theory, research, ethical leadership, health policy with global application in health care systems, principles of evidence-based practice, and leadership in advanced care management. Courses related to these topics were presented to advanced practice students as well as those in the nursing leadership and management track. Students had the opportunity to apply theories and concepts from the courses to their practica, thus solidifying the assimilation of leadership skills in the health care system and policy-making environments.

To gain an appreciation on the costs of health care in the United States, Nickitas (2013) cites examples of high-cost medical procedures compared to other Western countries. For example, U.S. costs of caesarian sections, colonoscopies, and other diagnostic tests far exceed the costs in other nations. She reports that the total cost of care in America is $2.7 trillion and that many of the costs may be attributed to insurance companies and hospitals generating revenue for their maintenance at the expense of the consumer. Such factors are important for nurses to be aware of when helping to shape policy as well as when providing services that may not be necessary and are costly.

The health insurance industry covers the vast majority of health care costs incurred in the current U.S. health care delivery system. Kelly (2013) presents an overview of the health insurance industry and its lack of competition in the market. The article traces the history of the skyrocketing costs of health care including the Medicare, Medicaid, and the VA systems. It illustrates the need for leaders in health care to influence health policies through legislative action. The implementation of the Patient Protection and Affordable Care Act (PPACA) of 2010 will cause major changes in the health care industry, resulting in a competitive health care marketplace. Updates on these issues and their effect on nursing are necessary in the preparation of professionals for the health care system.

CLINICAL PREVENTION AND POPULATION HEALTH

A primary resource when planning the curriculum that includes clinical prevention, population health, and health promotion is the Healthy People 2020 (2012) document that lists the 10-year national objectives for improving the health of all Americans. Implications for nursing education come from the document and include the need for knowledge of epidemiology, population health, determinants of health, and disparities to achieve health equity for all groups. Healthy People 2020, HHS announces new health promotion disease prevention agenda (2012) brought to the attention of its members the importance of the Healthy People 2020 agenda and the role of nursing in realizing its goals. An example of nursing responding to this agenda is presented in an editorial by Berg and Pace (2010) and followed by a series of articles focused on nurse practitioner services in women's health focused on health promotion, risk reduction, and prevention of diseases.

Majette (2011) reviews the U.S. Congress deliberations related to the development and enactment of the PPACA of 2010 as it relates to health promotion and prevention of disease. As an insider in the process, she identified specific content in the act that was discussed by Congress and addressed public health, wellness, and prevention recommendations from such entities as the Institute of Medicine (IOM) and national and international health and human rights organizations.

Diversity and Cultural Competence

When considering clinical prevention and population health, an important concept to include is diversity. Diversity is defined in its broadest sense not only in terms of race, ethnicity, culture, language, and gender but also in terms of the diversity of opportunities in nursing. Thus, when faculty develops the philosophy, it must consider these factors and how the curriculum will meet society's diverse health care needs from entry-level graduates who function in all settings to those in advanced nursing roles in primary and tertiary care settings. Nursing care requires cultural sensitivity and awareness of differences among groups, while cultural competence denotes the knowledge and skills required for delivering care in cross-cultural situations. Dudas (2012) conducted a review of the literature regarding cultural competence and its evolution in nursing education. She points out the increasing diversity in the student population, although it still lags behind that of the general population, and the need for integrating the concepts into the educational program related to cultural diversity and the development of cultural competence.

Adeniran and Smith-Glasgow (2010) discuss the need for nurse educators to recognize diversity in learners including culture, language, gender, and learning styles. Bednarz, Schim, and Doorenbos (2010) discuss strategies for working with the increasingly diverse nursing student population. Although many articles are in the literature discussing diversity and its integration into entry-level nursing programs, Comer, Whichcello, and Neubrander (2013) describe a master's level curriculum that prepares nurse leaders for the delivery of quality diverse cultural and linguistic services in the health care system.

An update on the standards for culturally competent care was developed through a review of the literature and relevant resources by Douglas et al. (2011). In addition to the review, the authors called for comments on the Internet from nurse clinicians and nurse educators worldwide to gather ideas. The findings and comments were synthesized into a table of worldwide nursing standards for the delivery of culturally competent care. The general categories for the standards include social justice, critical reflection, knowledge of cultures, cultural competence in health care systems and organizations, patient advocacy and empowerment, a multicultural workforce, education and training in culturally competent nursing care, cross-cultural communication and leadership, and evidence-based practice and research.

INTERPROFESSIONAL COMMUNICATION AND COLLABORATION

In the past, nursing and other health care disciplines recognized the need for interprofessional education, and with the complexity of the current U.S. health care system, it is an important concept to include in discussions and planning for the educational program. The AACN (2014a) and other professional education organizations support the IOM's (2010) recommendations that call for interprofessional collaboration to meet the health care needs of the population.

Thibault (2011) reviews the IOM (2010) recommendations regarding *The Future of Nursing* and the Josiah Macy Jr. Foundation's work to promote interdisciplinary education and its relationship to nursing's role in the delivery of health care. Thibault presents an overview of what interprofessional collaboration means and how the health care professions need to move out of their silos in order to deliver comprehensive and quality care to patients. He emphasizes the need for leadership from the top administrators in health care professions education; careful planning in advance of students' learning experiences; clinical experiences that take place over the continuum, that is, not in isolated experiences; interprofessional students experiences with new technologies such as patient simulations; and the need for faculty development to encourage commitment to interprofessional education and to promote new pedagogies involving interprofessional collaboration. Thibault reports that while the majority of projects sponsored by the Macy Foundation were between nursing and medicine, some of the projects involved other health care disciplines.

Several examples from the literature exemplify the collaboration among other disciplines and serve as models for developing curricular experiences that are interdisciplinary in nature. Milton (2012) offers definitions of interprofessional and interdisciplinary education and presents some ethical implications associated with the implementation of such programs from a nursing point of view.

Dacey, Murphy, Anderson, and McCloskey (2010) conducted a pilot study for undergraduate health psychology, pharmacology, premedicine, and nursing students to introduce them to each discipline and promote cross collaboration. While the sample was small, it was successful in developing the students' skills for patient-centered care and an appreciation for other health care professions. Sheu et al. (2010) studied student-run clinics for medical, nursing, and pharmacy students to deliver interprofessional services to poor and underserved people. Several instruments to measure interprofessional attitudes were utilized and while quantitative findings were mixed, they found that there was an increased appreciation for interprofessional learning among the student groups. Interestingly, nursing students scored higher on the Readiness for Interprofessional Learning Survey, to which the authors comment, "that they may enter school with a different perspective, or that unique characteristics of their curricula, such as earlier clinical exposure, may change their perspective" (p. 1068).

Matthews, Parker, and Drake (2012) describe a service-learning, interprofessional experience of communication disorders, nursing, physical therapy, and social work students who visited older adults in the community. The experience was very positive for clients as well as the students, who gained an appreciation for other disciplines' roles as well as skills in working with geriatric clients. A unique perspective to this project is the partnership developed between the school and the community in providing clinical experiences for the students.

PROFESSIONALISM, PROFESSIONAL VALUES, AND NURSING PRACTICE

Nursing has the largest number of professionals in the U.S. health care system and while it has many pathways for entry into professional practice, it meets the criteria of a profession. Criteria for a professional discipline require a specific body of knowledge with members who study and practice the discipline. It includes specific ethics, and theories, and it produces relevant research. Smith and McCarthy (2010) discuss the AACN *Essentials* documents (2014c) and the recommended standards for education at the various levels of professional nursing practice, that is, the generalist (baccalaureate), the advanced generalist (master's), and the advanced practice practioner (DNP). The article by Smith and McCarthy provides guidelines for determining the concepts of professionalism at certain curricular levels and what constitutes the discipline (profession) of nursing.

Miller (1988) presented a model of professionalism in nursing that had at its core, education in a university setting, and scientific knowledge as a basis for the discipline. She listed attributes of nursing professionalism as adherence to the ANA (2014) *Code of Ethics*, a community service orientation, professional organization participation, autonomy and self-regulation, publication and communication, the development and use of research, and continuing education and competence. All of these concepts can serve as discussion points when developing this thread in the curriculum. For ideas on presenting concepts related to professionalism, Rhodes, Schutt, Langham, and Bilotta (2012) use Miller's Wheel of Professionalism in Nursing for introducing professionalism to undergraduate nurses. They describe the learner-centered strategies for discussion of professionalism and its application to nursing.

SOCIAL JUSTICE AND ADVOCACY

Many of the standards for accreditation of nursing programs and requests for proposals for educational funding refer to the notion of inequality, health disparities, and access to health care. Certain populations and oppressed groups suffer the consequences of discrimination and unfair treatment in the health care system. Nursing as a prime caring profession must be cognizant of these injustices and have the power and strategies to advocate for their clients and themselves to provide quality health care for all. Social justice is an important concept often found in the missions and philosophies of educational programs; however, it is sometimes difficult to find evidence of its integration into the curriculum plan and its implementation.

Fahrenwald, Taylor, Kneip, and Canales (2007) present several characterizations of social justice from a nursing perspective and the importance of it to nursing education and practice. They review the complexities of social justice and the need to analyze it from many viewpoints and its role in the discipline of nursing. Traditionally, social justice is taught in public health courses; however, the authors point out that it transcends all specialties in nursing and needs to be integrated throughout the curriculum. In addition to analyzing the characteristics and concepts related to social justice, they advocate for its presentation in the nursing program through transformative learning activities. They believe that learners must participate in confronting issues related to social justice to become leaders in the health care system and advocates for the people who suffer health disparities and limited access to quality care. This idea applies to all concepts related to the philosophy that guide the curriculum and returns to the theories related to teaching and learning. Each concept discussed and integrated into the philosophy and program of study must be considered by faculty for how it will be presented to students and how students will interact with it to assimilate and practice what the program defines as expectations for its graduates.

Lathrop (2013) discusses the social determinants of health with an emphasis on socioeconomic status in the United States and cites statistics that demonstrate the effect of one's place in the economy on health outcomes. For example, the poorest people experience higher morbidity and mortality rates those who are economically advantaged. She goes on to say that nursing leaders, as advocates and representatives of the caring profession, should have a role in bringing attention to the social determinants of health to the nation and its policy makers. Additionally, she urges nurse educators to bring these issues into the curriculum and suggests ways in which students can participate as advocates for the economically and socially disadvantaged.

SCHOLARSHIP, RESEARCH, TRANSLATIONAL SCIENCE, AND EVIDENCE-BASED PRACTICE

Scholarship and Research

Scholarship and research provide the foundation for evidence-based practice. Both concepts appear in nursing curricula and should be addressed by faculty when developing or revising the philosophy of the educational program. Scholarship and research concepts begin at the associate degree level and continue in complexity to the PhD where new knowledge is tested and added to the body of scientific knowledge for the discipline. Faculties identify the scholarship and research competencies they expect of their graduates according to the level of the educational program and the practice areas or role functions that they expect their graduates to achieve. For example, associate degree programs expect their graduates to use evidence-based practice based upon credible, research-based nursing interventions and to challenge practices that lack data to support their use and do not result in quality patient outcomes.

Baccalaureate programs usually require a basic statistics course to support a separate nursing research course in the curriculum with expectations that graduates will understand the research process so that they can be discerning consumers of the research literature and use it to provide evidence-based practice. Writing assignments across the curriculum develop students' scholarly skills to review, analyze, and critique the literature in order to communicate professionally and apply evidence from the literature to practice. Greenwald (2010) describes the role of undergraduate research in light of faculty's own research needs and expectations and the development of scholarship skills in students. She reviews Boyer's (1990) statements of scholarship in academe and their relationship to research in nursing education.

Most graduate nursing programs require graduate level statistics and research in nursing courses. They usually have capstone options for theses, scholarly projects, professional papers, advanced practice projects, or research-focused dissertations. Many include comprehensive examinations in addition to the written paper or dissertation or sometimes as the only capstone requirement. The thesis at the master's level can serve as a pathway to doctoral studies and uses extensive reviews and analysis of the literature in addition to utilization of research processes to investigate a problem. Projects or other scholarly works and professional papers at the master's level include extensive reviews of the literature and their integration to support the project or paper. At the doctoral level, both research-intensive and applied research projects require supporting research and statistical analyses courses. The number and depth of knowledge and research contained in these courses depend upon the type of doctoral program. Research-based PhD or DNS dissertations synthesize knowledge of nursing science on a selected topic and generate new knowledge through quantitative, qualitative, or mixed method processes.

Regan and Pietrobon (2010) present ideas about scholarly writing and its application to the dissemination of research findings. They point out that graduate education programs often require scholarly and evidence-based written papers/dissertations that specify what format the content of the paper should take but fail to use a conceptual model for the writing format. They offer a conceptual model for scholarly writing composed of four principles and suggest a course revolved around them for students. The principles (rhetoric, ethnographic, recognition, and practice) offer different perspectives on style of writing according to the discipline and type of research reported upon.

Translational Science

Translational science is a relatively new discipline in health care and applies to the analyses of research and current practice and applies these analyses to practice. One of the newest institutes at the National Institutes of Health is the National Center for Advancing Translational Sciences (2014), which offers opportunities for health care professionals to apply research to practice. Grady (2010) offers a definition for translational research as it applies to nursing:

> Translational research addresses this gap between research and research application. It addresses the internal and external validity—to help scientists identify strategies that promote the ready translation of research findings into timely, effective, and efficient practice innovations across diverse

community and population based settings. The feedback loops inherent in the translational research process allow research to inform practice and practice to inform research, toward the goal of improving health care. (p. 165)

Applied practice or professional doctoral (DNP or clinical doctorate) projects translate existing knowledge and research on a selected topic to develop new evidence-based strategies for advanced practice and/or application to leadership roles that initiate change.

Evidence-Based Practice

Research and translational science are the base for evidence-based practice. Therefore, it is important for all levels of nursing education to graduate students who understand these concepts and discern between valid and reliable evidence-based nursing interventions and interventions that have no supportive data or rationale for their use. Evidence-based practice applies to all health care disciplines and its utilization has a major role in patient outcomes and quality care. As with the research process, evidence-based practice is leveled according to the type of nursing education program. Associate degree students should have theory and clinical experiences that demonstrate the use of evidence-based practice. Baccalaureate students further this knowledge by raising questions related to practice and seeking answers through literature review. Master's students apply evidence-based practice in advanced roles, raise questions, and investigate current research to inform their practice. Students in applied practice or professional doctoral programs synthesize this knowledge and generate new interventions for evidence-based practice. Theory-based doctoral students study the domain of evidence-based practice and develop new knowledge related to its use and value.

Stevens (2013) reviews the evolution and integration of evidence-based practice concepts into practice and education dating from the IOM's 2001 *Quality Chasm Report* to the present. She identifies from the literature several frameworks for faculty utilization in planning the curriculum for ensuring that evidence-based concepts are included. The major resources she lists include the AACN *Essentials* (2014c) that specify evidence-based practice across the levels of education, the Quality and Safety Education for Nurses (QSEN) Institute (2014), and the teaching IOM competencies by Finkelman and Kenner (2014). Scholarship, research, translational science, and evidence-based practice are important concepts to include in philosophical statements for nursing curricula. The concepts can be leveled according to type of program and the statements provide guidelines for how the concepts will be delivered and evaluated in the instructional program.

INFORMATION SYSTEMS AND PATIENT CARE TECHNOLOGY

Information systems and patient care technology are crucial components to include in the curriculum in order to keep abreast of expanding developments in the field and their impact on the delivery of health care, research and scholarly activities, and teaching and learning modalities. As with many other concepts in nursing education, the integration and use of information systems and technology are included in the AACN *Essentials* (AACN, 2014c) and the Accreditation Commission for Education in Nursing (ACEN) Standards and Criteria (2013).

Technology and informatics serve as platforms for the delivery of nursing education programs such as web-based, hybrid, and web-enhanced courses and they apply to the practice setting as students gain nursing competencies in the care of clients. In the clinical setting, students use personal digital assistants, patient information systems, computerized medical records, telemedicine/nursing, and high-tech devices for patient monitoring and care. It is important for faculty to be knowledgeable and competent in these skills in order assist students in the application of informatics and technology.

In response to the IOM *Future of Nursing* (2014) recommendations and the implementation of the Affordable Care Act (2014), Nguyen, Zierler, and Nguyen (2011) surveyed nursing faculty from the Western United States for their knowledge, skills, and use of informatics, simulation, telehealth, and technology. They found that more than half of the respondents were using distance education technologies, simulation, telehealth, and informatics in their teaching activities. Of those utilizing the technologies, two-thirds rated themselves as competent in teaching these skills, although the majority of faculty still felt the need for additional education and resources to support the implementation of these concepts into the program.

Flood, Gasiewicz, and Delpier (2010) surveyed the literature for instructional strategies related to informatics and technology in nursing programs. Based on their review and the need for integrating these skills throughout the undergraduate program, they developed a model for integrating the concepts into the undergraduate program. It is a useful model when considering how informatics and technology occur throughout the nursing education program. Faculty in graduate programs could pick up the threads to continue them into the master's and doctoral levels.

QUALITY HEALTH CARE AND PATIENT SAFETY

Quality health care and patient safety concepts are embedded in nursing knowledge and clinical practice. Based on the recommendations of the IOM (2001) regarding patient safety, these concepts are receiving increased emphasis in the education of health professionals and the delivery of health care. Increased acuity levels and patients with complex physiological and psychosocial challenges add to the challenges for providing safe and quality care. In addition, all of these factors call for interdisciplinary collaboration to ensure a safe and compassionate health care environment. The Agency for Healthcare Research and Quality (2014) lists quality indicators and prevention strategies for patient safety. A useful website for finding the latest information on quality health care and patient safety is www.ahrq.gov.

Barnsteiner, Disch, Johnson, McGuinn, and Swartwout (2013) report on the nationwide project sponsored by the Robert Wood Johnson Foundation to integrate the six core competencies for patient safety and quality of care. Regional institutes were held throughout the United States with more than 1,000 nursing faculty members attending. It was found that the institutes served to motivate and equip faculty with the tools needed to integrate QSEN competencies into the curriculum. A useful website with the QSEN competencies for prelicensure and graduate students can be found at the QSEN home page (2014; www.qsen.org). The ultimate goal is for improved patient safety outcomes and patient-centered quality care. The following citations provide additional information on quality health care and patient safety that educators may find useful: Debourgh (2012); Didion, Kozy, Koffel, and Oneall (2013); Disch (2012); Kelly and Starr (2013); and Piscotty, Grobbel, and Abele (2013).

ORGANIZATIONAL FRAMEWORKS AND CONCEPT MAPPING

Organizational Frameworks

Although accreditation is voluntary, most schools of nursing in the United States are accredited by a national organization, either the ACEN or the Commission on Collegiate Nursing Education (CCNE) (ACEN, 2013; CCNE, 2014). At one time, both accrediting bodies required or implied that organizational frameworks were necessary to design the educational program's objectives, content, and instructional design. It was common for schools of nursing to use theoretical or conceptual models from nursing or other related disciplines as organizational frameworks. These frameworks served a useful purpose to place certain theories, concepts, content, and clinical learning experiences into the curriculum. While they are no longer explicitly required in the standards for accreditation, both the ACEN (2013) and CCNE (2014) make reference to an organizational structure for the curriculum. Many of the concepts listed under the discussion of the philosophy in this text are included in the accreditation standards for the curriculum, for example, social justice, population health, cultural diversity, patient safety, quality health care, and so on. The accreditation standards/competencies for the ACEN and CCNE may be found at their websites (www.acenursing.net/manuals/SC2013.pdf and www.aacn.nche.edu/ccne-accreditation/about/mission-values-history).

A word of caution: Faculty should check the regulations of the governing body in which the school of nursing is located, such as State Boards of Nursing, when developing or revising the curriculum. Some of these agencies may require a conceptual or theoretic framework for the curriculum.

The organizational framework serves to logically order the delivery of the body of knowledge in the curriculum and provides a checklist of sorts that ensures that no concepts are omitted. CCNE (2014) states in its standards for accreditation that baccalaureate and graduate programs including the DNP should demonstrate evidence for integrating the essentials and competencies developed by the AACN for each level of education. Information on how to access these documents may be found at AACN's website (2014b; www.aacn.nche.edu/Education/curriculum.htm). Likewise, the National League for Nursing (NLN) (2014b), in collaboration with nurse educators, developed outcomes and competencies that provide guidelines for nursing education programs. Information on how to access the document may be found at www.nln.org/facultyprograms/competencies/graduates_competencies.htm.

Concept Mapping

The process of concept mapping is useful for ensuring that essential knowledge and skills are integrated into the curriculum. Concept mapping is a detailed analysis of a concept and its relationships within the curriculum that is depicted into a map with arrows signifying relationships. It should include the expected competencies for student achievement as well as the places in the curriculum where the concept in introduced, built upon, and mastered. Ervin, Carter, and Robinson (2013) conducted a review of the literature for reports on the use of concept mapping in curriculum development and evaluation. While they found few references, they identified some of the processes used to develop concept maps and some of the problems encountered when developing them. A useful website by Novak and Cañas (2013) that discusses in detail the process of concept mapping is found at http://cmap.ihmc.us/publications/researchpapers/theoryc-maps/theoryunderlyingconceptmaps.htm. Dearman, Lawson, and Hall (2011) describe the process a faculty of a baccalaureate program went through to map concepts in their curriculum using the AACN *Essentials* (2014b). The process included assessment and evaluation activities that were tied into the graduates' success rate on NCLEX (National Council of State Boards of Nursing, 2013) and a practice exam.

Once the mission and philosophy for the curriculum are finalized, faculty identifies the major theories, concepts, and skills it believes should be in the curriculum. As the implementation plan for the curriculum is developed or as faculty assesses the curriculum, the process of concept mapping helps to identify where these elements occur. A sample concept map is provided in the case study at the end of the chapter.

IMPLEMENTATION OF THE CURRICULUM

Overall Purpose and Goal of the Program

After the philosophy, mission, and organizing framework are chosen, the next logical step in curriculum development is to state the overall purpose or goal of the program. There are arguments against behavioral statements for goals as post-modernist and humanism philosophies take hold in the 21st century. The arguments against them relate to the lack of freedom they provide for the learner and for the teacher whose role is to empower the learner. At the same time, there are accountability issues that relate to graduates' competencies in meeting the health care systems' demands and the health care needs of the people they serve. Faculty must grapple with these issues as it develops statements on the purpose of the nursing program and the overall long-term goal for graduates. Whether the statement becomes global and idealistic or specific and stated in measurable terms depends upon the faculty's philosophy, values, and beliefs and subsequent statements and objectives that specify the graduates' learning outcomes.

In addition to a choice of the format of the statement of purpose or goal for a nursing program, that is, global or behavioral, there are certain components belonging to professional nursing education that faculty may wish to consider and include, if not explicitly, implicitly. Examples of concepts that might be empha- sized include statements on caring, health promotion and other types of nursing interventions, client systems, professional behaviors and competencies, the health care system, and so forth. Characteristics of the graduate that are unique to the specific school of nursing can be included (e.g., "a caring, compassionate health care provider").

The type of nursing education program influences the overall program purpose or goal statement. Levels of clinical competence and knowledge acquisition will differ among licensed practical/vocational nursing, diploma, associate degree, baccalaure- ate, master's, and doctoral programs. Programs with multiple layers of preparation including undergraduate and graduate education usually have a global statement of purpose with each program, adapting that statement to meet its specific level of edu- cation. Although the statements of purpose and overall goal can be succinct, they act as the guides for the end-of-program objectives (SLOs). The statement should reflect the faculty's mission statement, philosophy, and organizational framework.

STUDENT LEARNING OUTCOMES OR END-OF-PROGRAM AND LEVEL OBJECTIVES

As reiterated throughout this chapter, nursing programs must demonstrate that they meet the overall program mission, purpose, and goal. SLOs or end-of-program objectives reflect the organizing framework and define the specific expectations or competencies of graduates upon completion of the nursing program. In order to reach these objectives, intermediate level or semester objectives are developed in sequential order. For example, in a 2-year associate degree program, there are end- of-first-year and end-of-second-year expectations all of which lead to the end-of- program objectives. In a baccalaureate program, there may be freshman, sophomore, junior, and senior level objectives. Some programs prefer to divide the objectives into semesters and could be titled in that fashion, that is, first semester, second semester, third semester, and so on. Graduate programs may indicate junior or senior levels, semester levels, first year and second year, doctoral candidate, and so forth.

Chapter 4 of the text presents educational taxonomies such as the classics developed by Bloom et al. (1956). These taxonomies categorize domains of learn- ing and provide guidelines for writing objectives related to the domains. The major domains are cognitive, affective, psychomotor, and behavioral. Furthermore, these domains are divided into levels of development and difficulty. For example, in nurs- ing, the psychomotor skill of measuring blood pressure moves from recognition of the blood pressure measurement tools to mastery of the skill. At the same time, the student is utilizing the cognitive domain by first recalling the physiology of blood pressure and identifying the norms for blood pressure. The student continues to comprehend, apply, analyze, synthesize, and evaluate knowledge that results in nurs- ing diagnosis and actions such as referral of clients for management of abnormal findings, teaching clients how to manage hyper- and hypotension, or in the case of the advanced practitioner, prescribing interventions to control hypertension.

The classic taxonomies assist in the development of end-of-program, level (intermediate), and course objectives. To develop or assess end-of-program objectives, the first task is to look at the program mission, purpose, and overall goal. Faculty members discuss what they expect of their graduates at the end of the program to meet the overall goal. A list of these expectations is developed into end-of-program objectives, which are analyzed for their specificity to meet the overall goal and the selected organizing framework of the curriculum. For example, if the NLN (2014a) competencies for associate degree and diploma nursing are used for the curriculum's organizational framework, the end-of-program objectives should include a statement(s) reflecting the NLN competency: *Advocate for patients and families in ways that promote their self-determination, integrity, and ongoing growth as human beings* (www.nln.org/facultyprograms/competencies/comp_ad_dp.htm).

Level or semester objectives follow the end-of-program objectives and each of these steps may be viewed deductively or inductively to ensure that the total body of knowledge and skills expected at the end of the program are included in the curriculum plan. All levels of objectives provide the guidelines for planning, implementing, and evaluating the curriculum.

When developing objectives, there are basic components in them that provide ways in which to meet their expectations and to determine to what extent they are attained. The cardinal rule is that objectives must be learner-focused. Additional components include the content as it relates to the outcome, expected learner behavior and at what level, feasibility, and the time frame. The content of the objective is the knowledge and/or skills that students are expected to learn. An example of an end-of-program objective is "the graduate will provide competent, compassionate nursing care based on the assessment of clients and families across the life span." In this example, the content is nursing care, assessment, and clients and families. The behavior expected of the graduate is to "provide, competent, compassionate nursing care." This statement implies that the graduate will provide this care 100% of the time competently and also compassionately. Objectives like these require definitions of competence and compassion and how to measure consistency in these behaviors (100% of the time). Thus, faculty agrees upon definitions for these terms and prepares statements that describe them, usually in the philosophy and/or organizational framework. Based on these definitions, the faculty assesses the feasibility for accomplishing the objectives that includes the time frame (end of the program) and expected levels of performance and consistency. These are defined according to the type of program, that is, associate degree, baccalaureate, advanced practice, or other graduate level tracks. Additional considerations relate to the resources available for implementing the objectives, the abilities of the graduates to accomplish them, and at what level the objectives should be accomplished.

Level or semester objectives follow the same pattern as the SLOs. Faculty reviews each level for the progression of objectives toward the end-of-program objectives. Some programs start from basic knowledge and skills at the first level or semester to the complex knowledge and skills expected at the senior level of the program. Other programs expect mastery of specific knowledge and skills earlier in the program that are reinforced throughout the program and practiced after graduation. Still other programs use a combination of both. Decisions on the patterns of progression will depend upon the philosophy and organizational framework, including the developmental stage of the learner. These decisions should be documented with a rationale for their placement in the curriculum to aid in evaluation of the curriculum, total quality management of the program, and accreditation reports.

PROGRAM OF STUDY

The overall goal, SLOs, level objectives, and organizing framework serve as a master plan for placing content into the curriculum and developing a program of study. Faculty is responsible for developing the curriculum plan and revising it periodically as needed. The prerequisites for the program are examined for their logical location in the curriculum. Prerequisites for prelicensure nursing programs include the liberal arts; social, physical, and biological sciences; communications; mathematics; and other general education requirements.

Graduate nursing programs usually require a baccalaureate in nursing; although students with associate degrees in nursing and a baccalaureate in another discipline are sometimes admitted conditionally subject to completing prescribed courses in nursing that the faculty designates as requirements for meeting the equivalent of a baccalaureate in nursing. The same principles apply to nursing or other disciplines' doctorate programs. Each doctoral program will prescribe the courses or degree work necessary to meet the equivalent of their lower degree requirements.

Once the prerequisites are completed, the nursing curriculum plan has a progressive order for sequencing nursing courses. For example, a Nursing 101 Fundamentals of Nursing course is a prerequisite for Nursing 102 Nursing Care of the Older Adult and Nursing 501 Nursing Research is the prerequisite for Nursing 502 Master's Thesis. Co-requisites are courses that can be taught simultaneously and are complementary; for example, N301 Health Promotion of Children and Adolescents and N303 Nursing Care of Children and Adolescents. Again, the placement of courses depends upon the organizing framework with the course objectives and content leading toward the achievement of level objectives and eventually, the program outcomes.

The numbers of units or credits are assigned to each course keeping in mind the total allotted to the major. For associate degree in nursing programs, nursing credits average 30 semester credits with total degree requirements averaging 60 to 70 semester credits. It should be noted that some programs operate on quarter credits or units that are usually 10 weeks in length as contrasted to the usual semester length of 15 weeks. In that case, one-quarter credit or unit is equivalent to two thirds of a semester credit or unit.

Baccalaureate programs average 60 nursing credits with a total of 120 to 130 credits for the degree. The master's in nursing program ranges from 30 to 60 or more total credits depending upon the nature of the program, with advanced practice roles requiring the higher number of credits. Owing to the wide range of nursing credits and the many credits required for advanced practice at the master's level, the profession is moving toward advanced practice degrees at the doctoral level. The AACN recommended that the preparation of advanced practice nurses move to

the doctorate level by 2015 (AACN, 2014b). The majority of master
ate degree credits are in the nursing major with only a few from other
electives.

Content experts serve as guides for nursing course placements and once
the courses have been placed in logical sequence, the course descriptions are
written, usually by the content expert or the person who will serve as "faculty of
record" (in charge of the course). For example, the content expert for the course
"Nursing Care of Children and Adolescents" would probably be a faculty member certified as a clinical specialist or nurse practitioner in pediatrics. Course
descriptions are brief paragraphs with several comprehensive statements that
provide an overview of the content of the course. They do not contain student-
centered objectives.

Course objectives follow the course description, and are learner-centered,
based upon the content of the course, their place in the curriculum plan, relationship to the level and end-of-program objectives, and relevance to the organizational framework. Finally, an outline of the course content is listed and should be
tied to the objectives of the course. A course schedule is usually included and tied to
the content outline. See Figure 9.1 for a classic outline for a course syllabus.

Parent Institution Logo
School of Nursing
Type of Program
Course # and Title
Course Description:

Credits:

Pre or co-requisites:

Class Type: (lecture, seminar, laboratory, practicum)

Faculty Information:

Required and Recommended Texts:

Course Objectives:

Teaching and Learning Strategies: (include teacher and student expectations)

Attendance and Participation Requirements:

Evaluation Methods:

Assignments:

Course Content and Schedule:

Academic Dishonesty Statement:

Disability Statement:

FIGURE 9.1   The major components of a syllabus.

All of these components are subject to faculty approval as well as the parent institution. Once established, faculty members who are assigned to courses have the freedom to rearrange or update the content and to teach the courses in their preferred method. However, changes to the course title, credits, objectives, or descriptions must undergo the same approval processes as the original courses. Although this may appear stifling to academic freedom, it ensures the integrity of the curriculum.

Usually, new or revised course descriptions, objectives, and content outlines are presented to the program's curriculum committee for recommendations and approval, submitted to the total faculty for approval, and continue through the appropriate channels of the parent institution for final formal approval. Because of the many layers of approval, faculty must be mindful of the initial proposals so that they will not need frequent revision, as any changes to course titles, credits, descriptions, number of credits, and objectives are subject to the same review processes.

SUMMARY

Chapter 9 reviewed the components of the curriculum and the processes faculty undergo in developing or revising curricula. Assessing and revising (if necessary) each component of the curriculum in logical sequence helps to maintain its integrity and ensure its quality. Faculty members are experts in their discipline and are therefore, responsible for ensuring that essential knowledge as well as the latest breakthroughs in its science are in the curriculum. Curriculum development and revision processes must be based on information from evaluation activities; the latest changes in the profession, health care, and society; and forecasts for the future. Table 9.1 provides guidelines for assessing the key components of a curriculum or educational program.

TABLE 9.1	GUIDELINES FOR ASSESSING THE KEY COMPONENTS OF A CURRICULUM OR EDUCATIONAL PROGRAM	
COMPONENTS	QUESTIONS FOR DATA COLLECTION	DESIRED OUTCOMES
Mission	What are the major elements of the parent institution and subdivision (if applicable) missions? Are these major elements in the nursing mission? If not, give a rationale as to why. How does the nursing mission speak to its teaching, service, and research/ scholarship roles?	The nursing mission is congruent with that of its parent institution and if applicable, the academic subdivision in which it is located The mission reflects nursing's teaching, service, and research/scholarship role
Philosophy	Is the nursing philosophy congruent with that of the parent institution philosophy and subdivision (if applicable)? If not, give the rationale as to why they are not	The philosophy statement is congruent with that of the parent institution and academic subdivision (if applicable)

(continued)

TABLE 9.1	GUIDELINES FOR ASSESSING THE KEY COMPONENTS OF A CURRICULUM OR EDUCATIONAL PROGRAM (*continued*)	
COMPONENTS	**QUESTIONS FOR DATA COLLECTION**	**DESIRED OUTCOMES**
	What statements in the philosophy relate to the faculty's beliefs and values about teaching and learning, critical thinking, liberal arts and the sciences, the health care system, clinical prevention and population health, interprofessional collaboration, diversity and cultural competence, social justice, scholarship, research and evidence-based practice, information systems and technology, quality health care, and patient safety?	The philosophy reflects the faculty's beliefs and values on teaching and learning, critical thinking, etc.
Organizing Frameworks	What is the organizing framework for the curriculum and how does it reflect the mission and philosophy statements? To what extent does the framework appear throughout the implementation of the curriculum? Are its concepts readily identified in all of the tracks of the programs?	The curriculum has an organizing framework that reflects its mission and philosophy The concepts of the organizing framework are readily identified in all tracks of the nursing education program
Overall Purpose and Goal of the Program	To what extent does the overall goal or purpose statement reflect the mission, philosophy, and organizing framework? Is the statement broad enough to encompass all tracks of the nursing program? To what extent does the statement lead to the measurement of program outcomes?	The overall goal or purpose statement reflects that of the mission, philosophy, and organizing framework The overall goal or purpose includes all tracks of the nursing program The overall goal or purpose is stated in such a way that it is a guide for measuring outcomes of the program (program review)
Student Learning Outcomes or End-of-Program and Level Objectives	To what extent are the mission, overall goal or purpose, and organizational framework reflected in the objectives? How are the objectives arranged in logical and sequential order? Is each objective learner centered and does it include the content, expected level of behavior of the learner, feasibility, and time frame?	The objectives reflect the mission, overall purpose or goal, and organizing framework The objectives are sequential and logical The objective statements are learner centered and include the content, expected learner behavior and at what level, feasibility, and time frame
Implementation Plan	To what extent does the curriculum plan reflect the organizing framework, overall goal, end-of-program, and level objectives?	The implementation plan for the curriculum reflects the organizing framework, overall goal or purpose, end-of-program and level objectives

(*continued*)

TABLE 9.1	GUIDELINES FOR ASSESSING THE KEY COMPONENTS OF A CURRICULUM OR EDUCATIONAL PROGRAM (*continued*)	
COMPONENTS	QUESTIONS FOR DATA COLLECTION	DESIRED OUTCOMES
	Is there documentation of approval of the curriculum plan in the permanent records?	The curriculum plan and its prerequisites and courses have the approval of the appropriate governing bodies
	Does each track in the program have a curriculum plan that includes course descriptions, credits, pre- and co-requisites, objectives, and content outlines?	The implementation plan for each track includes all courses and credits, pre- or co-requisites, descriptions, objectives, and content outlines
Summary	Has each component of the curriculum been addressed?	Based on an analysis of the curriculum, each component is addressed
	To what extent is each component congruent with those of the parent institution? If not congruent, has the rationale for incongruence been addressed?	The curriculum components are congruent with the parent institution and with each other
	Are the components of the curriculum listed and do they flow in a logical and sequential order?	The components flow in a logical and sequential order
	To what extent does the implementation plan flow from the overall goal, SLOs, end-of-program objectives, and level objectives?	The implementation plan flows from the overall goal, SLOs, and level objectives
	To what extent is the implementation plan congruent with the organizing framework?	The implementation plan is congruent with the organizing framework. The curriculum reflects relevance to current nursing practice demands and the need for nurses and projected future changes in the health care system.
	To what extent is the curriculum relevant to current and future nursing practice demands and needs for nurses?	

CASE STUDY

The case study from Chapters 6 and 7 continues with a description of the processes faculty used in a fictional school of nursing to revise its RN to BSN program that accelerates into the MSN, to develop an entry-level MSN program and a BSN to DNP curriculum with a postmaster's track. The entry-level MSN will produce new RNs into the workforce, while the RN to MSN and the DNP program will produce advanced practice nurses and administrators for the evolving health care system. The decision to revise the curriculum and develop new programs was agreed upon by the faculty. Administrative units in the college were advised of the proposals and approved them and the State Board of Nursing approved the entry-level MSN tentatively, while awaiting the final proposal. The accrediting agencies were made aware of the proposed programs and are standing by for review and approval of the program proposals.

Since the school of nursing has an existing extended education RN to BSN program and there are three tracks in the MSN program, it is anticipated that it will take one academic year to develop the totally online RN to MSN program. The entry-level MSN program accelerates college graduates through baccalaureate level nursing courses into the MSN program. It is anticipated that it will be developed in tandem with the RN to MSN program. The school plans to admit the first classes for both tracks in the spring semester following completion of the curricula and approval of the State Board of Nursing and accrediting bodies. The postmaster's DNP program will be developed over 1 ½ academic years with the first class admitted in the fall of the second year. The BSN to DNP program will be developed within 2 academic years with the first class admitted in the fall of the third year. Eventually the family nurse practitioner (FNP) and adult/geriatric acute care nurse practitioner (ACNP) track will be phased out of the master's program and into the DNP program. The clinical nurse leader (CNL) master's track will continue but graduates of that track will be eligible to apply to the Nursing Administration and Health Systems track of the DNP.

MISSION

The faculty reviews the existing college and school of nursing mission statements found in the most recent accreditation reports as well as the college catalogue and recruiting materials. The college mission states: "The mission of the college is to educate students in the traditions of the liberal arts, sciences, and spiritual beliefs of its founding fathers to become intellectually and socially responsible, compassionate citizens and leaders in their communities and society." The school of nursing mission statement states: "The mission of the school of nursing is to prepare intellectually and socially aware, competent, and compassionate nurses and nurse leaders to meet the health care needs of their communities and society."

The faculty agrees that both missions are similar and contain elements of teaching, service, and research. Specifically, the school of nursing mission implies teaching and learning by the verb "prepare" and all that it entails including acquisition of knowledge and skills. The service element specifies that the graduates will provide competent and compassionate care to communities and society and the allusions to intellectual and social awareness imply research or, in this case, scholarship and evidence-based practice. Since the RN to MSN program is an adaptation of the existing RN to BSN program and operates within the mission, it is determined that it is not in conflict with the current college and school of nursing mission statements which, in turn, are congruent. The same is true for both the entry-level MSN and the DNP programs; in addition, both prepare nurse leaders.

PHILOSOPHY

The philosophy statement of the college is as follows: "The college fosters the liberal study of the arts and sciences, of humanity in its diverse historical and cultural forms, and of the insight derived from spiritual and religious study. Students and faculty interact in critical and creative thinking processes and effective communication to acquire the skills needed for active participation and leadership in transforming their communities and the world. Through faculty's research and scholarly activities and collaborative teaching and learning processes, students cultivate a global perspective that embodies the values of social justice and compassion and results in the responsible valuing and sharing of knowledge and skills as articulate and responsible citizens and leaders in their communities."

The school of nursing philosophy states: "Students and faculty of the school of nursing interact in teaching and learning processes that empower students to build upon a strong liberal arts and sciences foundation and assimilate the nursing knowledge and skills that lead to the provision of competent and compassionate nursing care and leadership in the health care system for the health promotion and prevention of disease for multicultural and ethnic persons, families, and populations. The liberal arts and sciences foundation, the nursing code of ethics, and professional standards guide the students and faculty in the teaching and learning processes to foster creative thought, critical thinking, clinical decision making, scholarship, evidence-based practice, and ethical and professional judgments."

An analysis of the philosophies of the college and school of nursing reveals that they are congruent. Although the nursing philosophy does not speak specifically to that of the college's statement on religious study, it incorporates the notion of spirituality and designates the study of the liberal arts and sciences including religious studies as the foundation for nursing knowledge and skills. The nursing statement includes the classic concepts related to nursing education and practice. The philosophy is broad enough to incorporate all levels of the nursing program.

ORGANIZING FRAMEWORK

The school of nursing uses the *Essentials* documents for the undergraduate and graduate programs published by the AACN (2014c) to serve as the organizing framework for the programs. Faculty members analyze the *Essentials* documents for their relationship to the mission and philosophy statements and find them to be congruent. For example, the baccalaureate *Essentials* (AACN, 2014c) have most of the same concepts discussed in the school's philosophy and state that it: "emphasizes such concepts as patient centered care, interprofessional teams, evidence based practice, quality improvement, patient safety, informatics, clinical reasoning/critical thinking, genetics and genomics, cultural sensitivity, professionalism, and practice across the life span in an ever-changing and complex health care environment" (p. 3). The DNP builds upon the undergraduate and master's programs and as stated by AACN (2014c): "One constant is true for all of these models. The DNP is a graduate degree and is built upon the generalist foundation acquired through a baccalaureate or advanced generalist master's in nursing" (p. 6).

OVERALL PURPOSE AND GOAL OF THE PROGRAM

The school of nursing's overall goal is: "The school of nursing prepares highly competent and compassionate nurses and nurse leaders to deliver professional nursing care and inter-professional health care for multicultural and ethnic people, families, aggregates, and populations in all settings."

The faculty agrees that the goal is broad enough to encompass the undergraduate and graduate programs. Some members raise the question about the term nurse leaders as it applies to the baccalaureate program; however, they agree that leadership in its broadest terms applies to those graduates as well as the graduates of the master's program. They point to the baccalaureate senior level nursing management course as well as the health policy course as foundations for preparing nurse leaders. The overall goal provides guidelines for the end-of-program objectives for all of the tracks and for evaluation of the outcomes of the program. By analyzing the mission and philosophy of the school, terms in the goal statement can be traced back to terms in those statements.

STUDENT LEARNING OUTCOMES (END-OF-PROGRAM) AND LEVEL OBJECTIVES

Both the accelerated RN to MSN program and the entry-level master's program are adaptations of the existing baccalaureate and master's programs. Therefore, the SLOs (end-of-program objectives) are the same as the existing master's program SLOs. Please see Table 9.2 for a listing of the SLOs and the level objectives related to social justice for each of the programs, that is, BSN, entry-level MSN, RN to MSN, MSN, and the DNP. Note the increasing depth in the SLOs from the BSN to the DNP and the alignment with the AACN *Essentials* documents. An analysis of the SLOs for all of these programs demonstrates that the SLOs are congruent with the mission, philosophy, conceptual framework, and overall goal. A model depicting the revised and new programs with their pathways for the school of nursing is presented in Figure 9.2.

TABLE 9.2   SAMPLE STUDENT LEARNING OUTCOMES RELATED TO SOCIAL JUSTICE ACROSS BSN, ENTRY-LEVEL MSN, RN TO MSN, MSN, AND DNP PROGRAMS

YEAR	BSN	ENTRY-LEVEL MSN	RN TO MSN	MSN	DNP
Liberal Arts and Sciences Prerequisites for Nursing	2 years of lower division studies	At least 4 years of previous study with a baccalaureate or higher degree *including* prerequisites for nursing in Liberal Arts and Sciences	RN with at least 2 years of prerequisites for nursing in the Liberal Arts and Sciences *and* ADN or diploma	BSN in nursing or its equivalent (4 years)	BSN or MSN

(*continued*)

TABLE 9.2	SAMPLE STUDENT LEARNING OUTCOMES RELATED TO SOCIAL JUSTICE ACROSS BSN, ENTRY-LEVEL MSN, RN TO MSN, MSN, AND DNP PROGRAMS (*continued*)				
YEAR	BSN	ENTRY-LEVEL MSN	RN TO MSN	MSN	DNP
1	Discuss social justice issues related to the health care delivery system and the role of nursing	Semester 1: Discuss social justice issues related to the health care delivery system and the role of nursing Semester 2: Participate in a nursing or community action group that seeks to address social justice issues	Participate in a nursing or community action group that seeks to address social justice issues	Analyze social justice issues as they apply to nursing and health policy actions for improving the health care delivery system	Evaluate social justice issues by assessing nursing and health care policies and nursing's role as a change agent, client advocate, and leader
2	Participate in a nursing or community action group that seeks to address social justice issues	Analyze social justice issues as they apply to nursing and health policy actions for improving the health care delivery system	Analyze social justice issues as they apply to nursing and health policy actions for improving the health care delivery system	Using a broad understanding of social justice issues, participate in nursing and health care policy actions to improve the health care delivery system	Act as a change agent, client advocate, and leader in the health care delivery system to address social justice issues
3	Continuing to DNP: Analyze social justice issues as they apply to nursing and health policy actions for improving the health care delivery system	Using a broad understanding of social justice issues, participate in nursing and health care policy actions to improve the health care delivery system	Using a broad understanding of social justice issues, participate in nursing and health care policy actions to improve the health care delivery system	Continuing to DNP: Evaluate social justice issues by assessing nursing and health care policies and nursing's role as a change agent, client advocate, and leader	
4	Using a broad understanding of social justice issues, participate in nursing and health care policy actions to improve the health care delivery system	Continuing to DNP: Evaluate social justice issues by assessing nursing and health care policies and nursing's role as a change agent, client advocate, and leader	Continuing to DNP: Evaluate social justice issues by assessing nursing and health care policies and nursing's role as a change agent, client advocate, and leader	Act as a change agent, client advocate, and leader in the health care delivery system to address social justice issues	

(*continued*)

TABLE 9.2 SAMPLE STUDENT LEARNING OUTCOMES RELATED TO SOCIAL JUSTICE ACROSS BSN, ENTRY-LEVEL MSN, RN TO MSN, MSN, AND DNP PROGRAMS (*continued*)

YEAR	BSN	ENTRY-LEVEL MSN	RN TO MSN	MSN	DNP
5	Continuing to DNP: Evaluate social justice issues by assessing nursing and health care policies and nursing's role as a change agent, client advocate, and leader. Act as a change agent, client advocate, and leader in the health care delivery system to address social justice issues	Act as a change agent, client advocate, and leader in the health care delivery system to address social justice issues	Act as a change agent, client advocate, and leader in the health care delivery system to address social justice issues		
6	Act as a change agent, client advocate, and leader in the health care delivery system to address social justice issues				

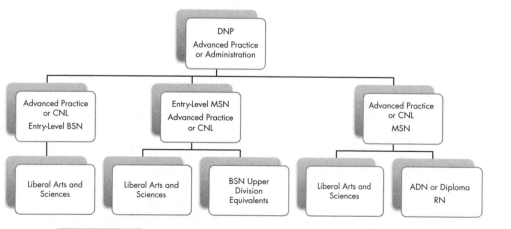

FIGURE 9.2 School of nursing proposed programs with pathways.

BSN PROGRAM

The BSN program is an upper-division-level program; thus students begin nursing courses in the junior year. There are two levels of objectives, level 1 and level 2, with the latter identical to the SLOs (end-of-program objectives). See Table 9.2 for a list of SLOs and level objectives. A sample syllabus from the BSN program appears at the end of this case study.

RN TO BSN TO MSN PROGRAM

In order to move into graduate level courses, RNs complete the equivalent of upper-division-level BSN courses having completed lower division courses in their entry-level nursing programs (ADN or diploma). It is planned that the accelerated RN to BSN to MSN program will take 3 years full time to complete (a part-time option will be available). The first year is one calendar year (three semesters) and students complete the equivalent of upper division nursing courses in the BSN program. Therefore, the level objectives for year 1 of the RN program are the same as the SLOs for the basic BSN. The RNs take many of the same courses that junior and senior students in the BSN program take, that is, pathophysiology, genetics, health assessment, interprofessional health care practice: communication and collaboration, introduction to nursing research, nursing leadership, community health nursing theory and practice, analysis of the health care system, and two upper division general education required core courses. A professional nursing course is the first course that RNs take to bridge concepts from lower division courses to upper division. A sample syllabus for it appears at the end of this case study.

After completing Level 1 courses, the RNs spend two semesters in the first level of the MSN program. They select the advanced practice option they wish to major in, that is, FNP or adult/geriatric ACNP, or the CNL program. The objectives for Level 2 of the RN to MSN program are the same as Level 1 of the MSN program. The Level 3 objectives for the RN to BSN to MSN program are the same as the SLOs of the MSN program (see Table 9.2).

MSN PROGRAM

The existing MSN program has three tracks, that is, FNP, ACNP, and CNL. The full-time program is 2 calendar years long with two summer terms and a part-time option will be available. All students have core courses in nursing theory, research, health care policy, and the advanced pathophysiology, pharmacology, and health assessment courses. Their specialty courses consist of three didactic courses with clinical preceptorships for each. Students complete 600 hours of supervised clinical practice by the end of the program. In addition, students complete either a thesis or project as a capstone experience. Like the BSN program, it has two levels, Level 1 with intermediate objectives and Level 2, which has objectives identical to the SLOs of the MSN program (see Table 9.2). A sample syllabus from the MSN program follows the summary.

ENTRY-LEVEL MSN PROGRAM

The entry-level master's program consists of three levels. The first level is the prelicensure content and is four semesters in length (including a summer session) ending with the SLOs of the BSN program. The second level is at the graduate level, meets graduate Level 1 objectives, and is another three semesters including summer. The third level is three semesters including summer. The level objectives for that year are the same as those of the MSN SLOs. The total program is eight full-time semesters for a total of 3.5 calendar years. A part-time option after completion of the BSN equivalents will be available. A sample syllabus from the entry-level MSN program, which is the same as a Level 2 SLO course in the MSN, follows the summary.

THE DNP PROGRAM

To guide the task force of faculty members who are developing the DNP program, the curriculum committee develops SLOs for the program. As with the other programs in the school, the organizational framework used for the DNP program is the AACN *Essentials of Doctoral Education for Advanced Nursing Practice* (2014c). Upon completion, the committee brings the objectives to the faculty as a whole for approval. Once approved, they go to the DNP task force for developing level objectives and the courses needed for students either from the BSN or postmaster's curricula to meet the objectives. See Table 9.2 for the list of the DNP SLOs.

A sample syllabus from the DNP program follows the summary. It is a course that occurs in the last semester of the DNP program.

SUMMARY

The faculty agrees that the level objectives for the RN to MSN, the entry-level MSN, and the DNP programs come from the SLOs (end-of-program objectives); are learner focused; contain the content of what is to be learned; and specify when they are to be completed and to what extent. The level objectives imply mastery of the content; they must be met by the end of course-work for each level, and are arranged in sequential order. All of the objectives are measurable and serve as guides for collecting data for formative (course, faculty, and level reviews) and summative (program review) evaluation.

Sample courses for the BSN, RN to MSN, the MSN, the entry-level MSN, and the DNP program follow. A concept map for one theme (interprofessional collaboration) that runs throughout the nursing program follows the sample courses (see Figure 9.3).

SAMPLE COURSES

BSN Level 1

Overarching Objective for Level 1 of the BSN Program
Discuss the professional role of nursing and its collaborative role with other health care disciplines.

Course Title: Nursing and Health Care: 3 credits theory
Prerequisite Courses: Completion of lower division level GE requirements, anatomy, physiology, chemistry, genetics, microbiology, nutrition, human development
Description: Introduces the nursing profession, its history, the science of nursing, current issues, and ethics. Discusses the role of the interprofessional health care team. Reviews the definitions of health and the health and illness continuum across the life span.
Objectives: At the end of the course, the student will:
1. Analyze the history of nursing and its impact on its status as a profession and a science.
2. Compare the definitions of a profession and an academic discipline to nursing.
3. Review the major health disciplines and their role in providing health care.
4. Formulate a definition of health and illness across a continuum and the life span for multicultural and ethnic people.
5. Examine selected issues in health care and nursing that have an impact on health care and the ethics for providing nursing care.
Content Outline:
• Nursing History
• Nursing as a Profession
• Nursing as a Science and an Academic Discipline
• The Interprofessional Health Care Team
• Health and Illness Definitions
• Diversity and the Delivery of Competent and Compassionate Nursing Care
• Health Care Issues and the Ethics of Nursing Care

RN to MSN Level 1 (Bridge course between Levels 1 and 2 of the BSN)

Overarching Objective From the SLOs BSN Program
Analyze the professional role of nursing and its collaborative role with other health care disciplines.

Course Title: The Nursing Profession: 3 credits theory
Prerequisite Courses: Graduation with a GPA of 3.0 from an associate degree program in nursing. Diploma graduates must have an overall 3.0 GPA from the diploma program and complete a portfolio to demonstrate equivalency to the ADN.
Description: Reviews nursing education and the profession, the science of nursing, current issues, and ethics. Discusses the role of nursing and collaboration with the interprofessional health care team. Analyzes health and the health and illness continuum across the life span as it applies to the nursing role.

Objectives: At the end of the course, the student will:

1. Analyze nursing education and its impact on its statu science
2. Analyze the nursing profession as an academic disciplii
3. Identify the major health disciplines and their relationsh viding health care
4. Discuss nursing's role in health and illness across its co ... and across the life span for multicultural and ethnic people
5. Analyze selected issues in health care and nursing that have an impact on health care and the ethics for providing nursing care

Content Outline:

- Nursing Education
- Nursing as a Profession
- Nursing as a Science and an Academic Discipline
- Interprofessional Collaboration
- Health and Illness
- Diversity and the Delivery of Competent and Compassionate Nursing Care
- Health Care Issues and the Ethics of Nursing Care

MSN Level 1

Overarching Objective From Level 1 of the MSN Program

Analyze the professional role of nursing and interprofessional collaboration in the delivery of health care through community service and scholarly activities.

Course Title: Advanced Practice and Leadership Roles in Nursing: 3 credits theory
Prerequisite Courses: Admission into the MSN program or completion of Level 1 courses for RN to MSN program or completion of Levels 1 and 2 of the entry-level MSN program.
Description: Reviews the evolution of advanced practice and leadership in nursing and its impact on issues facing the nursing profession and health care. Reviews evidence based advanced practice and leadership in nursing and their place in interprofessional collaboration and quality care in health care delivery system.
Objectives: At the end of the course, the student will:

1. Analyze advanced practice roles in nursing according to their history, regulating issues, ethics, and contributions to the health care system
2. Differentiate among the various levels of leadership roles in nursing and their influence on the delivery of health care
3. Debate evidence-based practice and how advanced practice nurses and the leadership of nursing can bring about change in the health care delivery system
4. Analyze communication and interpersonal relationships for effective collaborative interprofessional strategies
5. Analyze quality assurance methodologies and the role of advanced practice nurses to deliver safe and quality care to multicultural and ethnic clients

Content Outline:
- The history of Advanced Practice Nursing
- Regulation, Certification, and Licensure Issues for Advanced Practice Nursing
- Ethics for Advanced Practice Nurses
- Leadership Concepts Roles in Nursing From the Beginning to Executive Levels
- Evidence-Based Practice for Advanced Practice Nurses and Nurse Leaders
- Delivery of Culturally Competent Advanced Practice Nursing
- What it Takes for Interprofessional Collaboration
- Advanced Practice Nurses and Quality Care and Patient Safety

Entry-Level MSN (same end-of-program course for all tracks of the MSN program)

Overarching Objective From SLOs of the MSN Program
Value the professional role of nursing and interprofessional collaboration in the delivery of health care through community service and scholarly activities.

Course Title: Role Development for Advanced Practice: 2 credits seminar
Prerequisite Courses: Completion of Level 1 courses for the MSN program or its equivalent.
Description: Develops the role for ethical, advanced practice nursing, and leadership in nursing. Analyzes experiences from the clinical setting in evidence-based advanced practice and their effect on interprofessional collaboration, quality of care and patient safety, and changes in the health care delivery system. Discusses current issues in advanced practice roles in nursing.
Objectives: At the end of the course, the student will:
1. Analyze the phases of development to become an advanced practice nurse from novice to expert and the expectations placed upon self and the health care system for the novice advanced practice nurse
2. Analyze ethical dilemmas in advanced practice nursing
3. Analyze clinical experiences in the delivery of evidence-based advanced practice for multicultural and ethnic clients
4. Analyze clinical experiences in the role of the advanced practice nurse and effective strategies for interprofessional collaboration in the delivery of safe and quality health care
5. Present a persuasive case for a current issue in advanced practice nursing and how professional nursing can bring about change in the health care system
Content Outline:
- Theories and Concepts Related to Professional Socialization in Advanced Practice Roles
- Ethical Issues Confronting Advanced Practice Nurses in the Health Care System
- Leadership and Change Theories
- Evidence-Based Advanced Practice Nursing for Multicultural and Ethnic Clients
- Safe and Quality Care Through Effective Interprofessional Collaboration
- Current Issues in Advanced Practice Nursing
- The Art of Persuasion

DNP (One of the End-of-Program Courses)

Overarching Objective From the SLOs of the DNP Program
Assume leadership in health care systems through nursing and interprofessional collaboration in the delivery of health care through advanced practice, community service, and scholarly activities.

Course Title: Forum on the DNP Role: 2 credits seminar
Prerequisites: Completion of previous four semesters of course work in the DNP program.
Course Description: Evaluates the role of advanced practice and leadership in nursing to bring about change in the health care delivery system.
Objectives: At the end of the course, the student will:

1. Analyze the health care system and nursing profession for needed changes to deliver safe and quality health care to multicultural and ethnic clients
2. Synthesize evidence-based advanced practice strategies and interprofessional collaboration to demonstrate examples of their impact on changes in the health care delivery system
3. Evaluate leadership strategies that bring about change in the health care delivery system

Content Outline:
* Current State of the Health Care Delivery System Related to the DNP Role
* Current State of the Nursing Profession and its Educational System and the DNP Role
* Current State of Interprofessional Collaboration and the DNP Role
* Strategies for the Application of Change Theories to the Health Care System and Nursing Practice
* Leadership Strategies for Macrosystems and the DNP Role

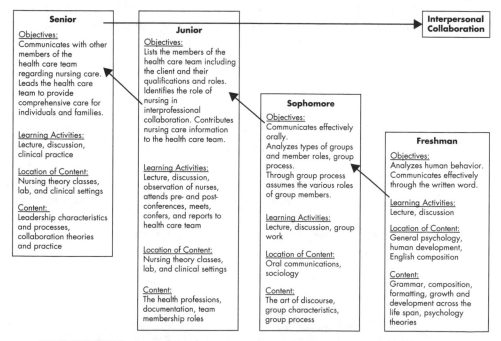

FIGURE 9.3   Concept map for interprofessional collaboration at the BSN level.

Figure 9.3 is an example of the beginning of a concept map for the theme of interprofessional collaboration that is threaded through the various levels of the BSN curriculum in the case study curriculum. To complete the concept map, faculty list the relevant course objectives and the learning activities that contribute to the objectives for the graduate level programs.

DISCUSSION QUESTIONS

1. Which component(s) of the curriculum do you believe has(have) the most impact on the implementation of the curriculum?
2. In which ways do you believe organizational frameworks serve to ensure quality of the educational program? Give an example of an organizational framework that illustrates your belief.
3. Why do you agree or disagree with the principle of faculty control of the curriculum?

LEARNING ACTIVITIES

STUDENT LEARNING ACTIVITIES

1. Using the "Guidelines for Assessing the Key Components of a Curriculum or Educational Program," assess the educational program in which you are enrolled for the components of the curriculum. Are they easily identified? What resources do you need to locate them?
2. Attend one or more Curriculum Committee meetings and identify which of the components of the curriculum are addressed. Observe faculty members' interactions, their commitment to curriculum development and evaluation, and the role they play in developing or revising the curriculum. Note evidence of the routes of approval for any changes to the curriculum.

NURSE EDUCATOR/FACULTY DEVELOPMENT ACTIVITIES

1. Using the "Guidelines for Assessing the Key Components of a Curriculum or Educational Program," assess the educational program in which you teach for the components of the curriculum. Are they easily identified? What resources do you need to locate them?
2. When you attend the next Curriculum Committee meeting, identify which of the components of the curriculum are addressed. Observe faculty members' interactions, their commitment to curriculum development and evaluation, and the role they play in developing or revising the curriculum. Note evidence of the routes of approval for any changes to the curriculum.

REFERENCES

Accreditation Commission for Education in Nursing. (2013). *Accreditation manual, standards and criteria*. Retrieved from http://www.acenursing.net/manuals/SC2013.pdf

Adeniran, R. K., & Smith-Galsgow, M. E. (2010). Creating and promoting a positive learning environment among culturally diverse nurses and students. *Creative Nursing, 16*(2), 53–58.

Aduddell, K. A., & Dorman, G. E. (2010). The development of the next generation of nurse leaders. *Journal of Nursing Education, 49*(3), 168–171.

Affordable Care Act. (2014). Health and human services. Retrieved from http://www.hhs.gov/healthcare/rights/index.html

Agency for Healthcare Research and Quality. (2014). *Home page. Department of health and human services*. Retrieved from http://www.ahrq.gov

American Association of Colleges of Nursing. (2010). *Fact sheet: The doctor of nursing practice*. Retrieved from http://www.aacn.nche.edu/Media/pdf/FS_dnp.pdf

American Association of Colleges of Nursing. (2014a). *AACN advances nursing's role in interprofessional education. News release*. Retrieved from http://www.aacn.nche.edu/news/articles/2012/ipec

American Association of Colleges of Nursing. (2014b). *AACN essential series*. Retrieved from http://www.aacn.nche.edu/Education/curriculum.htm

American Association of Colleges of Nursing. (2014c). *The essentials of baccalaureate education for professional nursing practice*. Retrieved from http://www.aacn.nche.edu/Education/bacessn.htm

American Association of Colleges of Nursing. (2014d). *Nursing fact sheet*. Retrieved from http://www.aacn.nche.edu/media-relations/fact-sheets/nursing-fact-sheet

American Nurses Association. (2014). *Code of ethics for nurses*. Retrieved from http://nursingworld.org/MainMenuCategories/ThePracticeofProfessionalNursing/EthicsStandards/CodeofEthics.aspx

Barnsteiner, J., Disch, J., Johnson, J., McGuinn, K., & Swartwout, E. (2013). The quality and safety education for nurses (QSEN) initiative began in 2005 and has rapidly gained traction in enhancing nursing curricula, practice-academic partnerships, and clinical practice. *Journal of Professional Nursing, 29*(2), 68.

Bednarz, H., Schim, S., & Doorenbos, A. (2010). Cultural diversity in nursing education: Perils, pitfalls, and pearls. *Journal of Nursing Education, 49*(5), 253–260.

Berg, J. A., & Pace, D. T. (2010). Health promotion/risk reduction and disease prevention in women's health. Editorial. *Journal of the American Academy of Nurse Practitioners, 22*, 57–59.

Beuttler, F. W. (2012). Moral philosophy in a social scientific age: A proposal to reintegrate the undergraduate curriculum. *Christian Higher Education, 11*(2), 81–93.

Bloom, B. S., et al. (Eds.). (1956). *Taxonomy of educational objectives: Handbook I, cognitive domain*. New York, NY: D. McKay.

Boyer, E. (1990). *Scholarship reconsidered: Priorities of the professoriate*. Princeton, NJ: Carnegie Foundation for the Advancement of Teaching.

Broussard, E. (2009). *The power of place on campus*. Washington, DC: The Chronicle of Higher Education.

Carnegie Foundation for Advancement of Teaching. (2014). *Classification descriptions*. Retrieved from http://classifications.carnegiefoundation.org/descriptions/index.php

Chan, Z. C. Y. (2013). A systematic review of critical thinking in nursing education. *Nurse Education Today, 30,* 236–240.

Colder, W. B. (2011). Institutional VVM statements on websites. *The Community College Enterprise, 17*(2), 19–27

Comer, L., Whichcello, R., & Neubrander, J. (2013). An innovative master of science program for the development of culturally competent nursing leaders. *Journal of Cultural Diversity, 20*(2), 89–93.

Commission on Collegiate Nursing Education. (2014). *About CCNE.* Retrieved from http://www.aacn.nche.edu/Accreditation/AboutCCNE.htm

Cox, B. E., McIntosh, K. L., Reason, R. D., & Terenzini, P. T. (2011). A culture of teaching: Policy, perception, and practice in higher education. *Research in Higher Education, 53,* 808–829.

Dacey, M., Murphy, J. I., Anderson, D. C., & McCloskey, W. W. (2010). An interprofessional service-learning course: Uniting students across educational levels and promoting patient-centered care. *Journal of Nursing Education, 49*(12), 696–699.

Dearman, V., Lawson, R., & Hall, H. R. (2011). Concept mapping a baccalaureate nursing program: A method for success. *Journal of Nursing Education, 50*(11), 656–659.

Debourgh, G. A. (2012). Synergy for patient safety and quality: Academic and service partnerships to promote effective nurse education and clinical practice. *Journal of Professional Nursing, 28*(1), 48–61.

DeBrew, J. K. (2010). Perceptions of liberal education of two types of nursing graduates: The essentials of baccalaureate education for professional nursing practice. *The Journal of General Education, 59,* 42–58.

DeSavo, M. R. (2010). Genetics and genomics resources for nurses. *Journal of Nursing Education, 49*(8), 470–474.

Didion, J., Kozy, M. A., Koffel, C., & Oneail, K. (2013). Academic/clinical partnership and collaboration in quality and safety education for nurses education. *Journal of Professional Nursing, 29*(2), 86–94.

Disch, J. (2012). What's QSEN? *Nursing Outlook, 60*(2), 58–59.

Douglas, M. K., Pierce, J. U., Rosenkoetter, M., Pacqulao, D., Callister, L. C., Hattar-Pollara, M., . . . Purnell, L. (2011). Standards of practice for culturally competent nursing care: Update. *Journal of Transcultural Nursing, 22*(4), 317–333.

Dudas, K. I. (2012). Cultural competence: An evolutionary concept analysis. *Nursing Education Perspectives, 33*(5), 317–321.

Elkins, D. J., Forrester, S. A., & Noël-Elkins, A. V. (2011). Student perceived sense of campus community: The influence of out-of-class experiences. *College Student Journal, 45*(1), 105.

Ervin, L., Carter, B., & Robinson, P. (2013). Curriculum mapping: Not as straightforward as it seems. *Journal of Vocational Education and Training, 65*(3), 309–318.

Fahrenwald, N. L., Taylor, J. Y., Kneip, S. M., & Canales, M. K. (2007). Academic freedom and academic duty to teach social justice: A perspective and pedagogy for public health nursing faculty. *Public Health Nursing, 24*(2), 190–197.

Finkelman, A., & Kenner, C. A. (2014). *Learning IOM: Implications of the IOM reports for nursing education.* Washington, DC: American Nurses Association.

Flood, L., Gasiewicz, N., & Delpier, T. (2010). Integrating information literacy across a BSN curriculum. *Journal of Nursing Education, 49*(2), 101–104.

Fuggazato, S. J. (2009). Mission statement, physical space, and strategies in higher education. *Innovative Higher Education, 34*(5), 285-298.

Grady, P. A. (2010). Translational research and nursing science. *Nursing Outlook, 58*(3), 164–166.

Greener, S. L. (2010). Plasticity. The online learning environment's potential to support varied learning styles and approaches. *Campus Wide Information Systems, 27*(4), 254–262.

Greenwald, D. (2010). Faculty involvement in undergraduate research: Considerations for nurse educators. *Nursing Education Perspectives, 31*(6), 368–371.

Healthy People 2020. (2012). HHS announces new health promotion, disease prevention agenda. *The American Nurse, 44*(1), 9.

The Human Genome Project. (2014). Retrieved from http://www.genome.gov/10001772

Improvement Science Research Network (ISRN). (n.d.). *ISRN resource list.* Retrieved from www.isrn.net/ISRNResourceList

Institute of Medicine. (2001). *Crossing the quality chasm: A new health system for the 21st century.* Committee on Quality of Health Care in America, Institute of Medicine. Washington DC: National Academies Press.

Institute of Medicine. (2010). *The future of nursing: Leading change, advancing health.* Washington, DC; National Academies Press.

Kelly, A. (2013). The cost conundrum: Financing the business of health care insurance. *Journal of Health Care Finance, 39*(4), 15–27.

Kelly, M. D., & Starr, T. (2013). Shaping service-academia partnerships to facilitate safe and quality transitions in care. *Nursing Economics, 31*(1), 6–11.

Lapum, J., Hamsavi, N., Veljkovic, K., Maohamed, Z., Pettinato, A., Sliver, S., & Taylor, E. (2012). A performative and poetic narrative of critical social theory in nursing education: An ending and threshold of social justice. *Nursing Philosophy, 13,* 27–45.

Lathrop, B. (2013). Nursing leadership in addressing the social determinants of health. Policy, *Politics & Nursing Practice, 14*(1), 41–47.

Lea, D. H., Skirton, H., Read, C. Y., & Williams, J. K. (2011). Implications for educating the next generation of nurses on genetics and genomics in the 21st century. *Nursing Scholarship, 43*(1), 3–12.

Logan, J. E., Pauling, C. D., & Franzen, D. B. (2011). Health care policy development: A critical analysis model. *Journal of Nursing Education, 50*(1), 55–58.

Majette, G. R. (2011). PPCA and public health. Creating a framework to focus on prevention and wellness and improve the public's health. *Journal of Law, Medicine, and Ethics, 39*(3), 366–379.

Matthews, R. L., Parker, B., & Drake, S. (2012). Healthy ager: An interprofessional service learning, town-and-gown partnership. *Nursing Education Perspectives, 33*(3), 162–165.

Meacham, J. (2008). What's the use of a mission statement? *Academe, 94*(1), 21–24.

Merriam-Webster. (2014). *Dictionary.* Retrieved from http://www.merriam-webster.com/dictionary/philosophy

Micari, M., & Pazos, P. (2012). Connecting to the professor: Impact of the student-faculty relationship in a highly challenging course. *College Teaching, 60*(2), 41–47.

Miller, B. K. (1988). A model for professionalism in nursing. *Today's OR Nurse, 19*(9), 18–23.

Milton, C. L. (2012). Ethical implications and interprofessional education. *Nursing Science Quarterly, 4,* 313–315.

Morphew, C. C., & Hartley, M. (2006). Mission statements: A thematic analysis of rhetoric across institutional type. *The Journal of Higher Education, 77(3),* 456–471.

National Center for Advancing Translational Sciences. (2014). *About NCATS.* Retrieved from http://www.ncats.nih.gov/about/about.html

National Council of State Boards of Nursing. (2013). 2010 NCLEX-RN *detailed test plan.* Retrieved from https://www.ncsbn.org/2010_NCLEX_RN_Detailed_Test_Plan_Educator.pdf

National League for Nursing. (2014a). *Competencies for graduates of associate degree and diploma programs.* Retrieved from http://www.nln.org/facultyprograms/competencies/comp_ad_dp.htm

National League for Nursing. (2014b). *NLN outcomes and competencies for graduates of nursing programs.* Retrieved from http://www.nln.org/facultyprograms/Competencies/graduates_competencies.htm

Nguyen, D. N., Zierler, B., & Nguyen, H. Q. (2011). A survey of nursing faculty needs for training in use of new technologies for education and practice. *Journal of Nursing Education, 50*(4), 181–189.

Nickitas, D. M. (2013). The cost of care in America: $2.7 Trillion. *Nursing Economics, 30*(4), 161, 170.

Novak, J. D., & Cañas, A. J. (2013). *The theory underlying concept maps and how to construct and use T=them. Technical report.* Retrieved from http://cmap.ihmc.us/Publications/ResearchPapers/TheoryCmaps/TheoryUnderlyingConceptMaps.htm

Nurses earn highest ranking ever, remain most ethical of professions in poll. (2013). *Georgia Nursing, 73*(1), 9.

Pavil, B. (2011). Fostering creativity in nursing students: A blending of nursing and the arts. *Holistic Nursing Practice, 25*(1), 17–25.

Piscotty, R., Grobbel, C., & Abele, C. (2013). Initial psychometric evaluation of the nursing quality and safety self-inventory. *The Journal of Nursing Education, 52*(5), 269–274.

The Princeton Review. (2001). *The best 331 colleges (2002 edition).* New York, NY: Princeton Review Publishing.

Pulcini, J. (2013). Update of the patient protection and affordable care act. *American Journal of Nursing, 113*(4), 25–27.

Quality and Safety Education for Nursing. (2014). *Funded by the Robert Wood Johnson foundation.* Retrieved from http://www.qsen.org

Quality and Safety Education in Nursing Institute. (2014). *About QSEN.* Retrieved from http://qsen.org/about-qsen

Regan, M., & Pietrobon, R. (2010). A conceptual framework for scientific writing in nursing. *Journal of Nursing Education, 49*(8), 437–443.

Rhodes, M. K., Schutt, M. S., Langham, G. W., & Bilotta, D. E. (2012). The journey to professionalism: A learner-centered approach. *Nursing Education Perspectives, 33*(1), 27–29.

Sheu, L., Lai, C. J., Coelho, A. D., Lin, L. D., Zheng, P., Hom, P., . . . O'Sullivan, P. S. (2010). Impact of student-run clinics on preclinical sociocultural and interprofessional attitudes: A prospective cohort anaylsis. *Journal of Health Care for the Poor and Underserved, 23*(3), 1058–1072.

Smith, M., & McCarthy, M. P. (2010). Disciplinary knowledge in nursing education. *Nursing Outlook, 58*(1), 44–51.

Stevens, K. R. (2013). The impact of evidence-based practice in nursing and the next big ideas. *Online Journal of Issues in Nursing, 18*(2).

Thibault, G. E. (2011). Interprofessional education: An essential strategy to accomplish the future of nursing goals. *Journal of Nursing Education, 50*(6), 313–317.

Tonkin, E., Calzone, K., Jenkins, J., Lea, D., & Prows, C. (2010). Genomic resources for nursing faculty. *Nursing Scholarship, 43*(4), 330–340.

Troxler, H., Jacobson Vann, J. C., & Oermann, M. H. (2011). How baccalaureate nursing programs teach writing. *Nursing Forum, 46*(4), 280–288.

U.S. Department of Health and Human Services. (2014). *About the law.* Retrieved from http://www.hhs.gov/healthcare/rights/index.html

U.S. Department of Health and Human Services, Health Resources and Services Administration. (2014). *Health professions. Nursing grant programs.* Retrieved from http://bhpr.hrsa.gov/nursing/index.html

VickyRN. (2014). Entry into practice: *Diploma programs for registered nursing.* Retrieved from http://allnurses.com/showthread.php?t=422071

Wolkowitz, A. A., & Kelley, J. A. (2010). Academic predictors of success in a nursing program. *Journal of Nursing Education, 49*(9), 498–503.

Curriculum Planning for Associate Degree Nursing Programs

Karen E. Fontaine

Upon completion of Chapter 10, the reader will be able to:

1. Apply the steps involved in curriculum development and evaluation to associate degree prelicensure nursing education programs
2. Analyze current regulatory, accreditation, political, and social factors that may affect the development and revision of associate degree prelicensure nursing education curricula
3. Provide examples of evolving pedagogies that can be used in curriculum development and evaluation for associate degree prelicensure nursing education programs
4. Describe current national issues that affect prelicensure associate degree in nursing (ADN) educational programs

Chapter 10 begins with the history of ADN prelicensure nursing education programs. A description of the current status of this type of nursing program is presented as well as the pressures on this type of program in the context of dramatic health care and education system changes. The process of developing and evaluating ADN education curriculum follows. Sample associate degree curricular components are included.

The development of curricula for associate degree prelicensure programs follows the steps that were previously outlined in Chapter 9. Attention to the process of curriculum development or revision helps ensure that graduates of any type of program meet desired outcomes. The forces that guide the curriculum are the same for all programs: National accreditation and state regulatory standards, social and political climates, the health care industry, economic situations, and the profession of nursing.

THE HISTORY OF ASSOCIATE DEGREE NURSING

The current model of ADN education providing entry into practice began after World War II when there was a nursing shortage. Haase (1990), in describing the sequence of events leading to the development of associate degree programs, states that in 1948, the Committee on the Functions of Nursing made a recommendation that nursing practice consist of two tiers of nurses, one professional and the other technical. An educational model for the community college setting was developed intended to educate a technical nurse, with a more limited scope of practice than a professional nurse, but broader than that of a practical nurse.

During the same post-wartime period, community colleges were expanding as a result of pressure from veterans and consequent increased funding. Several pilot studies implemented the above nursing education model in the community college setting, and found that there was little difference in the graduates of associate degree programs than those from the existing university and diploma educational systems (Haase, 1990). Although the model was subsequently implemented, the practice issue of technical versus professional nurse was not addressed. The model did, however, provide an evolutionary educational step by moving nursing education from the type of apprentice program (diploma) that was controlled by hospitals and physicians to the college and university system (Orsilini-Hain & Waters, 2009).

CURRENT STATUS OF ASSOCIATE DEGREE NURSING

Today's nursing workforce in the United States consists of four levels of basic or prelicensure nursing preparation: diploma, associate degree, baccalaureate, and entry-level master's. ADN programs provide the majority of nursing education, 45% (U.S. Department of Health and Human Services, 2010), comprising 60% of prelicensure programs (National League for Nursing [NLN], 2013), and graduating 63% of all registered nurses. Two thirds of all prelicensure RN enrollees are associate degree students (NLN, 2013).

Part of the attraction of ADN programs is that they are affordable and provide streamlined access to the nursing profession. The Urban Institute (2009) emphasized that many rural and underserved communities rely on community colleges for their nursing workforce. These programs also have the largest number of minorities, educating rural nurses in underserved areas, who are employed where they work (National Organization for Associate Degree Nursing [N-OADN], 2012). The NLN (2013) states that there has been a recent substantial increase in the percentage of associate degree students aged 30 years old, highlighting the maturity and second-degree nature of the students.

All nursing education programs are currently under great pressure to create a more educated nursing workforce due to health care reform. Associate degree programs, however, are also being forced to reduce credit requirements for the degree. These combined forces could result in a "perfect storm," threatening ADN education itself, according to Sportsman and Allen (2011).

A more educated nursing workforce is needed in the current health care environment because nurses are expected to fill roles that are increasingly complex, sophisticated, and expanded. The Institute of Medicine (IOM) called for 80% of nurses to hold a bachelor's nursing degree by 2020 (IOM, 2010). Leaders within the nursing profession call for an increase in the number of nurses prepared at the baccalaureate level due to the need to advance the profession. Donley and Flaherty (2008) state that advanced educational preparation is needed in order for nurses to sit in on policy discussions and as members of governing boards. Smith (2009) concurs, stating that because nurses are the least educated of the major health care professionals, they are currently less likely to be included in discussions on health care policy.

The pressure on nursing education to prepare nurses at a higher educational level comes from research into patient outcomes as well. In 2006, Murray (2006) stated that there was an accumulating body of research showing a positive relationship between increased nursing educational preparation and improved patient outcomes. A landmark study by Aiken, Clarke, Cheung, Sloane, and Silber (2003) found that a 10% increase in nurses with a bachelor's degree was associated with a 5% decrease in the likelihood of patients dying within 30 days of admission. There was also an increase in the odds of a patient being rescued from a life threatening event. Although the IOM (2010) concludes that the relationship between academic degree and patient outcomes is not established, Zimmerman, Miner, and Zittle (2010) list five research reports as evidence that there is a relationship between the level of nursing education and improved patient outcomes. The National Advisory Council on Nurse Education and Practice (2010) concurs.

Calls for a more educated nurse due to a revised health care system are occurring at the same time that ADN programs are being asked to reduce program length, change structure, and redesign curriculum and content. Recently, under pressure from the U.S. Department of Education, the Accreditation Commission for Education in Nursing (ACEN) revised its standards to require that ADN programs have a curriculum that allows students to complete all requirements, including prerequisites, within five semesters and between 60 and 72 credits (ACEN, 2013).

Most associate degree programs require at least 3 years of study, if not more. Credit creep can easily result when the inclusion of recommendations for content in genetics/genomics, gerontology, community health, perioperative care, pharmacology, bioterrorism, mass casualty response, health economics, cultural competence, health policy, palliative and end-of-life care, evidence-based practice, assessment, interprofessional team management, leadership, and informatics is implemented. There are also the multiple specialty standards from the American Nurses Association (2013) in pediatrics, oncology, critical care, and mental health/psychiatric practice to consider. Regulatory organizations such as the National Council of State Boards of Nursing and individual State Boards of Nursing also require specific content. Finally, general education and sciences courses may be either corequisite or prerequisite for admission into nursing programs.

The current pressures on ADN programs provide an opportunity to improve educational models, and clarify their purpose. There is widespread support for creating models within the nursing education system that honor and preserve the existing associate and baccalaureate nursing education programs and increase the percentage of bachelor of science in nursing (BSNs). The National Advisory Council on Nurse Education and Practice (2010), a group that advises the federal government and Congress, suggests that partnerships between ADN and BSN programs are methods for attaining the goal of increasing the proportion of BSNs in the workforce. Several states allow community colleges to confer baccalaureate degrees in nursing (Orsilini-Hain & Waters, 2009).

A curriculum that fosters dual enrollment of students from the start of their nursing education is suggested by Hall, Causey, Johnson, and Hayes, (2012). The IOM (2010) concurs, promoting a seamless transition for all levels of nursing into higher degree programs, believing that the capacity exists within the system. An example of such a transition is provided by the Oregon Consortium for Nursing Education (OCNE) whose member schools allow for seamless and automatic enrollment for ADN to BSN programs (Munkvold, Tanner, & Hendrickx, 2012). A shared pathway, combined with agreements among the community colleges and universities that participate in the consortium, creates the expectation and availability for students to continue their education and receive their BS degree (OCNE, 2013).

CURRICULUM REFORM IN ASSOCIATE DEGREE EDUCATION

Health care reform is driving the need for a changed nursing education model as care is moved from the hospital to different practice settings (IOM, 2010). The IOM believes that nursing students need to be to competent in such areas as health policy, financing, leadership, quality improvement, and systems thinking since graduates are called on to work within teams and lead care coordination efforts. No longer can nurses learn everything they need to know about content areas of maternity, mental health, pediatrics, and medical–surgical nursing.

Benner, Sutphen, and Day (2009), in a study of professional nursing education, found that schools of nursing were not current in responding to changes in the practice setting, nor were they successful in teaching nursing science, natural sciences, social sciences, technology, and the humanities. The authors issued a "call to action" for nursing education, stating that the profound changes in nursing practice demand equally profound changes in nursing education (Benner et al., 2009). Curricular reform is needed for all of nursing education, but the requirement is intensified for associate degree programs that must accomplish this with fewer credits and in a context of radical change.

COMPONENTS OF AN ASSOCIATE DEGREE CURRICULUM

Nursing programs exist within a context of regulation, accreditation, professional standards, and an educational milieu. Any nursing program that educates prelicensure candidates for registered nursing must adhere to regulations and standards. At the national level, the National Council of State Boards of Nursing (2012) developed a model nurse practice act that offers guiding principles to all state boards of nursing for regulation of education and practice. ADN programs are offered accreditation status by ACEN, which maintains and updates national accreditation standards. Current standards for associate degree programs can be found at www.acenursing.net/manuals/SC2013_ASSOCIATE.pdf.

Nursing programs that exist within a public or private educational institution may also need to meet regional accreditation standards for the parent institution, such as the Northwest Commission on Colleges and Universities or national accrediting agencies such as the Accreditation Commission for Independent Colleges and Schools. Both public and privately funded schools may belong to a larger national or statewide system that has additional requirements.

MISSION OR VISION

ACEN (2013) accreditation standards for ADN programs require that the nursing program's mission and/or philosophy reflect the governing organization's core values and be congruent with the outcomes, strategic goals, and objectives. When developing or revising the mission and philosophy statements, the faculty and leaders of the nursing program should develop the program's mission in relation to those of the institution. Recommended sources of guidance are other programs within a system or programs that are similar or have good reputations. An ongoing program evaluation process ensures that the mission statement is continuously evaluated, both for congruence and currency. A sample mission statement presented with permission from Western Nevada College in Carson City, Nevada, a state-funded community college, reflects the program's purpose. "The mission of the nursing program at Western Nevada College is to meet the nursing educational needs of the service area. The program prepares qualified students to function as entry-level registered nurses and to transfer to higher degree programs" (Western Nevada College, 2013). Samples of the curriculum from Western Nevada College will be used to illustrate a traditional model of ADN education in this chapter.

In an effort to meet the challenges posed by the IOM, Carnegie Foundation, and the NLN, the NLN Education Competencies Work Group (NLN, 2010) was formed. The group developed program outcomes and competencies for each type of educational program in nursing and an Education Competencies Model that can be used as a framework to develop curriculum. The model is also used in this chapter to illustrate the development of parts of a fictional ADN program's curriculum based on the model. A mission statement for a college based on the work of the NLN Education Competencies Model might be "to provide students with the knowledge, practice, and ethical comportment competencies needed to practice within the nursing profession."

PHILOSOPHY STATEMENTS

The philosophy flows from the mission statement and reflects the beliefs of the program's faculty and staff about nursing, nursing education, students, teaching and learning, critical thinking, and evidence-based practice. These are generally longer statements that help guide curricular development and content. Table 10.1 offers sample philosophy statements from the fictional ADN program that were developed based on the NLN Education Competencies Model (NLN, 2010).

TABLE 10.1   PHILOSOPHY OF A FICTIONAL ADN PROGRAM BASED ON THE NLN EDUCATION COMPETENCIES MODEL

COMPONENT	DEFINITION
Person	A person is an individual with biological, psychological, social, cultural, spiritual, and developmental dimensions. A person's health is influenced by his or her constant interaction with the environment and has the potential to flourish.
Environment	Environment impacts the person through interaction with internal and external components.
Health	Health consists of wellness and illness dimensions with both subjective and objective aspects, but is always seen from the perspective of the person
Nurse	The nurse functions within an interprofessional practice model to provide nursing care, education, and leadership utilizing clinical decision making as an integral process. Nurses affirm and embrace the value of each person respecting the dignity, behaviors, environment, social norms, cultural values, physical characteristics, and religious beliefs and practices of each limitation. They reach out to those who are vulnerable. Nurses continually update knowledge and skills. They are committed to continuous growth with a goal of excellence within themselves and the environment in which they practice.
Nursing	Nursing is a dynamic, evolving art and science discipline that involves the application of knowledge, skills, and attitudes based in the behavioral and biological sciences. Nursing is a caring profession that promotes health, healing, and hope in response to human conditions. Professional nursing practice is based upon standards of practice and an ethical and legal framework.
Learning	Learning is a continuous process that involves changes in knowledge, practice, and ethical behavior. Teaching and learning are shared processes that support personal and professional development and stimulate inquiry. The student is a self-directed learner who is committed to lifelong learning.

Source: NLN (2010).

ORGANIZATIONAL FRAMEWORK

Curriculum components common to the various types of educational programs of nursing were described previously in Chapter 9. Although an organizational framework based on a nursing theorist is not required by accrediting bodies, it can be useful to illustrate or diagram how the curricular components interact and fit together.

Applying a simple house analogy can also be used to help explain the function, structure, and purpose for each part of a curriculum and how they work together. The foundation of a house can be seen as the mission and vision, providing support to the overall curriculum. The infrastructure, sewer, water, and fire and police services in the construction analogy, and the parent institution and the social and political setting in a college setting, are dependent on location and the resources available. These must be considered when building the curriculum.

Next is the building frame, providing support for the roof, ceilings, and walls. This is the organizational framework of the curriculum that provides a common theme and envelops the curriculum in form and structure. The rooms in the building are thus the courses and content, such as gerontology, family health, wellness, illness, or diversity. All of the disparate rooms in the structure have ceilings, floors, and a common purpose—the curriculum threads, or concepts that run throughout the program (see Figure 10.1).

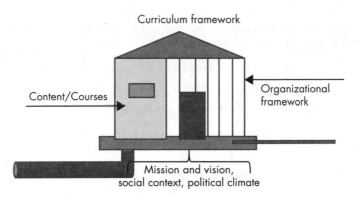

FIGURE 10.1 Curriculum framework.

Many programs have core values, defining fundamental beliefs that go beyond the philosophy of nursing, health, environment, teaching, and learning. The NLN Work Group defined seven core values as fundamental to nursing: caring, diversity, ethics, excellence, holism, integrity, and patient-centeredness (NLN, 2010). They are illustrated at the foundation of the model, showing that nursing must be grounded in these fundamental values.

STUDENT LEARNING OUTCOMES

Establishing learner outcomes and assessing whether students achieve those outcomes are required by accrediting agencies. According to ACEN (2013), student learning outcomes (SLOs) are used to organize the curriculum, guide the delivery of instruction, direct learning activities, and evaluate student progress. SLO statements are broad and describe desired and expected behaviors of the program's graduates and differ from program outcomes such as first time NCLEX-RN® graduate pass rates, retention rates, employment rates, and program satisfaction. The SLOs should be reflected in level and course objectives.

Quality and Safety Education for Nurses (QSEN) provides an example of competencies that can be used to embed safety and quality outcomes within a curriculum for nurses. QSEN developed a comprehensive listing of the knowledge, skills, and attitudes (KSAs) necessary to continuously improve the quality and safety of the care that nurses provide (QSEN, 2010).

Table 10.2 offers sample SLOs for a fictional associate degree program, which were based on the NLN Education Competencies Model (NLN, 2010) and the QSEN project (QSEN, 2014).

TABLE 10.2   NURSING PROGRAM STUDENT LEARNING OUTCOMES BASED ON THE NLN EDUCATION COMPETENCY MODEL

Cares for patients and families while facilitating self-determination, integrity, and growth as a human being

Acknowledges the patient as the source of control and forms a partnership based on patient preferences, values, and needs

Makes clinical judgments in practice, substantiated with evidence and science to provide safe, quality care

Minimizes risk of harm to patients individually and by using appropriate systems

Uses information and technology to communicate, manage knowledge, avoid error, and support decision making

Implements individual practices that reflect personal and professional integrity, responsibility, and ethical practices

Works within nursing and interprofessional teams, using open communication, mutual respect, and shared decision making

Uses the evidence that underlies clinical nursing practice to question assumptions and change practice

Uses data to monitor the outcomes of care and implements improvement methods to continuously improve the quality and safety of health care systems

Integrates best current evidence with clinical expertise and patient/family preferences and values

Source: NLN (2010).

PROGRAM OF STUDY CONCEPTS

In response to the transformational movement called for in nursing education, there is a trend in toward the adoption of a concept-based curriculum (Faison & Montague, 2013). As the IOM points out, "There simply are not enough hours in the day or years in an undergraduate program to continue compressing all available information into the curriculum" (IOM, 2010, p. 191). Stating that new approaches should be developed, they recommend the presentation of concepts that have application to different contexts rather than having students memorize facts and information for each condition (IOM, 2010).

Derived from middle-range theories, concepts help to shape and frame knowledge gained (OCNE, 2013). They are embedded within each course and guide the focus of care and the related evidence-based interventions. Benner (2013) recommends providing a definition for each concept and then introducing it with a real patient condition that evolves from practice—an exemplar. Repetition of the concept by different exemplar conditions in increasing complexity helps the student apply the understanding to practice. Benner states that new concepts should be introduced with new exemplars and then the relationship between concepts be explored in order to teach students to use creative thinking in practice. She explains that in order to use content knowledge well, clinicians have to be able to grasp the nature of the clinical situation and recognize the knowledge, evidence, and theories that are most pertinent to that situation.

Selecting the concepts to be used for a revised curriculum is not an easy task for faculty. The concepts should reflect those large ideas or related groups of processes that are important and relevant to nursing and current health care problems. Exemplars chosen should be based on hospital discharge data, prevalence of diseases or conditions, and public and community health concerns.

Several good resources are available that offer examples and help in selecting those most important for each individual program. The North Carolina Curriculum Improvement Project (2008) developed a website that provides extensive resource documents, including concepts and exemplars and the rationale for inclusion. In addition, the authors describe the integration of these within the curriculum. Several textbooks are also available to support concept-based teaching and learning.

PROGRAM OF STUDY

There are many practical matters to consider in developing and revising nursing programs of study. Course sequencing, program length, prerequisite and corequisite courses, and admission criteria should be based on national and regional standards as well as any respective State Board of Nursing regulations. ACEN (2013) standards require that the nursing program length must meet state and national standards, and best practices. The parent college or university establishes requirements for corequisite and general education courses that must be included within the program of study.

ADN programs were designed at inception to require only 2 years of instruction (Orsilini-Hain & Waters, 2009). However, additive curricula and the increasing complexity of nursing practice expanded the curricula, which now must be re-evaluated in order to serve its graduates. In revising curriculum, each program needs to determine what students need in order to be successful in their program's nursing curriculum, and course SLOs need to flow from program SLOs. The nursing faculty must create or revise a curriculum that includes classroom, laboratory, simulation, and clinical experiences, while ensuring that the students meet the program objectives and SLOs.

A typical program of study is presented by Western Nevada College in Carson City, Nevada. It is a state supported associate degree program, accredited by the ACEN and the regional accrediting body, the Northwest Commission on Colleges and Universities. Table 10.3 illustrates the program of study.

TABLE 10.3 ASSOCIATE OF APPLIED SCIENCE IN NURSING PROGRAM OF STUDY, WESTERN NEVADA COLLEGE, CARSON CITY, NEVADA

TOTAL REQUIREMENTS: 71 UNITS (CREDITS)		
PREREQUISITE COURSES*		**21 UNITS (CREDITS)**
BIOL 223**	Human Anatomy and Physiology I	4
BIOL 224**	Human Anatomy and Physiology II	4
BIOL 251	General Microbiology	4
ENG 101	Composition I	3
MATH 120	Fundamentals of College Mathematics	3
or MATH 126	Precalculus I	
or higher MATH course		
PSY 101	General Psychology	3
or SOC 101	Principles of Sociology	

*Chemistry: Show evidence of completion of high school chemistry from a regionally accredited school within the past 3 years or completion of CHEM 121 (4 units) or CHEM110 (4 units) within 10 years of program application. ** BIOL 223 and BIOL 224 must be completed at the same college or university at an institution if not completed within the Nevada System of Higher Education. Science prerequisites must be completed no more than 10 years prior to the semester of application to the nursing program.

FIRST YEAR: FALL SEMESTER COURSES		13 UNITS (CREDITS)
ENG 102*	Composition II	3
NURS 136	Foundations of Nursing Theory	3
NURS 137	Foundations of Nursing Laboratory	1
NURS 138	Foundations of Nursing Clinical	2
NURS 147	Health Assessment Theory	2
NURS 148	Health Assessment Laboratory	1
NURS 152	Foundations of Pharmacology in Nursing I	1

*Indicates corequisite. Corequisite courses must be completed by the end of the fourth semester of the nursing program.

FIRST YEAR: SPRING SEMESTER COURSES		14 UNITS (CREDITS)
NURS 149	Mental Health and Illness Theory	3

(*continued*)

TABLE 10.3	ASSOCIATE OF APPLIED SCIENCE IN NURSING PROGRAM OF STUDY, WESTERN NEVADA COLLEGE, CARSON CITY, NEVADA (*continued*)

TOTAL REQUIREMENTS: 71 UNITS (CREDITS)		
NURS 151	Mental Health and Illness Clinical	1
NURS 153	Foundations of Pharmacology in Nursing II	1
NURS 165	Medical–Surgical Nursing I Theory	3
NURS 166	Medical–Surgical Nursing I Laboratory	1
NURS 167	Medical–Surgical Nursing I Clinical	2
PSY 101*	General Psychology	3
or SOC 101*	Principles of Sociology	

*Indicates corequisite. Corequisite courses must be completed by the end of the fourth semester of the nursing program.

SECOND YEAR: FALL SEMESTER COURSES		12 UNITS (CREDITS)
NURS 263	Nursing Care Childbearing Family Theory	2
NURS 264	Nursing Care of the Childbearing Family Laboratory	1
NURS 265	Nursing Care of the Childbearing Family Clinical	1
NURS 270	Advanced Clinical Nursing I Theory	3
NURS 271	Advanced Clinical Nursing I Clinical	2
U.S./Nevada Constitutions Course (PSC 103, HIST 111, or CH 203 recommended)*		3

*See the Associate of Applied Science page for more information on courses fulfilling the general education requirement.

SECOND YEAR: SPRING SEMESTER*		11 UNITS (CREDITS)
NURS 266	Pediatric Nursing Theory	2
NURS 267	Pediatric Nursing Laboratory	1
NURS 268	Pediatric Nursing Clinical	1
NURS 276	Advanced Medical–Surgical Nursing II Theory	3

(*continued*)

TABLE 10.3	ASSOCIATE OF APPLIED SCIENCE IN NURSING PROGRAM OF STUDY, WESTERN NEVADA COLLEGE, CARSON CITY, NEVADA (*continued*)	
TOTAL REQUIREMENTS: 71 UNITS (CREDITS)		
NURS 277	Advanced Medical–Surgical Nursing II Clinical	2
NURS 284	Role of the ADN Manager of Care	2

*Indicates corequisites. Co-requisite courses must be completed by the end of the fourth semester of the nursing program.
Source: Western Nevada College (2013). Used with permission.

ASSESSMENT

The achievement of SLOs must be evaluated by the faculty as a means of determining the quality of instruction and overall improvement needs (ACEN, 2013). Through regular and systematic assessment, each program must demonstrate that students who complete their programs, no matter where or how they are offered, have achieved these outcomes. For nursing programs, this means that each course within a nursing curriculum must have course and content learning outcomes or objectives that guide the delivery of content. These are the important and measureable behaviors or competencies for students of the course.

Level objectives for each semester or year are developed to assess the expected performance at specific points. All objectives and program learning outcomes are measureable so that they can be assessed at each step within the program. If results are less than expected, curriculum and instructional changes should be made that are based on evidence. ACEN (2013) standards and criteria can be used to establish a method of curriculum review that offers evaluation of both student learning and of the curriculum itself. Table 10.4 offers some sample course objectives for one course that relates to the program SLOs for the fictional program.

TABLE 10.4	STUDENT LEARNING OUTCOMES FOR A FICTIONAL HEALTH ASSESSMENT COURSE
AT THE COMPLETION OF THE COURSE THE STUDENT WILL BE ABLE TO:	

Perform a health history that includes the patient's developmental status, culture, family, values and other unique human needs
Apply therapeutic communication techniques during assessment demonstrating patient centeredness
Identify physical and clinical data that enable the nurse to make judgments based on evidence in order to plan care
Discuss the ways that informatics and technology can help communicate assessment findings within the interprofessional team
Identify the data that would be gathered during evaluation of the care plan in order to establish whether there have been improved health outcomes for a patient
Interpret assessment findings in order to develop additional questions for the nurse and other needs for additional data
Illustrate components of assessment findings that the nurse could use as a stimulus for further interprofessional collaboration

SUMMARY

This chapter applied the components of the curriculum to an ADN program. Details specific to ADN regulations and accreditation standards as well as community college education were provided. Examples were given using an existing curriculum in use at a public, state supported communities college as well as a fictional program using the NLN Nursing Education Competencies Model (2010). Curriculum development and evaluation, no matter what the setting, is a responsibility of the faculty members. They are responsible for the development, implementation, and ongoing evaluation process. The examples provided here and the needs assessment process described in Chapters 6 and 7 can provide guidance for use by ADN programs and faculty.

LEARNING ACTIVITIES

STUDENT LEARNING ACTIVITIES

1. Define the term "concept" and discuss various concepts that might be used to develop an organizing framework for an ADN program, and the process that could be used to apply the framework.
2. Explore the ACEN standards for ADN programs, Standard 4, which can be found at www.acenursing.net/manuals/SC2013_ASSOCIATE.pdf. Discuss how the Standard 4 criterion can be used to evaluate curriculum. Here are sample evaluation criteria derived from the criterion.
   a. Are current professional standards, guidelines, or competencies used to guide the curricular design and incorporated into the curriculum?
   b. Are the SLOs used to organize the curriculum, guide delivery of courses, and direct learning activities?
   c. Are evaluation methodologies varied and appropriate to measure attainment of learning outcomes?
   d. Is there regular review by the faculty of the curriculum for rigor and currency?
   e. Do the general education courses enhance nursing knowledge?
   f. Does the curriculum address best practices?
   g. Does the curriculum include diverse concepts and experiences?
   h. Does the program of study provide time for student to learn and achieve the outcomes?
   i. Are the clinical learning experiences appropriate for students to achieve the identified outcomes/competencies? Reflective of best practices and national safety standards?
   j. Are the contracts for clinical experiences current and designed to protect students?
   k. Are the delivery methodologies congruent with the curricular design?

NURSE EDUCATOR/FACULTY DEVELOPMENT ACTIVITY

1. Compare your associate degree curriculum with standards presented by your state's Nurse Practice Act or Board of Nursing.

REFERENCES

Accreditation Commission for Education in Nursing. (2013). *NLNAC 2013 standards and criteria associate.* Retrieved from http://www.acenursing.net/manuals/SC2013_ASSOCIATE.pdf

Aiken, L. H., Clarke, S. P., Cheung, R., B., Sloane, D., M., & Silber, J., H. (2003). Educational levels of hospital nurses and surgical patient mortality. *Journal of the American Medical Association, 290*(12), 1617–1623. Retrieved from http://www.ncbi.nlm.nih.gov/pubmed/14506121

American Nurses Association. (2013). *Scope and standards of practice.* Retrieved from http://www.nursingworld.org/scopeandstandardsofpractice

Benner, P. (2013). *Re-conceptualizing the curricular and pedagogical uses of concepts in nursing education.* Retrieved from http://www.educatingnurses.com/articles/re-conceptualizing-the-curricular-and-pedagogical-uses-of-concepts-in-nursing-education

Benner, P., Sutphen, M., Leonard, V., & Day, L. (2009). *Educating nurses: A call for radical transformation.* San Francisco, CA: Jossey-Bass.

Donley, R., & Flaherty, M. J. (2008). Revisiting the American Nurses Association's first position on education for nurses: A comparative analysis of the first and second position statements on the education of nurses. OJIN: *The Online Journal of Issues in Nursing, 13(2).*

Faison, K., & Montague, F. (2013). Paradigm shift: Curriculum change. *The ABNF Journal, 24*(1), 21–22.

Haase, P. T. (1990). *The origins and rise of associate degree nursing education.* Durham, NC: Duke University Press.

Hall, V. P., Causey, B., Johnson, M. P., & Hayes, P. (2012). Regionally increasing baccalaureate-prepared nurses: Development of the RIBN model. *Journal of Professional Nursing. 28*(6), 377–380.

Institute of Medicine. (2010). *The future of nursing: Leading change, advancing health report recommendations.* Retrieved from http://www.iom.edu/media/Files/Report-percent20Files/2010/The-Future-of-Nursing/Futurepercent20ofpercent20Nursingpercent202010percent20Recommendations.pdf

Munkvold, J., Tanner, C. A., & Henrinckx, H. (2012). Factors affecting the academic progression of associate degree graduates. *Journal of Nursing Education, 51*(4), 232–235.

Murray, C. (2006). Advancing the profession of nursing: A new approach. *Journal of the New York State Nurses Association,* Fall/Winter 2006, *37*(2), 22–25.

National Advisory Council on Nurse Education and Practice. (2010). *Addressing new challenges facing nursing education- solutions for a transforming healthcare environment.* Eighth Annual Report to the Secretary of the U.S. Department of Health and Human Services and the U.S. Congress. Rockville, MD: Health Resources and Services Administration, U.S. Department of Health and Human Services.

National Council of State Boards of Nursing. (2012). *Nurse practice acts guide and govern nursing practice.* Retrieved from https://www.ncsbn.org/2012_JNR_NPA_Guide.pdf

National League for Nursing. (2010). *Outcomes and competencies for graduates of practical/vocational, diploma, associate degree, baccalaureate, master's practice doctorate and research doctorate programs in nursing.* New York, NY: Author.

National League for Nursing. (2013). *Annual Survey of Schools of Nursing, Fall 2012.* Retrieved from http://www.nln.org/researchgrants/slides/pdf/AS1112_F01.pdf

National Organization for Associate Degree Nursing. (2012). *Academic progression: N-OADN position statement.* Retrieved from https://www.noadn.org/component/option,com_docman/Itemid,250/task,doc_download/gid,399

North Carolina Curriculum Improvement Project. (2008). *Curriculum files.* Retrieved from http://adn-cip.waketech.edu/curriculumfiles.html

Oregon Consortium for Nursing Education. (2013). *Organization of the OCNE curriculum.* Retrieved from http://ocne.org/curriculum-org.html

Orsilini-Hain, L., & Waters, V. (2009). Education evolution: A historical perspective of associate degree nursing. *Journal of Nursing Education, 48*(5), 266–271.

Quality and Safety Education for Nurses. (2014). *Project overview.* Retrieved from http://qsen.org/about-qsen/project-overview

Smith, T. (2009). A policy perspective on the entry into practice issue. OJIN: *The Online Journal of Issues in Nursing, 15*(1).

Sportsman, S., & Allen, P. (2011). Transitioning associate degree in nursing students to the Bachelor of Science in nursing and beyond: a mandate for academic partnerships. *Journal of Professional Nursing, 6,* e20–e27.

Urban Institute. (2009). *Public policy for a dynamic and complex market: The nursing workforce challenge.* Retrieved from http://www.urban.org/publications/411933.html

U.S. Department of Health and Human Services. (2010). *Registered nurse population: Findings from the 2008 national sample survey of registered nurses. Retrieved from* http://bhpr.hrsa.gov/healthworkforce/rnsurveys/rnsurveyfinal.pdf

Western Nevada College. (2013). *Nursing program/degree, associate of applied science.* Retrieved from http://www.wnc.edu/academics/degrees/aas/nur

Zimmerman, D. T., Miner, D. C., & Zittle, B. (2010). Advancing the education of nurses a call for action. *The Journal of Nursing Administration, 40*(12), 529–533.

Curriculum Planning for Baccalaureate Nursing Programs

Peggy Wros

Pamela Wheeler

Melissa Jones

OBJECTIVES

Upon completion of Chapter 11, the reader will be able to:

1. Summarize current trends in prelicensure baccalaureate nursing education
2. Describe the integration of the *Essentials of Baccalaureate Education for Professional Nursing Practice* as a foundation for developing a bachelor of science in nursing (BSN) curriculum
3. Explain the process of developing or revising an existing BSN curriculum
4. Summarize innovation in nursing education, including models of clinical instruction and interprofessionalism
5. Develop a plan for collaboration with a community/service organization to create an academic-practice partnership model for clinical education
6. Analyze the relationship between generic, accelerated bachelor of science in nursing (ABSN), and registered nurse to BSN (RN to BSN) programs
7. Evaluate the challenges for graduate residency programs that facilitate transition into practice
8. Design a curriculum plan and program of study for a baccalaureate program in your institution

OVERVIEW

Chapter 11 provides an overview of the process of curriculum development for baccalaureate nursing programs. It reviews the utilization of the American Association of Colleges of Nursing (AACN) *Essentials of Baccalaureate Education for Professional Nursing Practice* (2008b) in curriculum development and discusses fast track programs and RN to BSN programs. This chapter summarizes the advantages and challenges related to residency/externship programs for the new graduate. The following outlines the content of the chapter.

- When is it time for curriculum change?
  - The baccalaureate essentials
  - Recommendations for curriculum reform
  - Advances in educational technology
  - The learning-centered paradigm
- Curriculum development
  - Conceptual framework
  - Curriculum outcomes
  - Identifying courses
- BSN curriculum design: Special considerations
  - Content overload in nursing curricula
  - The inclusive curriculum: Paying attention to diversity
  - Interprofessional education (IPE): Preparing for collaborative practice
  - Transformative approaches to clinical education
- Completing the curriculum development process
- Transition to practice
- Alternative baccalaureate pathways
  - Accelerated baccalaureate programs
  - Baccalaureate completion programs
- Summary

WHEN IS IT TIME FOR CURRICULUM CHANGE?

Nursing is at the crossroads of major societal changes in health care reform, technology, and educational accountability, and the Institute of Medicine (IOM) has recommended an increase in the number of baccalaureate prepared nurses (IOM, 2010). The population of the United States is becoming more diverse, the income gap is widening, and baby boomers are aging. Veterans are returning from war and the country is experiencing a prolonged recovery from the economic recession. All of these factors affect the kind of programs that are offered at schools of nursing, the content of the curricula, and the way that faculty teach in nursing education.

In order to prepare graduates of prelicensure nursing education programs for practice in an ever-changing health care environment, baccalaureate nursing curricula must be revised or updated on a regular basis. Nursing schools rely on a robust evaluation plan to provide information that guides curriculum revision. In addition, there are compelling factors external to individual nursing programs that influence the need for curricular change within baccalaureate nursing programs across the country. These are reflected in the *Essentials of Baccalaureate Education for Professional Nursing Practice* (AACN, 2008b) and include expressed concern with the quality of prelicensure nursing education by health care organizations, advances in education and health technology, and educational research that identifies more effective teaching–learning strategies.

THE BACCALAUREATE ESSENTIALS

The *Essentials* (AACN, 2008b) reflect current priorities in: (1) health care, including expanded emphasis on quality and safety, patient technology, patient-centered care, population health, health care regulation, and globalization; (2) nursing education, with a focus on the liberal arts and information management; and (3) professional nursing practice, which is grounded in evidence-based practice, interprofessional communication and collaboration, and enduring social values. See Table 11.1 for a list of the *Essentials* (AACN).

TABLE 11.1   *THE ESSENTIALS OF BACCALAUREATE EDUCATION FOR PROFESSIONAL NURSING PRACTICE*

Essential I: Liberal Education for Baccalaureate Generalist Nursing Practice
- A solid base in liberal education provides the cornerstone for the practice and education of nurses

Essential II: Basic Organizational and Systems Leadership for Quality Care and Patient Safety
- Knowledge and skills in leadership, quality improvement, and patient safety are necessary to provide high-quality health care

Essential III: Scholarship for Evidence-Based Practice
- Professional nursing practice is grounded in the translation of current evidence into one's practice

Essential IV: Information Management and Application of Patient Care Technology
- Knowledge and skills in information management and patient care technology are critical in the delivery of quality patient care

Essential V: Health Care Policy, Finance, and Regulatory Environments
- Health care policies, including financial and regulatory, directly and indirectly influence the nature and functioning of the health care system and thereby are important considerations in professional nursing practice

Essential VI: Interprofessional Communication and Collaboration for Improving Patient Health Outcomes
- Communication and collaboration among health care professionals are critical to delivering high-quality and safe patient care

Essential VII: Clinical Prevention and Population Health
- Health promotion and disease prevention at the individual and population level are necessary to improve population health and are important components of baccalaureate generalist nursing practice

Essential VIII: Professionalism and Professional Values
- Professionalism and the inherent values of altruism, autonomy, human dignity, integrity, and social justice are fundamental to the discipline of nursing

Essential IX: Baccalaureate Generalist Nursing Practice
- The baccalaureate graduate nurse is prepared to practice with patients, including individuals, families, groups, communities, and populations across the life span and across the continuum of health care environments
- The baccalaureate graduate understands and respects the variations of care, the increased complexity, and the increased use of health care resources inherent in caring for patients

---

Source: AACN (2008b).

The *Essentials* (AACN, 2008b) are supported by landmark documents such as IOM reports (2001, 2003) and related Quality and Safety Education for Nurses (QSEN) competencies that include indicators for patient-centered care, teamwork and collaboration, evidence-based practice, quality improvement, safety, and informatics (Cronenwett et al., 2007). Other compelling and influential documents that impact nursing curricula include Healthy People 2020 (U.S. Department of Health and Human Services [HHS], 2011), the professional nursing study supported by the Carnegie Foundation for the Advancement of Teaching (Benner, Sutphen, Leonard, & Day, 2010), and numerous research and position papers authored by a variety of key health care and educational organizations. The *Essentials* (AACN) are the foundation for BSN curriculum development and will be referenced frequently throughout the discussion in this chapter.

RECOMMENDATIONS FOR CURRICULUM REFORM

There is significant concern with the preparedness of entry-level nurses to provide quality care within the complex and changing health care environments in which they practice. In addition, the shortage of nursing faculty and reduced capacity of clinical sites compel nurse educators to reconsider more traditional models of prelicensure clinical education. A national survey conducted by the National League for Nursing indicated that barriers to clinical education include lack of integration between theory and clinical components of the curriculum, inadequate preparation of clinical preceptors, and outdated clinical practice skills of supervising faculty (Jacobson & Grindel, 2006). The IOM (2001, 2010) clearly recommends a mandate for change in health care education, compelling schools of nursing to focus on patient-centered quality and safety in the health care system. Benner et al. (2010) describe a practice–education gap, which must be addressed by improving the quality of nursing education. The American Organization of Nurse Executives (AONE) (2004) took the position that the nurse of the future will need different skills, baccalaureate preparation will be necessary to meet the demands of practice, and BSN education must be "reframed" in order for graduates to be prepared. Additional reports from practice settings indicate that new graduates of prelicensure programs are not adequately prepared for nursing practice and therefore require additional development of clinical skills and professional competencies postgraduation (Forbes & Hickey, 2009; Hickey, 2009; Hofler, 2008).

ADVANCES IN EDUCATIONAL TECHNOLOGY

Advances in educational technology and web-based learning radically altered the process of prelicensure nursing education and affect the structure of the curriculum. As digital natives, students are often more technologically competent than faculty and expect current learning technology to be incorporated into the curriculum for interactive learning (Bleich, 2009; Skiba, 2007). Computer-based simulations such as the virtual neighborhood or community (Curran, Elfrink, & Mays, 2009; Giddens, 2007) and interactive avatars (Kidd, Knisley, & Morgan, 2012; Skiba, 2009) are examples of innovations that are woven throughout the structure of the curriculum. Applications are available for teaching students to use electronic health records (Gardner & Jones, 2012; Johnson & Bushey, 2011). Distance education and high-fidelity simulation learning strategies have been expanded and integrated into BSN programs.

Distance Education

Online learning is increasingly integrated into nursing education, although application of web-based approaches varies widely between nursing programs. Quality standards, such as Quality Matters (www.qualitymatters.org), have been developed for online education and faculty development and instructional design support are essential to ensure the effective delivery of online coursework (Anderson & Tredway, 2009; Little, 2009). The web-enhanced classroom can be used to supplement learning through online activities such as discussion boards, resource-sharing, exams, videos, or other virtual programming (Creedy et al., 2007). While specific nonclinical courses may be taught online or offered as an alternative method of delivery in prelicensure programs, they may be the primary pedagogy for baccalaureate completion programs (Anderson & Tredway, 2009). Distance applications include electronic classrooms and videoconferencing that facilitate inclusion of rural students and teaching across college campuses, or to facilitate supervision for students involved in off-site practicum experiences. New software applications are proliferating and significantly expand the resources available for educators. The availability of distance education technologies and the related philosophy of an academic institution toward their use as a teaching–learning methodology have significant implications for the curriculum development.

High-Fidelity Simulation

While nursing educators have long employed low- and mid-fidelity simulation in nursing skills labs, high-fidelity simulation has become the "gold standard" as schools of nursing incorporate this teaching strategy into curricula to prepare students for clinical experiences and to supplement or replace clinical hours. Using this technology, faculty can create standardized and realistic clinical learning activities that ensure that all students get experience with critical patient-care situations in a variety of health care settings, including mental health and community, in a low-risk and supportive environment (Nehring, 2008). High-fidelity simulation has the potential to improve student knowledge, skill performance, clinical reasoning and judgment, role identity, and self-confidence (Cordeau, 2012; Harder, 2010; Ironside, Jeffries, & Martin, 2009; Sinclair & Ferguson, 2009). Simulated learning experiences can be developed to support the progressive achievement of curriculum outcomes by intentionally spiraling core concepts and skills throughout the curriculum in increasingly more complex scenarios (Dubose, Sellinger-Karmel, & Scoloveno, 2010). Interprofessional simulations can provide an opportunity for students to learn about teamwork and collaboration and the roles of other health care professions (Baker et al., 2008; Buckley et al., 2012; McGuire-Sessions & Gubrud, 2010; Reese, Jeffries, & Engum, 2010; Riesen, Morley, Clendinneng, Ogilvie, & Murray, 2012; Scherer, Myers, O'Connor, & Haskins, 2013).

It must be noted, however, that there is little evidence regarding how high-fidelity simulation compares to traditional clinical approaches, and it is fairly costly and time intensive for faculty (National Council of State Boards of Nursing [NCSBN], 2009). Depending on the goal of instruction, lower fidelity simulation can be an effective alternative (Sharpnack & Madigan, 2012). Simulation using live actors as standardized patients is also a powerful strategy with the potential to change attitudes, beliefs, and behaviors among student participants (Bornais, Raiger, Krah, & El-Masri, 2012; Luctkar-Flude, Wilson-Keates, & Larocque, 2012; Noone, Sideras, Gubrud-Howe, Voss, & Mathews, 2012; Ward, Cody, Schaal, & Hojat, 2012).

The focus in simulation in nursing education has been primarily on learning, including prebriefing and debriefing, with less emphasis on more high-stakes summative evaluation (Cordeau, 2012). In planning for use of simulation in a curriculum, schools are advised to check with their State Board of Nursing regarding regulations for percentage or replacement of clinical hours with high-fidelity simulation (Nehring, 2008). In order to make the best use of this technology, simulation must be approached with vision and intention in the curriculum development process (Harder, 2010).

THE LEARNING-CENTERED PARADIGM

There have been significant advancements in educational research that improve understanding of how students learn. For over a generation, college educators have developed innovative approaches to interactive learning in higher education and there is a significant body of knowledge that provides evidence for the effectiveness of these practices (American Association of Colleges and Universities, 2007). Over a decade ago, Weimer (2002) described a paradigm shift in learning-centered education in which the power in the classroom is shared between teacher and students, content becomes less important than the reflective construction of knowledge, teachers become coaches, students assume responsibility for their learning, and authentic learning assessment is incorporated into the curriculum.

Nurse educators have made a case for moving away from the traditional content-laden behaviorist paradigm to a constructivist learning-centered model in which students are active participants. The traditional lecture and testing approach to instruction has been expanded to include narrative pedagogies, such as storytelling, reflective journaling, and literature interpretation (Brown, Kirkpatrick, Mangum, & Avery, 2008; Diekelman, 2005), cooperative or team-based learning (Andersen, Strumpel, Fensom, & Andrews, 2011; Hanson & Carpenter, 2011), and problem-based learning (Williams, 2001; Yuan, Williams, & Fin, 2007). Faculty are "flipping the classroom" by assigning readings and online lectures as homework and focusing on discussion and application of concepts in class (Bergman & Sams, 2012; Missildine, Fountain, Summers, & Gosselin, 2013). The Carnegie Foundation's nursing education study supports significant innovation in prelicensure nursing education and recommends expansion of authentic pedagogies that focus on patient experiences, such as clinical simulation scenarios, unfolding case studies, and clinical conferences focused on reflection about student experiences (Benner et al., 2010). These recommendations call for significant changes not only in the structure and organization of the program of study but also the way the curriculum is delivered. As an example, Nielsen, Noone, Voss, and Mathews (2013) describe a model of clinical learning activities that take into consideration the developmental needs of the learner.

Nursing educators are being challenged to seize the opportunity and challenge of developing new programs of study for prelicensure students for the 21st century and beyond. The creative wisdom of nursing faculty, grounded in educational expertise and experience and in collaboration with practice partners, has the potential to shape a more effective, relevant, and responsive system of nursing education.

CURRICULUM DEVELOPMENT

The curriculum reflects the heart and soul of a nursing faculty. For each school, at least some of the current faculty were most likely involved in developing the existing curriculum and are invested in its success. The curriculum expresses the faculty's values and beliefs about nursing and education, and reflects their professional identity. Faculty members have educated and mentored many students through the program and their courses have been the core of their daily work—in some cases, for many years. The curriculum is familiar and comforting. These factors mean that curriculum change is one of the most challenging undertakings for any faculty. It may prove difficult to build consensus about a new program based on different values and priorities among a diverse group of faculty members. Some faculty members have kept up with best practices and innovation in nursing education, while others are content with the status quo. Ideally curriculum revision is driven by the faculty and begins with an agreement by the faculty as a whole to enter into the process.

Once a decision has been made to revise an existing curriculum or develop a new curriculum, next steps include selecting a work group or committee, developing a plan, and exploring best practices in nursing education. The composition of the group that will be leading the work of developing the curriculum is of primary importance to the success of the endeavor, and the members should be selected with intention. A strong team includes a diverse group of tenured and untenured faculty with various areas of expertise and backgrounds that are committed to the goal, motivated to do the difficult work of curriculum development, and able to work collaboratively through the process of change (Mawn & Reece, 2000). In addition to faculty with passion for curriculum, a balanced group includes both faculty members with current practice experience and those with expertise by virtue of their long teaching careers. Nursing students bring a unique and practical perspective to the work and their participation enriches the curriculum development process. As the group organizes, a discussion about roles within the committee and ground rules facilitates the process. One strategy recommended by Hull, St. Romain, Alexander, Schaff, and Jones (2001) is for one member of the committee to assume the role of facilitator to make sure that the ground rules are followed and to mediate the inevitable conflicts. An early discussion of bias, territoriality concerns, and "sacred cows" contributes to the process. Other suggestions include a tentative plan and timeline to help the group to stay on schedule, and a plan for communicating the progress of the curriculum revision and points for feedback from the faculty as a whole.

The initial preparatory work of the curriculum development group is to review program evaluation data and plan a variety of strategies to identify best practices in nursing education. The extent of this effort will depend on the time elapsed since the last curriculum revision and the extent of the planned revision. The following information and documents will inform the committee and provide data for difficult discussions and decision making.

- The *Essentials* (AACN, 2008b) document is foundational and should be made available to all members from the beginning. The document includes rationale, performance indicators, and sample content for each essential that are helpful in understanding the scope of each statement for application to a particular program of study
- A comprehensive search of the literature identifies best practices and innovation in nursing education; synthesizing the information for the faculty as a whole facilitates shared understanding (Forbes & Hickey, 2009; Hull et al., 2001)
- A review of professional standards such as the American Nurses Association *Code of Ethics* (2005) and various published competencies for BSN graduates is important. Based on current issues and priorities in nursing practice, specific baccalaureate level competencies have been developed for quality and safety (Cronenwett et al., 2007); cultural competency (AACN, 2008a); genetics and genomics (AACN, 2006); geriatric nursing care (AACN & John A. Hartford Foundation, 2010), and end-of-life care (AACN, 1998)
- A survey of other regional and national programs provides examples of model programs of study. Programs that have been recently updated and incorporate innovation, have similar missions, and have been recently accredited may be of most value
- Focus groups or surveys of stakeholders including students, faculty, and clinical or community partners provide invaluable information regarding expectations and priorities and create an inclusive process. These surveys provide meaningful local information about what was working and not working in the old curriculum, suggested changes or direction, new information and trends to be aware of, and priority knowledge and skills to include in the new curriculum

Information in this chapter is relevant to the development or revision of curricula for several types of baccalaureate programs that will be addressed, including 4-year traditional collegiate nursing programs, transfer programs in which students complete prerequisites and general education courses before entering the nursing program, accelerated (or fast-track) bachelor's degree programs, and RN completion programs. If a school has more than one type of program, there must be consistency and congruency among programs. The suggested approach is to start with development of the generic prelicensure program and then develop modifications based on the core curriculum model. Examples of documents that describe the recent curriculum revision at Linfield-Good Samaritan School of Nursing (LGSSON) at Linfield College are presented throughout the chapter and supplemented by descriptions of innovations from other BSN programs.

The process of curriculum development is an iterative process of discovery, and the components of the curriculum package generally remain flexible until all parts are completed to allow for new insights and learning of the curriculum development team and the faculty. The curriculum development process begins with values clarification and development of a mission, vision, philosophy, and a specific goal or purpose of the program (as described in Chapter 9). These statements must be consistent with that of the parent institution and underlie all nursing programs at the school.

CONCEPTUAL FRAMEWORK

The conceptual framework (theoretical or organizational model) guides the development of the program of study and makes it unique; it unifies the curriculum and creates a coherent approach across courses and levels (Ervin, Bickes, & Schim, 2006). While there are some curricular elements that are common among schools based on the *Essentials* (AACN, 2008b), others define the particular identity of the program based on the characteristics of the parent institution and the philosophy of the nursing program. Traditional academic nursing frameworks no longer reflect the complexity of nursing education or practice. The use of a single theorist is an outdated approach and most nursing programs have an eclectic model that reflects their values and priorities (McEwen and Brown, 2002). The meta-paradigm for nursing that includes the key concepts of person, environment, health, and nursing is no longer an adequate foundation for an educational program (Webber, 2002). Theoretical models for BSN programs have shifted away from nursing process to critical thinking (McEwen & Brown, 2002) and reflect alternatives for the biomedical model that more closely reflect nursing concepts and values. If the theoretical model is basic and broad, it is possible for it to encompass and support a variety of views of practice and education that may be held by faculty (Ervin et al., 2006) and allow for new developments in nursing and health care (Newman, 2008).

The LGSSON Theoretical Model for Community-Based Nursing Education is grounded in the *Baccalaureate Essentials* and serves as an organizational structure for the curriculum. Figure 11.1 is a visual model of the LGSSON theoretical framework and reflects the school's community-based philosophy. The outer circles provide context for the curriculum. The concepts of *global community* and *social justice* are a reflection of the mission statements of both the college and school of nursing. *Health promotion, illness prevention, and treatment* are not only a focus for global health, but priorities for *local communities* and health care reform. Within the school's *community of learning*, the focus is on *learner-centered education*, which drives how students and faculty are engaged together on a journey of inquiry. The innermost circles of the model describe the content and approaches that structure the curriculum. *Professional education* reflects recommendations by the Carnegie Foundation for the Advancement of Teaching (Benner et al., 2010). The *curricular themes* of communication, community, diversity, ethics, health, and stewardship are foundational curricular concepts that are spiraled throughout the program of study and focus student outcomes. The *modes of inquiry* emphasize how the curricular themes and professional knowledge are acquired. For example, the faculty utilizes a clinical reasoning model that draws on evidence-based, reflective practice. Clinical praxis seminars are facilitated in such a way that reflective inquiry becomes a way of learning with the students. The *liberal education* circle again reflects the mission of the college and the school of nursing. This model was developed and approved by the faculty as a whole following extensive discussions.

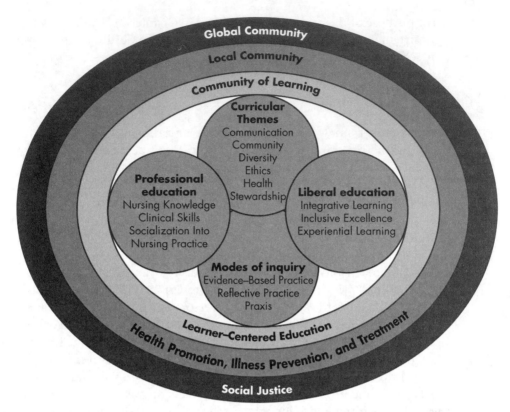

FIGURE 11.1   Linfield-Good Samaritan School of Nursing Theoretical Model for Community-Based Nursing Education.

CURRICULUM OUTCOMES

The next step in the BSN curriculum development process is to identify level and terminal or end-of-program outcomes/student learning outcomes (or objectives or competencies), which must be directly related to the *Essentials* (AACN, 2008b) in the context of the school's philosophy. Mapping is a strategy for ensuring that all elements of the *Essentials* (AACN) are included (see Chapter 9). Whether a school uses outcomes, objectives, or competencies to create the curricular structure, the term must be defined, used consistently, and leveled across the program. The outcomes form the backbone of the curriculum and will be the foundation for program evaluation. Student learning outcomes (end-of-program outcomes) can be developed by reviewing each essential and writing outcome statements that address the key concepts. This task can be completed either by the curriculum development group or be more inclusive and involve the faculty as a whole by assigning a small group of individuals to write outcomes for specific *Essentials* (AACN). When all outcome statements are reviewed and analyzed as a package, there will most likely be overlap and areas that need to be strengthened in preparing the final document. As the outcomes statements are combined and synthesized, some may address more than one essential, but all *Essentials* (AACN) must be addressed. When the terminal outcomes are identified, the level outcomes are developed and spiraled to show students' progression through the program. Table 11.2 gives an example of curriculum outcomes as they relate to the *Essentials* (AACN).

TABLE 11.2	MAPPING OF CURRICULUM OUTCOMES AND ESSENTIALS
CURRICULUM OUTCOMES	ESSENTIALS
1. Engages in ethical reasoning and actions that demonstrate caring and commitment to social justice in the delivery of health care to individuals and populations	I: Liberal Education for Baccalaureate Generalist Nursing Practice V: Health Care Policy, Finance, and Regulatory Environments VII: Clinical Prevention and Population Health VIII: Professionalism and Professional Values
2. Uses a range of information and clinical technologies to achieve health care outcomes for clients	II: Basic Organizational and Systems Leadership for Quality Care and Patient Safety III: Scholarship for Evidence-Based Practice IV: Information Management and Patient Care Technology IX: Baccalaureate Generalist Nursing Practice
3. Communicates effectively and collaboratively to provide client-centered nursing care in various health care communities	I: Liberal Education for Baccalaureate Generalist Nursing Practice VI: Interprofessional Communication and Collaboration for Improving Health Outcomes VIII: Professionalism and Professional Values IX: Baccalaureate Generalist Nursing Practice
4. Applies principles of stewardship and leadership skills to support quality and safety within complex organizational systems	II: Basic Organizational and Systems Leadership for Quality Care and Patient Safety
5. Provides effective nursing care that incorporates diverse values, cultures, perspectives, and health practices	I: Liberal Education for Baccalaureate Generalist Nursing Practice VII: Clinical Prevention and Population Health VIII: Professionalism and Professional Values IX: Baccalaureate Generalist Nursing Practice
6. Incorporates a liberal arts–based understanding of global health care issues to promote health, prevent disease, and facilitate healing of clients across the life span	I: Liberal Education for Baccalaureate Generalist Nursing Practice VII: Clinical Prevention and Population Health IX: Baccalaureate Generalist Nursing Practice
7. Applies sound clinical judgment and evidence-based practice in the provision of holistic nursing care	I: Liberal Education for Baccalaureate Generalist Nursing Practice III: Scholarship for Evidence-Based Practice IV: Information Management and Patient Care Technology IX: Baccalaureate Generalist Nursing Practice
8. Integrates knowledge of health care policy, populations, finance, and regulatory environments that influence system level change within professional nursing practice	II: Basic Organizational and Systems Leadership for Quality Care and Patient Safety V: Health Care Policy, Finance, and Regulatory Environments

Source: Linfield-Good Samaritan School of Nursing Curriculum Committee. Used with permission (2008).

There has been a resurgence in the use of competencies to structure curricula. Goudreau et al. (2009) identify the second-generation competency-based approach as grounded in a constructivist model that supports learning-centered approaches. Competencies are not constrained by the language of Bloom's taxonomy but are statements of "complex know-hows" specific to the discipline that "allows one to deal with different situations by drawing on concepts, knowledge, information, procedures, and methods" (Goudreau et al., 2009, p. 3). For example, the 10 competencies developed by the Oregon Consortium for Nursing Education (OCNE) are not grounded in the behaviorist tradition but reflect the complexity and integration of empirical knowledge and practical knowing (Gubrud-Howe et al., 2003). The OCNE competency statements can be viewed at http://ocne.org/Curriculum%20Competency%20Approved%205-11-2012.pdf.

IDENTIFYING COURSES

In the next step, essential knowledge, skills, and attitudes that students will need to accomplish related to each outcome are identified. This is the content that is organized into coherent and logical groupings, which become courses. There are many possible ways to cluster the information and the faculty should be guided by their previous research and philosophical work. The identification of new courses can be an exciting and creative activity but has the potential to be a phase of the curriculum development process that creates conflict. Issues of territoriality and "sacred cows" may assert themselves; it is sometimes difficult to think creatively and safer to regress to what is known (the old model). At this juncture, decisions must be made about which concepts to integrate and which to organize into a separate course. In the creation of a working course template, a program of study by term begins to emerge. Table 11.3 shows the courses in the plan of study for the generic BSN curriculum at LGSSON.

TABLE 11.3　GENERIC BSN PROGRAM OF STUDY

SEMESTER 1: FOUNDATIONS FOR COMMUNITY BASED NURSING PRACTICE	CREDITS	SEMESTER 2: CHRONIC HEALTH	CREDITS
Foundations of Community-Based Nursing Practice	4	Nursing Care of Children, Adults, and Older Adults With Chronic Conditions	3
Professional Communication in Diverse Communities	2	Clinical Pathophysiology and Pharmacology for Nursing Practice I	2
Scholarship of Nursing			
Integrated Experiential Learning I	3	Mental Health and Illness Across the Life Span	2
(1 didactic; 1 clinical)	6	Integrated Experiential Learning II (clinical)	6
		Elective or General Education	3
Total	15		13-16
SEMESTER 3: ACUTE HEALTH	CREDITS	SEMESTER 4: STEWARDSHIP FOR HEALTH	CREDITS
Nursing Care of Children, Adults, and Older Adults With Acute Conditions	3	Leading and Managing in Nursing	3
Transitions and Decisions: Pregnancy, Birth, and End-of-Life Care	2	Population-Based Nursing in a Multicultural and Global Society	2
Clinical Pathophysiology and Pharmacology for Nursing Practice II	2	Integrated Experiential Learning IV (clinical)	8
Integrated Experiential Learning III (clinical)	6	Elective NCLEX-RN® preparation course	1
Elective or General Education	3		
Total	13–16		13–14

Note: All courses are didactic except for the integrated experiential learning courses.
Source: Linfield-Good Samaritan School of Nursing. Used with permission.

A program that relies on the biomedical model will tend toward a traditional course structure that adheres more closely to medical specialties, for example, pediatric nursing, psychiatric nursing, and medical-surgical nursing. A program organized according to a nursing framework may have more integrated courses, for example, a course focusing on chronicity in which students explore health issues and concerns of clients with chronic illness, including physical and mental health problems across the life span and the entire health trajectory from prevention to end of life. The theoretical model should provide a framework for making decisions about the program of study. Once the program of study is drafted, faculty teams may begin work on course development.

BACCALAUREATE CURRICULUM DESIGN: SPECIAL CONSIDERATIONS

The nursing education literature identifies curriculum design issues and trends that must be considered as the faculty moves forward with development of the prelicensure program of study. These include the historical overloading of content in nursing curricula, the mandate for IPE, consideration of the needs of an increasingly diverse student body, and changes in clinical education.

CONTENT OVERLOAD IN NURSING CURRICULA

Advances and trends in nursing science compel additions to the nursing curriculum in the areas of quality and safety, informatics, diversity and cultural competence, genetics and genomics, evidence-based practice, transitional and population-based care and, most recently, veterans health care (Allen, Armstrong, Conard, Saladiner, & Hamilton, 2013). While these subjects are important for preparing baccalaureate nurses of the future, how can faculty possibly add this content to an already packed curriculum? Nursing education has historically been plagued with "content overload." As health care and nursing practice change, nurse educators typically keep adding information to courses without taking anything out (Ironside, 2004; Tanner, 2007). As a result, both students and faculty are chronically overloaded and overworked, with little time for reflection and real learning.

In order to facilitate meaningful learning, nursing faculty must reorient the curriculum from what the students need to know to how students think in their developing nursing practice (Ironside, 2004; Tanner, 2006). Learning-centered approaches (Benner et al., 2010; Diekelman, 2005; Ironside, 2006) address issues of overload at the course level but there are also curricular strategies to safeguard against it. Candela, Dalley, and Benzel-Lindley (2006) described learning-centered education as an approach to control content and suggested a systematic process for categorizing the importance of curricular content and eliminating all but the most essential. Giddens (2007) studied skills utilized by practicing nurses and determined that only a core set of skills taught in physical assessment classes were used in practice. Subsequently, Giddens and Eddy (2009) evaluated the content taught in physical assessment courses in associate degree in nursing (ADN) and BSN programs. Based on an apparent disconnect between skills taught in nursing education and those used in practice, they recommended that faculty teach fewer skills and only those most frequently used in practice. In similar fashion, nursing courses commonly teach management of clients with an exhaustive list of clinical disorders, many of them rare; in sorting essential content, only the most commonly encountered disorders should be used as exemplars within a nursing framework. Tanner (2007) suggests that faculty cover fewer topics more in depth to facilitate understanding of concepts most important for nursing practice.

The concept-based model for curriculum development is another way to reduce content saturation. In this approach, nursing faculty identifies, classifies, and defines concepts that subsequently provide the organizational framework for the curriculum and are threaded through courses (Giddens & Brady, 2007; Giddens, Wright, & Gray, 2012). For example, at LGSSON, the faculty identified six major themes that reflected the mission, vision, and philosophy of the school and were incorporated into the theoretical framework: communication, community, diversity, ethics, health, and stewardship. Essential concepts were identified for each of the themes and the concepts within each theme were spiraled from less to more complex and then leveled across four semesters. Although the emphasis on the themes varied from semester to semester and new information for each theme was introduced each semester, the expectation was that knowledge and skills were cumulative throughout the program. Examples of the leveling of the concepts within three of these themes are provided in Table 11.4.

TABLE 11.4 COMMUNITY-BASED CURRICULUM FRAMEWORK: CONCEPTUAL ORGANIZATION; EXAMPLARS OF CONCEPTS IDENTIFIED WITHIN CURRICULUM THEMES: COMMUNICATION, DIVERSITY, STEWARDSHIP (THREE OF SIX THEMES)

CURRICULUM THEMES	SEMESTER 1: FOUNDATIONS FOR COMMUNITY-BASED NURSING PRACTICE	SEMESTER 2: CHRONIC HEALTH	SEMESTER 3: ACUTE HEALTH	SEMESTER 4: STEWARDSHIP FOR HEALTH
Communication Continuum: Student, client, family/group, team	Therapeutic use of self-emotional intelligence Documentation Scholarly writing Interpersonal communication interviewing Therapeutic communication	Interdisciplinary communication Collaboration Advocacy Family dynamics Group dynamics	Making a case	Conflict management Delegation Teambuilding
Diversity Continuum: Cultural self Intercultural Multicultural International	Cultural identity Cultural diversity Difference Cultural competence Racism Privilege Intercultural communication Spirituality Holism	Culturally adaptive care Cultural health beliefs Integrative health care Cultural humility	Cultural advocacy Cultural relativism	Intercultural bridging Immigration Global health disparities Organizational cultural competence Universal cultural values

(continued)

| TABLE 11.4 | COMMUNITY-BASED CURRICULUM FRAMEWORK: CONCEPTUAL ORGANIZATION; EXAMPLARS OF CONCEPTS IDENTIFIED WITHIN CURRICULUM THEMES: COMMUNICATION, DIVERSITY, STEWARDSHIP (THREE OF SIX THEMES) (*continued*) |

CURRICULUM THEMES	SEMESTER 1: FOUNDATIONS FOR COMMUNITY-BASED NURSING PRACTICE	SEMESTER 2: CHRONIC HEALTH	SEMESTER 3: ACUTE HEALTH	SEMESTER 4: STEWARDSHIP FOR HEALTH
Stewardship Continuum: Professional nurse Organizational systems Professional leadership	Evolution of nursing professionalism Self-care Lifelong learning Practice regulation	Care delivery Client outcomes	Organizational systems Cost consciousness Quality improvement/ patient safety	Stewardship: Leadership management organizational culture change Mentorship Continuous quality improvement Risk management Health care regulation Health care economics

Source: Linfield-Good Samaritan School of Nursing. Used with permission.

| TABLE 11.5 | ORGANIZATION OF CURRICULUM CONCEPTS INTO THEORY COURSES FOR THE FINAL TWO SEMESTERS |

SEMESTER 3 (FALL): ACUTE HEALTH	SEMESTER 4 (SPRING): STEWARDSHIP OF HEALTH
Nursing Care of Children, Adults, and Older Adults with Acute Conditions: Acuity, crisis, trauma, clotting, perfusion, hemostasis, homeostasis, fluid and electrolytes, immunity, inflammation, infection, oxygenation, cell growth and regulation, hormonal regulation, generalizing experiences, adapting practice, cultural advocacy, organizational systems, QI/patient safety, cost consciousness, making a case, resource connecting, evidence-based client care: acute *Transitions and Decisions: Pregnancy, Birth, and End-of-Life Care*: Family coping, pregnancy, childbirth, midwifery, death and dying, loss and grief, good nurse, quality of life, self-determination, comfort care, moral distress, health care ethics, case analysis, health care ethics, genetics/genomics, cultural relativism *Clinical Pathophysiology and Pharmacology II*: Inflammation/immunity/infection; alterations in cell growth; alterations in fluid, electrolyte, and acid-base balance; alterations in ventilation and diffusion; alterations in perfusion Integrated Experiential Learning III (6 credits)	*Leading and Managing in Nursing*: Leadership, management, teambuilding, conflict management, organizational culture, organizational systems, health care economics, mentorship, quality improvement, risk management, health care regulation, organizational ethics, organizational cultural competence, collective action, health policy, responsible action, change, evidence-based organizational change, delegation *Population-Based Nursing in a Multicultural and Global Society*: Healthy communities, epidemiology, immigration, community education, community outreach, environmental health, sustainability, emergency preparedness, universal cultural values, global health, global consciousness, global nursing ethics, global health disparities, complex health situations, evidence-based aggregate care Integrated Experiential Learning IV (7–8 credits)

Source: Linfield-Good Samaritan School of Nursing, with permission.

Within each semester, concepts from all themes were organized into courses; as an example, the conceptual organization of the theory courses from the final two semesters of the program are shown in Table 11.5. By identifying more abstract concepts instead of content for each course, the faculty member is free to update and prioritize course content as it changes over time. For example, the concept of "environmental health," which is introduced in semester 4, does not specify specific content and allows the teacher to vary explanatory models and exemplars according to current research and community priorities.

THE INCLUSIVE CURRICULUM: PAYING ATTENTION TO DIVERSITY

There is a national call to increase the enrollment of students from underrepresented populations in schools of nursing, and recent reports show that some progress is being made (Budden, Zhone, Moulton, & Cimiotti, 2013; U.S. Department of HHS, 2010). Learning-centered education generally addresses diverse learning styles and there is a growing body of literature regarding effective teaching and assessment strategies for nursing students from underrepresented populations (Bosher & Pharris, 2009). However, schools of nursing typically have not considered the needs of students who are minorities, low income students, first in family to attend college, or multilingual, nonnative-English speakers in developing the plan of study or the curriculum structure. Ideally, the curriculum should be creative, flexible, and reflect the multicultural perspectives of our pluralistic society (Warda, 2008). If diversity and cultural competence are part of the mission or philosophy of the school, related concepts should be included in the theoretical framework, made explicit in program and level outcomes, and reflected in concepts/content threaded throughout the curriculum (Crow, 1997). For example, at tribal colleges, curriculum is structured to focus on important elements of the Native American culture.

The American Association of Colleges and Universities (2014) promotes *inclusive excellence*, a commitment to diversity and equity based on the understanding that becoming an educated person in a pluralistic society includes developing the ability to communicate and interact with individuals and populations that are different from ourselves (Williams, Berger, & McClendon, 2005). This philosophy presupposes a broad definition of diversity, and compels faculty members to facilitate the success of all students, including those with diverse backgrounds and learning styles. Swaner and Brownell (2008) recommend high-impact strategies for the success of underrepresented minority students, including learning communities, service learning, undergraduate research, first-year seminars, and capstone projects that could readily be incorporated into the structure of nursing programs. Faculty may not be aware of how programmatic organization affects students differentially. For example, the practice of "front-loading" theory in a curriculum or a particular course prior to engagement in clinical practice disadvantages tactile and kinesthetic learners and this is the preferred learning style for many English as a second language (ESL) students (Reid, 1987). In a theory-first model, students who are having difficulty with theory miss the opportunity to reinforce classroom learning in the most effective way possible—through hands-on learning in the real world

(Bosher, 2007). These learners would best achieve academically in a curriculum model that more closely integrated theory and clinical experience.

Other ways of demonstrating inclusiveness in curriculum planning include pre-entry nursing courses, parallel academic support courses, culture-focused or special interest general education courses or electives, and international experiences as part of the program of study. The co-curriculum can play an important role in supporting and validating underrepresented students on the campus. Other ideas include development of clinical models that facilitate clinical experiences with diverse populations and intentionally threading exemplars throughout the curriculum that address health care issues experienced by particular ethnic, cultural, or minority groups. Another strategy is to institute a curriculum requirement that ensures that students have a variety of experiences with populations or clients that are different from themselves. One promising practice in nursing education identified in a study of California nursing programs included organizing and scheduling the program of study to accommodate working students, which could include options for evening and/or part-time coursework (Buchbinder, 2007). And finally, admission and progression requirements for incoming students that support or, conversely, disadvantage those who were educated in another country or are multilingual nonnative English speakers will shape the student body and affect the quality of learning for all the students. A diverse student body has been shown to be associated with improved outcomes among all students (IOM, 2004).

INTERPROFESSIONAL EDUCATION: PREPARING FOR COLLABORATIVE PRACTICE

In response to quality and safety standards in health care and a vision for accessible, patient-centered care, AACN collaborated with leadership from other professional organizations to develop competencies for interprofessional practice (Interprofessional Education Collaborative Expert Panel, 2011), which have been integrated into the *Baccalaureate Essentials* (AACN, 2008b). The World Health Organization (2010, p. 7) stated that IPE "occurs when students from two or more professions learn about, from and with each other to enable effective collaboration and improve health." Health professions schools are developing models for IPE in classroom, simulation, and, more recently, clinical and community settings.

IPE models have been studied in undergraduate nursing programs (Hudson, Sanders, & Pepper, 2013). The University of Florida requires an interdisciplinary family health course in which student teams make visits to volunteer families in the community, and the University of Washington developed the co-curricular SPARX program (Bridges, Davidson, Odegard, Maki, & Tomkowiak, 2011). Salfi, Solomon, Allen, Mohaupt, and Patterson (2012) described a framework for IPE in which students developed competencies throughout the curriculum beginning with learning about their own profession and culminating in their effective participation on the health care team. Shiyanbola, Lammers, Randall, and Richards (2012) implemented an IPE program with students from five health care profession programs, including nursing, that focused on care of an underserved diabetic population. At Oregon Health and Sciences University (OHSU), interprofessional student groups are working with a nursing faculty in residence and collaborating with community partners to address social determinants of health for some of the most vulnerable and marginalized clients, families, and populations in target neighborhoods. Details can be found at www.ohsu.edu/i-can.

Although there are significant logistical, cultural, and historical barriers to IPE and practice, the benefits of IPE for prelicensure students are many, including: greater understanding of roles and contributions of other health care professionals and dynamics within the health care team; development of professional pride and identity; importance of effective interprofessional communication and reflective practice; knowledge of patient conditions and increased comfort with targeted patient populations; improved cultural sensitivity; building of professional networks; and an improved sense of collaboration and cooperation (Angelini, 2011; Bridges et al., 2011; Buckley et al., 2012; Mellor, Cottrell, & Moran, 2013; Shiyanbola et al., 2012); Each school has unique opportunities and, going forward, IPE/interprofessional collaborative practice must be considered as an integral element of every baccalaureate curriculum.

TRANSFORMATIVE APPROACHES TO CLINICAL EDUCATION

One of the most challenging aspects of curriculum revision is designing an approach to students' clinical experiences that reflects the school's theoretical model and integrates new learning pedagogies in the context of local realities regarding the availability of qualified clinical faculty and clinical sites. While clinical experience is essential in preparation for practice, what constitutes clinical experience? What kinds of clinical learning activities and how much time in what kind of health care settings is most effective for BSN students to meet generalist competencies and transition successfully into practice? The National League for Nursing Think Tank on Transforming Clinical Nursing Education (2008) made recommendations for the ideal clinical education model that described integrative experiences, including cross-disciplinary experiences; new relationships within learning communities, including innovative relationships with clinical partners; and reconceptualized learning experiences in which all students don't have clinical experiences in traditional rotations. While there are scarce data about the effectiveness of either traditional or new clinical models, it is incumbent on nurse educators to develop and test models and approaches and contribute to the database. Each school of nursing needs to develop an approach that best utilizes its resources and fits its theoretical model.

Clinical models: The traditional clinical education model in which a nursing faculty member provides direct supervision and oversight for a small group of students on a hospital unit is no longer practical or effective for several reasons:

- Shortened patient lengths of stay make it difficult for students to collect information from the medical record and prepare for patient care prior to the clinical experience and often patients are discharged sooner than anticipated
- Students miss experiences when they're dependent on clinical faculty and obligated to wait for them before engaging in particular skills or situations

- Students spend too much of their clinical time in repetitive tasks and not enough on higher level thinking activities (Ironside & McNelis, 2009)
- The total patient care model for a limited number of patients does not provide the breadth of experiences with authentic nursing activities required for preparation for generalist practice
- The traditional role that faculty plays in sequentially supervising skills (like passing medications) isn't responsive to the rapidly changing and competing demands of clinical practice and doesn't focus on development of students' clinical thinking skills
- Given the reduced capacity of clinical sites, faculty logistically can't attend to all students with placements at a variety of community clinical sites or even on different units at a hospital

In response to the changing reality, MacIntyre, Murray, Teel, and Karshmer (2009) made recommendations to strengthen academic–practice relationships and create new models for clinical education that:

1. Re-envision nursing student-staff nurse relationship
2. Reconceptualize the clinical faculty role
3. Enhance development for school-based faculty and staff nurses working with students
4. Reexamine the depth and breadth of the clinical component
5. Strengthen the evidence for best practices in clinical nursing education (p. 448)

The need for new clinical models was driven in large part by the lack of availability of clinical sites and increased enrollments in nursing programs in response to the projected nursing shortage. Nursing faculty members were challenged to find meaningful and predictable clinical experiences for students in health care facilities where there is less staff caring for higher acuity patients. As previously discussed, many schools are using simulated learning activities in the classroom and the learning lab to prepare students for clinical experiences and, in some cases, to substitute for clinical hours (NCSBN, 2009). According to Benner et al. (2010), students learn better when they are in a classroom that integrates theory and clinical. Based on the results of the professional nursing education study, Benner et al. (2010) recommend that BSN curricula integrate three apprenticeships into the program of study: nursing knowledge, learned skills and clinical reasoning, and ethical comportment and formation. In this model, apprenticeships refer to situated learning and meaningful integration of theory and practice in which students learn through experiences within a "community of practice" (Benner et al., 2010, p. 25). Noone (2009) suggests that educators develop curricula in which all three apprenticeships are integrated within each course.

In lieu of the traditional model, the OCNE, which includes the five campuses of OHSU School of Nursing (SON) and nine community colleges, developed a new approach to expand clinical capacity that proposed five elements of clinical learning that defined a set of activities, which build on one another throughout the curriculum. The new model includes focused direct client care; concept-based experiences; case-based experiences; intervention skill-based experiences; and integrative experiences (Gubrud-Howe & Schloesser, 2008; Nielsen et al., 2013). In this approach, traditional comprehensive patient care is only one strategy among others that supports students to meet course outcomes. At LGSSON, overcrowding and complex scheduling of limited lab space and decreasing (and sometimes competing) clinical opportunities resulted in the development of an integrated experiential learning (IEL) model. Concepts introduced in multiple co-requisite theory courses in a particular semester are applied and synthesized in a single course that includes field experiences, lab, simulation, and clinical experiences. Each clinical course includes some experience with clients in a primary, secondary, and tertiary site according to the theoretical model.

The University of Delaware developed a nurse residency model, which is a senior-year clinical immersion experience that meets 3 days per week during the last semester along with clinical integration seminars. What is unique about this model is that during the first 3 years of the program, students do not have traditional acute care clinical experiences. Students instead demonstrate readiness by successful completion of didactic courses and progressive development of knowledge and competence through lab and simulation, field experiences, teaching assistantships, and a work requirement (Diefenbeck, Plowfield, & Herrman, 2006; Herrman & Diefenbeck, 2009). In this innovative approach, practice is decoupled from theory in coursework, and the definition of clinical education is expanded to include alternative experiences. In the context of the new definition, the total number of clinical hours increased in the residency model although less faculty resources were required (Diefenbeck et al., 2006).

Another approach to clinical education relies on community partnerships in which student cohorts stay primarily in one health care system so that they don't spend precious learning time repeatedly reorienting to different organizations (Joynt & Kimball, 2008). For example, the University of North Florida's BSN program utilizes a clinical model in which the school partners with communities to develop ongoing relationships in service oriented to the community's specific issues and agendas. Students are assigned to a home base during their first year and participate in collaborative activities during their entire nursing program. While students have other clinical experiences, the long-term relationship with the community agency and gradual progression of clinical experiences results in positive learning experiences for students (Kruger, Roush, Olinzock, & Bloom, 2010).

The University of North Florida partnership model exemplifies service learning, in which academic learning objectives are met through academic-practice partnerships that focus on meeting identified community needs (Kruger et al., 2010). The "bucket list" approach provides authentic learning in less-structured community environments and improves quality of population health experiences (Broussard, 2011). Service learning affects outcomes related to cultural competency, critical thinking, and civic engagement (Nokes, Nickitas, Keida, & Neville, 2005), and increases student participation in health policy (O'Brien-Larivee, 2011). Service learning has been shown to increase leadership and social justice skills among nursing students (Groh, Stallwood, & Daniels, 2011) as well as attitudes regarding marginalized and vulnerable populations (Loewenson & Hunt, 2011; Simpson, 2012). AACN and AONE published guiding principles for academic–practice partnerships (AACN-American Organization of Nurse Executives Task Force on Academic-Practice Partnerships, 2012).

The dedicated education unit (DEU) is another education–practice collaborative model that relies on ongoing partnerships with clinical agencies. In this model, nurses, faculty, and students working together create an optimal teaching environment, while continuing the commitment to quality patient care. Staff nurses on identified patient care units assume the direct teaching role with support from faculty who facilitate development of the staff nurses' expertise in teaching. Since the unit is utilized exclusively by students from the partner school, the nurses become adjunct faculty members and are oriented to the curriculum and specific learning outcomes (Moscato, Miller, Logsdon, Weinberg, & Chorpenning, 2007). The DEU model utilizes scarce faculty resources in an efficient manner that significantly increases the capacity for student placements (Moscato et al., 2007).

Lourdes University implemented a clinical education model that incorporated several of the elements described above. Students enroll in multiple didactic courses and an integrated clinical course. They remain in a single clinical site for one to two semesters. Students in acute care are placed on education resource units, which have similarities to DEUs but are focused on the QSEN competencies and also cultivate nurse mentors within the partner hospital (Didion, Kozy, Koffel, & Oneail, 2012).

These innovative approaches to clinical education are grounded in new pedagogy, and make creative use of scarce resources to help students achieve curriculum outcomes. They rely on more focused clinical experiences that maximize faculty resources, collaborative relationships with clinical agencies, and student learning potential. Evaluation of the effectiveness of models such as these, including cost/benefit, will inform and influence the quality of nursing education in the future.

COMPLETING THE CURRICULUM DEVELOPMENT PROCESS

Concurrent with the development of the program of study, additional work must be completed as part of the comprehensive curriculum package. A glossary defines terms that have special meaning within the mission, vision, and philosophy; theoretical model; and curriculum plan, including concepts that provide the organizational framework for the curriculum. Prerequisites including humanities, science, and social science courses that serve as the foundation for the nursing coursework must be identified and negotiated with various other departments. These include college-wide requirements such as general education. Progression issues must be considered, including minimum grade point average for admission into the school of nursing, a description of how students will progress from semester to semester, and prerequisites and co-requisites for each course. The curriculum development group will need to work with the administrative team to cost out the curriculum, including faculty and other resources that will be needed to manage the new curriculum. Often old and new curricula will be offered simultaneously for a period of time until the students in the old program graduate, which may require additional resources. The curriculum package must be approved by the nursing faculty and be directed through academic channels for approval. The new curriculum must be submitted to the State Board of Nursing and the national accrediting body.

TRANSITION TO PRACTICE

Transition of new BSN graduates into clinical practice is recognized as an issue since *Reality Shock* was first published (Kramer, 1974). Internships or integrative clinical experiences prior to graduation have been shown as one curriculum strategy that contributes to the socialization of graduate nurses into practice (Nielsen et al., 2013; Paul et al., 2011). Recommendations from national reports about transition from the academic environment to the nursing practice environment showed significant support for the formation of academic and service partnerships to develop standardized residency programs (Benner et al., 2010; IOM, 2010; Spector & Echternacht, 2010). The Commission on Collegiate Nursing Education (2008) implemented accreditation for postbaccalaureate nurse residency programs.

The goal of transition programs is primarily to facilitate professional formation and socialization into the culture of the health care organization, assist the new graduate to develop clinical competency, improve recruitment retention, and reduce orientation costs for the employer. Programs may be situated prior to graduation or following, and include educational and psychosocial support strategies such as mentoring, preceptor training, clinical coaching, expanded orientation, clinical and professional skill development, classes, and other learning and support activities targeted at the needs of the developing professional (Bratt, 2009; Olson-Sitki, Wendler, & Forbes, 2012).

A model residency program that promotes point-of-care leadership was developed and evaluated by the University Health System Consortium and AACN. This curriculum focuses on three content areas: leadership, patient safety, and professional role. Among other findings, an evaluation demonstrated that the residents' perceptions of confidence and competence, capacity to organize and prioritize, and ability to communicate and provide leadership improved significantly. In addition, retention rates of new graduates improved (Goode, Lynn, & McElroy, 2013).

Other postgraduation programs show similar results, and are reported to be particularly successful in building capacity and community for rural hospitals (Bratt, 2009). In one study, less satisfaction was documented among non-White program participants, indicating that additional research is needed to understand the needs of minority nurses (Altier & Krsek, 2006). One major challenge in residency program management is preparing and maintaining committed and effective mentor/preceptors (Eigsti, 2009; Fitzgerald, 2009). Achievement of quality indicators is important in order to justify program continuation in the climate of scarce resources; evaluation should include not only the cost-benefit analysis related to retention of new graduates but factors such as quality indicators of professional achievement of nurse residents (Bratt, 2009).

ALTERNATIVE BACCALAUREATE PATHWAYS

Accelerated Baccalaureate Programs

The first ABSN programs were initiated in the early 1970s and grew rapidly in number since the 1990s. In 2011, there were 231 established ABSN programs with

33 more under development (AACN, 2012). The continuing development of these programs was in response to the projected shortage of nurses and is viewed as a viable option to help meet the future need for more nurses (AACN, 2013a; Cangelosi, 2007; Penprase & Koczara, 2009). ABSN programs offer students who completed a bachelor's degree in another discipline the opportunity to obtain a degree in nursing in a shorter time frame than those in traditional baccalaureate nursing programs. Graduates from ABSN programs are highly valued by employers because of their maturity, ability to learn quickly, and clinical skills (AACN, 2012).

Description of the ASBN Program

Accelerated programs are generally offered as intensive full-time courses of study with no breaks between semesters or terms. Most programs are 11 to 18 months in length (AACN, 2012). ABSN students are admitted upon completion of program prerequisites, although the liberal arts and general education requirements are usually waived (Basilio, 2013).

It is difficult to identify a standardized design model for accelerated programs. In any given nursing program, curriculum outcomes should be the same for the traditional and accelerated programs of study. However, course structure and pedagogical approaches may vary. Some schools maintain accelerated and traditional students as separate cohorts, while others integrate them at some point during their educational process. ABSN programs of study may conform to the standard undergraduate academic schedule or define their own without breaks. By building on prior learning, students in ABSN programs are able to complete the same curriculum outcomes in a program with fewer overall credits. While the number of didactic or theory hours/courses may differ between the traditional BSN and the ABSN program at a given school, the number of clinical hours generally remains the same (AACN, 2012).

ABSN Students as Experienced Learners

Students in ABSN programs choose to return to school for a variety of reasons. Some indicate that they always wanted to be a nurse and look forward to the flexibility and practicality such a career might offer (Raines, 2013; Wright, 2012). Others experienced job loss and seek a profession where they can find consistent employment, while others envision nursing as a profession where they can "make a difference" (Raines, 2009, p. 2).

Students in accelerated programs have been characterized as adult learners (Raines, 2009) who return to school with high expectations of themselves (Raines & Sipes, 2007). Because many had a career following their first degree, they bring an increased depth of life experience and knowledge that broadens their perspectives and enriches their learning (Korvick, Wisener, Loftis, & Williamson, 2008). They are eager to learn (Hegge & Hallman, 2008) and expect to be actively engaged in their learning (Teeley, 2007). The critical thinking skills of ABSN students, when compared to those of traditional students, are higher (Cangelosi, 2007), which enables them to understand complex information faster and move through a nursing curriculum more quickly (Raines & Sipes, 2007). In a study conducted by Korvick et al. (2008), students in an accelerated program performed better academically than those in a traditional program. They also had a higher first-time NCLEX-RN® pass rate than traditional graduates (Brewer et al., 2009; Korvick et al., 2008; Raines & Sipes, 2007).

Having successfully completed a prior baccalaureate, students in accelerated programs are experienced learners who understand the challenges of college and have learned how to effectively navigate the system. These skills, grounded in their previous college experiences, help them to cope with the rigors of a professional program. Not only are they self-directed learners and highly motivated (Walker et al., 2007), they are also critical consumers of education and clear in what they want from their second degree: the knowledge and skill sets to become effective nurses in a program that is well-organized, relevant, and considerate of their learning styles.

As mature and motivated as ASBN students might be, they have reported high levels of stress (Neill, 2011; Penprase & Koczara, 2009) when challenged by the expectations of the student role and balancing the demands of family, work, and finances. An orientation to the challenges and demands of an accelerated program may be important for student success (Kohn & Truglio-Londigran, 2007). Utley, Phillips, and Turner (2007) describe a model developed and implemented to help those enrolled in an ABSN program to understand the culture of nursing and begin their socialization into the profession. The model describes various phases students might experience and find challenging, and identified strategies that will help them to be successful in their educational process. Neill conducted an extensive review of research-based literature to determine what other factors facilitated students' success in ABSN programs. Students indicated that support from family as well as cohort-specific peers were important to successfully navigate their programs of study (Kemsley, McCauslan, Feigenbaum, & Riegle, 2011; Neill, 2011). Supportive faculty who drew upon their students' life experiences and helped them navigate specific courses also facilitated their success (Neill, 2011). Students identified faculty who challenge them to use their critical thinking when dealing with complex client situations and who facilitate learning in a nonthreatening manner as essential to their learning. In addition, having clinical experiences on units where the staff is supportive and the time spent is of high quality is very helpful to their learning (Wright, 2012).

In addition to having high expectations of themselves, ABSN students have high expectations of their faculty and the learning environment. They enjoy the opportunity to ask questions in the classroom (Lindsey, 2009) and benefit from learning strategies that employ interaction between themselves as well as faculty (Kohn & Truglio-Londrigan, 2007). They are more apt to question assignments that are perceived as busy work (Lindsey, 2009), which may lead faculty members to feel as if they are being challenged. Clinical experiences are highly anticipated as a means to learn (AACN, 2012) and students report that they learn from the stories faculty members tell regarding their own clinical experiences (Walker et al., 2007). Although ABSN students look to their faculty to determine what they need to know (Teeley, 2007; Walker et al., 2007), they prefer a more collegial relationship with faculty, who serve as guides to and facilitators of learning. Kohn and

Truglio-Londrigan note that it is important to match students in ABSN programs with faculty who have an affinity for and an interest in teaching adult learners.

Students in accelerated programs do well in learning environments that are dynamic. Courses in which technology such as web-based teaching modalities, simulation, and case studies are integrated as well as face-to-face classroom activities serve them well (Hegge & Hallman, 2008; Teeley, 2007; Walker et al., 2007). Hegge and Hallman discuss the need for an environment in which collaborative learning occurs, noting that it lends itself to fostering students' "self-esteem, academic excellence, and social support" (p. 554).

Sample ABSN Program

At LGSSON, a comprehensive curriculum redesign was initiated in 2008, with implementation in 2011. During the planning phase, the intent was to develop a modified curriculum with fewer didactic credits delivered over a shorter period of time for the ABSN program. However, faculty struggled with the workload of developing different yet parallel courses for the generic and the ABSN programs as the implementation phase neared. A decision was made to have one common curriculum, with the ABSN program of study conducted over a 15-month period and the traditional program of study completed in four semesters over 2 academic years.

TABLE 11.6 ACCELERATED BSN PROGRAM OF STUDY (15 MONTHS)

SUMMER SEMESTER 1 (11 WEEKS)	FALL SEMESTER 2 (15 WEEKS)	SPRING SEMESTER 3 (15 WEEKS)	SUMMER SEMESTER 4 (11 WEEKS)
Foundations of Community-Based Professional Nursing: 4 credits Professional Communication in Diverse Communities: 2 credits Scholarship of Nursing: 3 credits Integrated Experiential Learning I: Foundations 6 credits (1 didactic; 5 clinical)	Nursing Care of Children, Adults, and Older Adults With Chronic Conditions: 3 credits Clinical Pathophysiology and Pharmacology for Nursing Practice I: 2 credits Mental Health and Illness Across the Life Span: 2 credits Integrated Experiential Learning II: Chronic Care: 6 credits (clinical) Elective: 3 credits	Nursing Care of Children, Adults, and Older Adults With Acute Conditions: 3 credits Transitions and Decisions: Pregnancy, Birth, and End-of-Life Care: 2 credits Clinical Pathophysiology and Pharmacology for Nursing Practice II: 2 credits Integrated Experiential Learning III: Acute Care: 6 credits (clinical) Elective: 3 credits	Leading and Managing in Nursing: 3 credits Population-Based Nursing in a Multicultural and Global Society: 2 credits Integrated Experiential Learning IV: 8 credits (clinical) Elective: 3 credits
15 credits	13–16 credits	13–16 credits	13–16 credits

Note: All courses are didactic except for the integrated experiential learning courses.
Source: Linfield-Good Samaritan School of Nursing. Used with permission.

Students in the two programs share some courses, and others are taught separately. The ABSN cohort is admitted at the beginning of every summer session with the students graduating at the end of the following summer (see Table 11.6). While the curriculum for most accelerated programs varies somewhat from the generic program, each school must create a curriculum that takes into account its own structure and resources when planning and delivering multiple programs of study simultaneously.

As engaged and motivated adult learners, ABSN students and graduates can offer important insights as part of the planning group during curriculum redesign initiatives. For example, during the curricular redesign process at LGS-SON, students in the ABSN program were surveyed to determine their perspectives and suggestions regarding the scheduling of the ABSN curriculum. When asked how important it was to maintain a continuous program of study without breaks, 97 of 107 students (91%) responded that it was either "important" or "very important." Many of the students took time off from previous careers to return to school and were anxious to complete the program to restore their income and spend more time with their families. Based in part on the survey results, the decision was made to implement the compressed 15-month program of study with minimal breaks.

ABSN Graduates

In a study by Raines (2007), ABSN program graduates were asked a series of questions about satisfaction with their program of study and if they felt it prepared them adequately for practice. A year later, they were surveyed again. The average scores at both times were above the mean and were even higher 1 year after graduation. This type of study is one way to evaluate the outcomes of accelerated programs and provides evidence that the graduates value the preparation provided by an accelerated curriculum. Raines (2010) conducted a study that in part, surveyed the perceptions of expert nurses who had worked with ABSN students in practice. These nurses indicated that the students were competent and "ready to become professional colleagues in the nursing practice setting" (Raines, 2010, p. 167).

Weathers and Hunt Raleigh (2013) compared retention rates and performance evaluation ratings by nurse managers of traditional and ABSN graduates after 1 year of practice and found that the retention rate was higher for ABSN graduates, as were the performance ratings. Rafferty and Lindell (2011) analyzed the responses of nurse managers who compared the clinical performance of traditional students with that of ABSN graduates. In their study, results indicated that the respondents saw no statistically significant differences in their clinical competencies, which the authors note supports the idea that ABSN programs produce comparably performing graduates in a shorter time frame.

Raines (2013) studied ABSN graduates 5 years after entering the workforce. She found that 91% (N = 54) were in practice, with 94% reporting they were *extremely satisfied* or *satisfied* with their careers. Two were inactive due to family caregiving responsibilities. Many (34.5%) had completed or were enrolled in graduate programs, including both doctor of nursing practice and PhD programs. Findings such as these demonstrate that ABSN programs are producing graduates who remain in the workplace and also pursue advanced degrees soon after graduation.

There is a growing body of literature about ABSN programs and their graduates. It is incumbent on nurse educators to continue to study this population to determine which educational approaches are most effective and facilitate the greatest learning. It is important to continue to evaluate the postgraduation experiences of these graduates, both in the workplace as well as during and after graduate education.

BACCALAUREATE COMPLETION PROGRAMS

Baccalaureate completion programs, also called RN to BSN programs, are designed for RNs who are graduates of accredited associate degree or hospital-based diploma programs and who seek a BSN degree. Based on research demonstrating improved performance on quality and safety outcomes when nurses are educated at the baccalaureate level or higher, AACN maintains that the BSN degree should be the minimum educational requirement for professional nursing practice (AACN, 2009). The BSN has become the preferred preparation for practice in health care settings including Magnet hospitals and organizations that require the baccalaureate for specific nursing roles (AACN). Nurses who seek positions in case management, public health and community-based settings, and leadership find that the BSN is an essential requirement for employment.

Nurses who enroll in RN to BSN programs have a variety of life and work experiences, in addition to experiences in previous educational programs. They are often motivated to enroll in RN to BSN programs and achieve the higher degree in order to secure employment, advance their careers, or fulfill their personal goals (Megginson, 2008). The BSN degree is the gateway to graduate education and subsequent roles in advanced practice, nursing education, and research. The purpose of the completion program is to assist students to develop higher level critical thinking skills, broaden their scope of practice, and understand the social, cultural, economic, and geopolitical context of health care in order to assume expanded professional roles (AACN, 2009).

Academic Progression for Nurses

Based on increasing demands in health care and the need for high-quality health outcomes across all care settings, the IOM (2010) recommended that the nursing education system be improved to support nurses' achievement of higher levels of education. Subsequently, the IOM challenged nurse leaders to work together to increase the number of baccalaureate-prepared nurses from 50% to 80% by the year 2020. As a result, academic nurse leaders recognized the need to develop collaborative relationships between community colleges and higher degree programs. Certain states have mandated articulation agreement requirements that facilitate academic progression for nurses. For example, the Administrative Rule Division 21 requires that all prelicensure programs in Oregon have an articulation agreement in place to facilitate progression to a baccalaureate or higher degree nursing program (Ingwerson, 2012).

Articulation agreements are renewable agreements negotiated to ensure equivalency between college and university courses, support educational mobility, and facilitate the seamless transfer of academic credit between ADN and BSN programs (AACN, 2013b). Articulation agreements address the needs of students and programs by facilitating a more streamlined progression experience. Students benefit from transferring credit between institutions, making informed decisions about course selection, and experiencing the collaboration across nursing programs (AACN, 2013b; Ingwerson, 2012; Spencer, 2008). Some agreements have been as specific as offering dual enrollment in the associate and baccalaureate programs upon admission to the associate degree program (Ingwerson, 2012). Dual enrollment provides students with additional benefits such as academic advising and support as well as more diverse course offerings.

RN to BSN Program of Study

The mission, vision, philosophy, theoretical model, and student learning outcomes for an RN to BSN program are often the same as the generic BSN program at a particular school, although the program of study may look very different. See Table 11.7 for an example of an RN to BSN program of study. Program credits and length are variable between schools, and the design of the curriculum often offers part-time and online options in order to meet the needs of working nurses.

TABLE 11.7 RN TO BSN PROGRAM OF STUDY

SEMESTER 1: FOUNDATIONS FOR COMMUNITY BASED NURSING PRACTICE	CREDITS	SEMESTER 2: STEWARDSHIP OF HEALTH	CREDITS	SEMESTER 3: STEWARDSHIP OF HEALTH EXPERIENTIAL LEARNING	CREDITS
Transition to Professional Nursing Practice*	6	Scholarship of Nursing	3	Integrated Experiential Learning IV (clinical)	8
Professional Communication in Diverse Communities	2	Leading and Managing in Nursing	3		
		Population-Based Nursing in a Multicultural and Global Society	2		
	8		8		8

*Includes 32 credits for prior learning after completion of the first RN to BSN class.
Source: Linfield-Good Samaritan School of Nursing Curriculum Committee. Used with permission.

Credit for Prior Learning

As the nursing workforce is challenged to meet the increasingly complex needs of the current and future health care system, nursing programs across the country are challenged to encourage RNs to return to school for BSN completion. Nursing programs responded to this challenge by acknowledging that the RN holds knowledge, skills, and abilities related to prior work experience that can be applied to the current degree they are seeking. It is typical for RN to BSN completion programs to require introductory courses that are designed to validate this prior knowledge and to "bridge" or "transition" the RN from diploma or associate degree preparation. In addition to providing an opportunity to validate prior knowledge and skills, these introductory courses offer learning experiences, such as professional portfolio activities, that assist with the role transition and socialization to the BSN level of preparation. The nurse is granted credit for selected prelicensure courses offered at the upper division level once the transition course is successfully completed.

For example, at the LGSSON RN to BSN program, credit for prior learning equates knowledge demonstrated through experience with Linfield College courses and awards 32 semester credits of nursing coursework that includes many of the clinical courses in the generic curriculum. Course outcomes and related learning assessments in the transition course focus on evaluation of the nursing knowledge, skills, and professionalism that the nurse brings to the program from prior work experience and demonstration of readiness for subsequent courses in the curriculum.

Curriculum Strategies

The RN to BSN curriculum addresses nurses' need for socialization, preparation for graduate study, career growth, and leadership development (Spencer, 2008). In the typical RN to BSN curriculum, the nurse is prepared for an expanded professional role through coursework focused on enhancing professional communication, theoretical perspectives, community and population-based nursing care, and leadership. The senior practicum hours are spent working with nurse preceptors in acute care settings as well as in community-based settings where the nurses build on previous knowledge and enhance their effectiveness across the continuum of care. Many programs incorporate professional projects designed to meet the needs of the clinical agency from an evidence-based perspective, while other activities include projects related to nursing leadership, health promotion, disease prevention, and the care of vulnerable populations.

With a growing awareness about the positive outcomes associated with advancing to higher levels of education and increasing encouragement from employers who provide tuition support for RN to BSN programs, more and more nurses are returning to school to complete a baccalaureate degree (Raines & Taglaireni, 2008). In order to meet the demand for BSN completion, nursing programs responded by offering curricula delivered through online and distance learning, the traditional classroom setting, or by using combined methods such as hybrid or web-enhanced approaches (AACN, 2009; Talbert, 2009). Distance education provides

RN to BSN students, who are usually employed and juggling multiple roles, with greater accessibility to attend class at times of the day that meet their needs. Nurses attending online completion programs also benefit from geographic flexibility, self-directed learning and motivation, professional socialization, and peer support.

Clinical Experiences

The increasing enrollment in RN to BSN programs creates additional strain on scarce clinical practicum sites and faculty. However, the fact that RN to BSN students are licensed, as compared to the BSN student, allows for placement of licensed nurses in a variety of traditional and nontraditional clinical sites. This ability generates opportunities for students to provide nursing care in settings in which they can begin to view caring in new ways, awakening a sense of advocacy, civic responsibility, and concern for political action (Hunt, 2007). A sense of responsibility is gained from various types of experiential and service learning experiences that extend beyond the singular nurse–client relationship to embrace the client's family, community, and society (Hunt, 2007). Clinical experiences designed for service in community-based settings assist the nurse in adopting a broader, global view of nursing practice.

RN to BSN students benefit from being able to explore areas of interest for their clinical experiences as well as collaborating with faculty to identify creative ways to meet their goals for learning. There is the potential for deep engagement and mutuality for preceptors and staff in clinical sites within the student's community. RN to BSN students often choose experiences in public and community health, school-based health settings, correctional nursing, mental and behavioral health centers, addiction treatment and homeless shelters, geriatric settings, and home health and hospice settings. In addition, RN to BSN students are uniquely suited for participation in global health care delivery when interested in opportunities for international travel and meeting the needs of the vulnerable and underserved.

International clinical placements and studies abroad are recognized as broadening students' cultural understanding and prepare them for authentic relationships in the professional clinical setting (Edgecombe, Jennings, & Bowden, 2013). Students have the opportunity to explore diverse cultures and communities as well as gain knowledge of different health care systems. RN to BSN students who complete international clinical experiences have described meaningful learning that took place related to awareness of diversity and cultural competence in nursing, enhanced skills in intercultural communication, an increased awareness of social and political injustices, and a greater understanding of poverty.

Inexperienced RN to BSN Students

As the trend toward hiring "BSN preferred" nurses continues, it is anticipated that more nurses will enter RN to BSN completion programs immediately following graduation from associate degree and diploma programs. In order to meet admission requirements for RN to BSN completion programs, applicants must pass the

NCLEX examination for licensure and obtain an RN license. Since the RN to BSN curriculum builds upon the prior work experience of the RN, nurses just beginning nursing practice require special consideration related to their relative lack of clinical experience. There may be new graduate nurses who have not found nursing jobs following completion of their initial degree and have no work experience, which challenges some of the assumptions of many RN to BSN programs. Depending on the structure of the curriculum, inexperienced RN to BSN students may have difficulty engaging in classroom activities designed for experienced RNs to apply new knowledge and insights to their current practice. In the clinical setting, the less experienced RN requires additional oversight and support by faculty and preceptors, beyond what is usually provided for licensed students.

Despite some of the challenges for new graduate nurses who enter completion programs, RN to BSN programs provide valuable experiences for students. Completion programs have demonstrated an impact on the socialization and resocialization of nurses (Clark, 2004) and the development of professional values of nurses (Kubsch, Hansen, & Huyser-Eatwell, 2008). Students benefit from learning collaboratively with nurses who have varied years and types of clinical experiences.

Research suggests that RN students, in their quest for higher education, seek to attain professional credibility, career mobility, personal achievement, and longevity in nursing (Megginson, 2008). The RN to BSN completion programs provide a rich and supportive environment for nurses returning to school. Nursing faculty members have the opportunity to mentor and role model professional behaviors that assist in building positive connections and influence the learning of their students.

SUMMARY

Robust baccalaureate nursing education programs are foundational to the health of the profession and the population and as preparation for graduate nursing education. Curriculum development and revision is both a challenge and an opportunity to shape the future. Collaboration with stakeholders including other health care professionals, consumers of health care, and health care service organizations is essential in order to innovate and find local solutions in a new age of health care reform. It is incumbent upon nurse educators to try new curricular approaches, evaluate their efficacy, and share the results with the professional community.

The authors would like to acknowledge the Curriculum Committee at LGS-SON for their hard work and commitment in developing their revised curriculum and their willingness to share their work with the nursing community.

DISCUSSION QUESTIONS

1. Identify your primary partners in service or education. What is the nature of those relationships and how could they be expanded to create innovative clinical experiences for nursing students?
2. What are the most common groups of underrepresented students in your region? How could your curriculum be changed to be more inclusive of these groups?

3. What are the barriers to prelicensure graduates' successful transition into practice? Describe strategies in your curriculum that help to mediate "reality shock." What are some new ideas that could be developed?
4. How will health care reform affect your prelicensure program? Interview the chair of the undergraduate curriculum committee at your school to determine if there is a plan for curriculum revision.
5. Using the Candela, Dalley, and Benzel-Lindley (2006) approach for categorizing content, review a course in the BSN curriculum and identify which content (knowledge, skills, and attitudes) is most essential?
6. Create an innovative clinical education model that meets the criteria outlined by MacIntyre et al. (2009).
7. How could IPE be integrated into the curriculum at your college or university?

LEARNING ACTIVITIES

NURSE EDUCATOR/FACULTY DEVELOPMENT ACTIVITIES

1. Map your curriculum outcomes according to the AACN *Essentials* (2008b). What changes need to be made to update your program?
2. Create a visual representation of your school's theoretical model.
3. Invite a colleague to coffee and discuss the "sacred cows" at your institution that could be barriers to innovative curriculum revision.

REFERENCES

Allen, P. E., Armstrong, M. L., Conard, P. L., Saladiner, J. E., & Hamilton, M. J. (2013). Veterans' health care consideration for today's nursing curricula. *Journal of Nursing Education, 52*(11), 634–640.

Altier, M. E., & Krsek, C. A. (2006). Effects of a 1-year residency program on job satisfaction and retention of new graduate nurses. *Journal for Nurses in Staff Development, 22*(2), 70–77.

American Association of Colleges and Universities. (2007). *College learning for the new global century. A report from the National Leadership Council for Liberal Education & America's Promise.* Washington, DC: AACN. Retrieved from http://www.aacu.org/leap/documents/GlobalCentury_final.pdf

American Association of Colleges and Universities. (2014). *Board statement on diversity, equity, and inclusive excellence.* Retrieved from http://www.aacu.org/about/statements/2013/inclusiveexcellence.cfm

American Association of Colleges of Nursing. (1998). *Peaceful death: Recommended competencies and curricular guidelines for end-of-life nursing care.* Retrieved from http://www.aacn.nche.edu/elnec/publications/peaceful-death

American Association of Colleges of Nursing. (2006). *Essential nursing competencies and curricula guidelines for genetics and genomics.* Retrieved from http://www.aacn.nche.edu/Education/pdf/Genetics%20%20Genomics%20Nursing%20Competencies%2009-22-06.pdf

American Association of Colleges of Nursing. (2008a). *Cultural competency in baccalaureate nursing education.* Retrieved from http://www.aacn.nche.edu/Education/pdf/competency.pdf

American Association of Colleges of Nursing. (2008b). *The essentials of baccalaureate education for professional nursing practice.* Retrieved from http://www.aacn.nche.edu/Education/pdf/BaccEssentials08.pdf

American Association of Colleges of Nursing. (2009). *Degree completion programs for registered nurses: RN to master's degree and RN to baccalaureate programs.* Retrieved from http://www.aacn.nche.edu/media-relations/fact-sheets/degree-completion-programs

American Association of Colleges of Nursing. (2012). *Fact sheet: Accelerated baccalaureate and master's degrees in nursing.* Retrieved from http://www.aacn.nche.edu/media-relations/AccelProgsGlance.pdf

American Association of Colleges of Nursing. (2013a). *Accelerated programs: The fast-track to careers in nursing.* Washington, DC: Author. Retrieved from http://www.aacn.nche.edu/publications/issue-bulletin-accelerated-programs

American Association of Colleges of Nursing. (2013b). *Articulation agreements among nursing education programs.* Retrieved from http://www.aacn.nche.edu/media-relations/fact-sheets/articulation-agreements

American Association of Colleges of Nursing–American Organization of Nurse Executives Task Force on Academic-Practice Partnerships. (2012). *Guiding principles.* Retrieved from http://www.aacn.nche.edu/leading-initiatives/academic-practice-partnerships/GuidingPrinciples.pdf

American Association of Colleges of Nursing & the John A. Hartford Foundation Institute for Geriatric Nursing. (2010). *Older adults: Recommended baccalaureate competencies and curricular guidelines for geriatric nursing care.* Washington, DC: Author. Retrieved from http://www.aacn.nche.edu/geriatric-nursing/AACN_Gerocompetencies.pdf

American Nurses Association. (2005). *Code of ethics for nurses with interpretive statements.* Silver Spring, MD: Author.

American Organization of Nurse Executives. (2004). *Guiding principles for the role of the nurse in future health care delivery.* Retrieved from http://www.aone.org/aone/resource/practiceandeducation.html

Andersen, E. A., Strumpel, C., Fensom, I., & Andrews, W. (2011). Implementing team based learning in large classes: Nurse educators' experiences. *International Journal of Nursing Education Scholarship, 8*(1), 1–16.

Anderson, G. L., & Tredway, C. A. (2009). Transforming the nursing curriculum to promote critical thinking online. *Journal of Nursing Education, 48*(2), 111–115.

Angelini, D. (2011). Interdisciplinary and interprofessional education. *Journal of Perinatal & Neonatal Nursing, 25*(2), 175–179. doi:10.1097/JPN.Ob013e3182ee7a

Baker, C., Pulling, C., McGraw, R., Dagnone, J. D., Hopins-Russeel, D., & Medves, J. (2008). Simulation in interprofessional education for patient-centred collaborative care. *Journal of Advanced Nursing, 62,* 372–379.

Basilio, N. O. (2013). *Accelerated nursing programs.* Washington, DC: AACN. Retrieved from www.aacn.nche.edu/education-resources/accelerated-article

Benner, P., Sutphen, M., Leonard, V., & Day, L. (2010). *Educating nurses: A call for radical transformation.* San Francisco, CA: Jossey-Bass.

Bergman, J., & Sams, A. (2012). *Flip your classroom.* Eugene, OR: International Society for Technology in Education.

Bleich, M. R. (2009). Technology: An imperative for teaching in the age of digital natives [Editorial]. *Journal of Nursing Education, 48*(2), 63.

Bornais, J. A. K., Raiger, J. E., Krahn, R. E., & El-Masri, M. M. (2012). Evaluating undergraduate nursing students' learning using standardized patients. *Journal of Professional Nursing, 28*(5), 291–296.

Bosher, S. (2007). *Recommendations for meeting the needs of ESL nursing students.* Unpublished report for Linfield-Good Samaritan School of Nursing, Linfield College, Portland, Oregon.

Bosher, S. D., & Pharris, M. D. (2009). *Transforming nursing education: The culturally inclusive environment.* New York, NY: Springer Publishing.

Bratt, M. M. (2009). Retaining the next generation of nurses: The Wisconsin nurse residency program provides a continuum of support. *The Journal of Continuing Education in Nursing, 40*(9), 416–425.

Brewer, C. S., Kovner, C. T., Poornima, S., Fairchild, S., Kim, H., & Djukic, M. (2009). A comparison of second-degree baccalaureate and traditional-baccalaureate new graduate RNs: Implications for the workforce. *Journal of Professional Nursing, 25*(1), 5–14.

Bridges, D. R., Davidson R. A., Odegard, P. S., Maki, I. V., & Tomkowiak, J. (2011). Interprofessional collaboration: Three best practice models of interprofessional education. *Medical Education Online, 16,* 1–10.

Broussard, B. B. (2011). The bucket list: A service-learning approach to community engagement to enhance community health nursing clinical learning. *Journal of Nursing Education, 50*(1), 40–43.

Brown, S. T., Kirkpatrick, M. K., Mangum, D., & Avery, J. (2008). A review of narrative pedagogy strategies to transform traditional nursing education. *Journal of Nursing Education, 47*(6), 283–286.

Buchbinder, H. (2007). *Increasing Latino participation in the nursing profession: Best practices at California nursing programs.* Los Angeles, CA: Tomás Rivera Policy Institute.

Buckley, S., Hensman, M., Thomas, S., Dudley, R., Nevin, G., & Coleman, J. (2012). Developing interprofessional simulation in the undergraduate setting: Experience with five different professional groups. *Journal of Interprofessional Care, 26,* 362–369.

Budden, J. S., Zhong, E. H., Moulton, P., & Cimiotti, J. P. (2013). Highlights of the national workforce survey of registered nurses. *Journal of Nursing Regulation, 4*(2), 5–13.

Candela, L., Dalley, K., & Benzel-Lindley, J. (2006). A case for learning-centered curricula. *Journal of Nursing Education, 45*(2), 59–66.

Cangelosi, P. R. (2007). Accelerated second-degree baccalaureate nursing programs: What is the significance of clinical instructors? *Journal of Nursing Education, 46*(9), 400–405.

Clark, C. (2004). The professional socialization of graduating students in generic and two-plus-two baccalaureate completion nursing programs. *Journal of Nursing Education, 43*(8), 346–351.

Commission on Collegiate Nursing Education. (2008). *Standards for accreditation of postbaccalaureate nurse residency programs.* Washington, DC: CCNE. Retrieved from www.aacn.nche.edu/Accreditation/PubsRes.htm

Cordeau, M. A. (2012). Linking the transition: A substantive theory of high-stakes clinical simulation. *Advances in Nursing Science, 35*(3), E90–E102.

Creedy, D. K., Mitchell, M., Seaton-Sykes, P., Cooke, M., Patterson, E., Purcell, C., & Weeks, P. (2007). Evaluating a web-enhanced bachelor of nursing curriculum: Perspectives of third-year students. *Journal of Nursing Education, 46*(10), 460–467.

Cronenwett, L., Sherwood, G., Barnsteiner, J., Disch, J., Johnson, J., Mitchell, P., . . . Warren, J. (2007). Quality and safety education for nurses. *Nursing Outlook, 55,* 122–131.

Crow, K. (1997). Interpreting transcultural knowledge into nursing curricula: An American Indian example. In A. I. Morey & M. K. Kitano (Eds.), *Multicultural course transformation in higher education* (pp. 211–228). Boston, MA: Allyn & Bacon.

Curran, C. R., Elfrink, V., & Mays, B. (2009). Building a virtual community for nursing education: The town of Mirror Lake. *Journal of Nursing Education, 48*(1), 30–35.

Didion, J., Kozy, M. A., Koffel, C., & Oneail, K. (2012). Academic/clinical partnership and collaboration in quality and safety education for nurses' education. *Journal of Professional Nursing, 29*(2), 88–94. Retrieved from http://dx.doi.org /10.1016/j.profurs.2012.12.004

Diefenbeck, C. A., Plowfield, L. A., & Herrman, J. W. (2006). Clinical immersion: A residency model for nursing education. *Nursing Education Perspectives, 27*(2), 72–79.

Diekelman, N. (2005). Engaging the students and the teacher: Co-creating substantive reform with narrative pedagogy. *Journal of Nursing Education, 44*(6), 249–252.

Dubose, D., Sellinger-Karmel, L. D., & Scoloveno, R. L. (2010). Baccalaureate nursing education. In W. M. Nehring & F. R. Lashley (Eds.), *High-fidelity simulation in nursing education* (pp. 189–209). Sudbury, MA: Jones & Bartlett.

Edgecombe, K., Jennings, M., & Bowden, M. (2013). International nursing students and what impacts their clinical learning: Literature review. *Nurse Education Today, 33*(2), 138-142.

Eigsti, J. E. (2009). Graduate nurses' perceptions of a critical care nurse internship program. *Journal for Nurses in Staff Development, 25*(4), 191–198.

Ervin, N. E., Bickes, J. T., & Schim, S. M. (2006). Environments of care: A curriculum model for preparing a new generation of nurses. *Journal of Nursing Education, 45*(2), 75–80.

Fitzgerald, B. (2009). Educating novice perioperative nurses. *Perioperative Nursing Clinics, 4*, 141–155.

Forbes, M. A., & Hickey, M. T. (2009). Curriculum reform in baccalaureate nursing education: Review of the literature. *International Journal of Nursing Education Scholarship, 6*(1), 1–16.

Gardner, C. L., & Jones, S. J. (2012). Utilization of academic electronic medical record in undergraduate nursing education. *Online Journal of Nursing Informatics, 16*(2), 31–37.

Giddens, J. F. (2007). The neighborhood: A web-based platform to support conceptual teaching and learning. *Nursing Education Perspectives, 28*(5), 251–256.

Giddens, J. F., & Brady, D. P. (2007). Rescuing nursing education from content saturation: The case for a concept-based curriculum. *Journal of Nursing Education, 46*(2), 65–69.

Giddens, J. F., & Eddy, L. (2009). A survey of physical examination skills taught in undergraduate nursing programs: Are we teaching too much? *Journal of Nursing Education, 48*(1), 24–29.

Giddens, J. F., Wright, M., & Gray, I. (2012). Selecting concepts for a concept-based curriculum: Application of a benchmark approach. *Journal of Nursing Education, 51*(9), 511–515.

Goode, C. J., Lynn, M. R., & McElroy, D. (2013). Lessons learned from 10 years of research on a post-baccalaureate nurse residency program. *Journal of Nursing Administration, 43*(2), 73–79.

Goudreau, J., Pepin, J., Dubois, S., Boyer, L., Larue, C., & Legault, A. (2009). A second generation of the competency-based approach to nursing education. *International Journal of Nursing Education Scholarship, 6*(1).

Groh, C. J., Stallwood, L. G., & Daniels, J. J. (2011). Service-learning in nursing education: Its impact on leadership and social justice. *Nursing Education Perspectives, 32*, 400–405.

Gubrud-Howe, P., & Schloesser, M. (2008). From random access opportunity to a clinical education curriculum [Editorial]. *Journal of Nursing Education, 47*(1), 3–4.

Gubrud-Howe, P., Shaver, K. S., Tanner, C. A., Bennett-Stillmaker, J., Davidson, S. B., Flaherty-Robb, M. . . . Wheeler, P. (2003). A challenge to meet the future: Nursing education in Oregon, 2010. *Journal of Nursing Education, 42*(4), 163–167.

Hanson, M. J. S., & Carpenter, D. R. (2011). Integrating cooperative learning into classroom testing. *Nursing Education Perspectives, 32*, 270–273.

Harder, B. N. (2010). Use of simulation in teaching and learning in health sciences: A systematic review. *Journal of Nursing Education, 49*(1), 23–28.

Hegge, M. J., & Hallman, P. A. (2008). Changing nursing culture to welcome second-degree students: Herding and corralling sacred cows. *Journal of Nursing Education, 47*(12), 552–556.

Herrman, J. W., & Diefenbeck, C. (2009). The nurse residency model: A clinical immersion model for curriculum change. *Dean's Notes, 30*(4), 1–2.

Hickey, M. T. (2009). Preceptor perceptions of new graduate nurse readiness for practice. *Journal for Nurses in Staff Development, 25*(1), 35–41.

Hofler, L. D. (2008). Nursing education and transition to the work environment: A synthesis of national reports. *Journal of Nursing Education, 47*(1), 5–12.

Hudson, C. E., Sanders, M. K., & Pepper, C. (2013). Interprofessional education and prelicensure baccalaureate nursing students: An integrative review. *Nurse Educator, 38*(2), 76–80.

Hull, E., St. Romain, J. A., Alexander, P., Schaff, S., & Jones, W. (2001). Moving cemeteries: A framewok for facilitating curriculum revision. *Nurse Educator, 26*(6), 280–282.

Hunt, R. (2007). Service-learning: An eye-opening experience that provokes emotion and challenges stereotypes. *Journal of Nursing Education,46*(6), 277–281.

Ingwerson, J. (2012). Articulation agreements support moving forward. *Oregon State Board of Nursing Sentinel,31*(2), 8–9.

Institute of Medicine. (2001). *Crossing the quality chasm*. Washington, DC: National Academies Press.

Institute of Medicine. (2003). *Health professions education: A bridge to quality*. Washington, DC: National Academies Press.

Institute of Medicine. (2004). *In the nation's compelling interest: Ensuring diversity in the health care workforce*. Washington, DC: National Academies Press.

Institute of Medicine. (2010). *The future of nursing: Leading change, advancing health*. Washington, DC: National Academies Press.

Interprofessional Education Collaborative Expert Panel. (2011). *Core competencies for interprofessional collaborative practice: Report of an expert panel*. Washington, DC: Interprofessional Education Collaborative. Retrieved from http://www.aacn.nche. edu/education-resources/ipecreport.pdf

Ironside, P. M. (2004). "Covering content" and teaching thinking: Deconstructing the additive curriculum. *Journal of Nursing Education, 43*(1), 5–12.

Ironside, P. M. (2006). Using narrative pedagogy: Learning and practicing interpretive thinking. *Journal of Advanced Nursing, 55*(4), 478–486.

Ironside, P., Jeffries, P., & Martin, A. (2009). Fostering patient safety competencies using multiple-patient simulation experiences. *Nursing Outlook, 57*(6), 332–337.

Ironside, P., & McNelis, A. (2009). NLN clinical education survey. In N. Ard & T. M. Valiga (Eds.), *Clinical nursing education: Current reflections* (pp. 25–38). New York, NY: National League for Nursing.

Jacobson, L., & Grindel, C. (2006). What is happening in pre-licensure RN clinical nursing education: Findings from the faculty and administrator survey on clinical nursing education. *Nursing Education Perspectives, 27*(2), 108–109.

Johnson, D. M., & Bushey, T. I. (2011). Integrating the academic electronic health record into nursing curriculum: Perparing student nurses for practice. *Computers, Informatics, Nursing, 29*(3), 133–137.

Joynt, J., & Kimball, B. (2008). *Blowing open the bottleneck: Designing new approaches to increase nurse education capacity*. Retrieved from http://championnursing.org/sites/ default/files/1695_BlowingOpentheBottleneck.pdf

Kemsley, M., McCausland, L., Feigenbaum, J., & Riegle, E. (2011). Analysis of graduates' perceptions of an accelerated bachelor of science program in nursing. *Journal of Professional Nursing, 27*(1), 50–58.

Kidd, L. I., Knisley, S. J., & Morgan, K. I. (2012). Effectiveness of a second life simulation as a teaching strategy for undergraduate mental health nursing students. *Journal of Psychosocial Nursing, 50*(7), 28–37.

Kohn, P. S., & Truglio-Londrigan, M. (2007). Second-career baccalaureate nursing students: A lived experience. *Journal of Nursing Education, 46*(9), 391–399.

Korvick, L. M., Wisener, L. K., Loftis, L. A., & Williamson, M. L. (2008). Comparing the academic performance of students in traditional and second-degree baccalaureate programs. *Journal of Nursing Education, 47*(3), 130–141.

Kramer, M. (1974). *Reality shock: Why nurses leave nursing.* St. Louis, MO: Mosby.

Kruger, B. J., Roush, C., Olinzock, B. J., & Bloom, K. (2010). Engaging nursing students in a long-term relationship with a home-based community. *Journal of Nursing Education, 49*(1), 10–16.

Kubsch, S., Hansen, G., & Huyser-Eatwell, V. (2008). Professional values: The case for RN-BSN completion education. *The Journal of Continuing Education in Nursing, 38*(8), 375–384.

Lindsey, P. (2009). Starting an accelerated baccalaureate nursing program: Challenges and opportunities for creative educational innovations. *Journal of Nursing Education, 48*(5), 279–281.

Little, B. B. (2009). The use of standards for peer review of online nursing courses: A pilot study. *Journal of Nursing Education, 48*(7), 411–415.

Loewenson, K. M., & Hunt, R. J. (2011). Transforming attitudes of nursing students: Evaluating a service-learning experience. *Journal of Nursing Education, 50*(6), 345–349.

Luctkar-Flude, M., Wilson-Keates, B., & Larocque, M. (2012). Evaluating high-fidelity human simulators and standardized patients in an undergraduate nursing health assessment course. *Nurse Education Today, 32*, 448–452.

MacIntyre, R. C., Murray, T. A., Teel, C. S., & Karshmer, J. F. (2009). Five recommendations for prelicensure clinical nursing education. *Journal of Nursing Education, 48*(8), 447–453.

Mawn, B., & Reece, S. M. (2000). Reconfiguring a curriculum for the new millennium: The process of change. *Journal of Nursing Education, 39*(3), 101–108.

McEwen, M., & Brown, S. C. (2002). Conceptual frameworks in undergraduate nursing curricula: Report of a national survey. *Journal of Nursing Education, 41*(1), 5–14.

McGuire-Sessions, M., & Gubrud, P. (2010). Interdisciplinary simulation center. In W. M. Nehring & F. R. Lashley (Eds.), *High-fidelity patient simulation in nursing education* (pp. 303–322). Sudbury, MA: Jones & Bartlett.

Megginson, L. (2008). RN-BSN education: 21st century barriers and incentives. *Journal of Nursing Management, 16*, 47–55.

Mellor, R., Cottrell, N., & Moran, M. (2013). "Just working in a team was a great experience…"—Student perspectives on the learning experiences of an interprofessional education program. *Journal of Interprofessional Care, 27*, 292–297.

Missildine, K., Fountain, R., Summers, L., & Gisselin, K. (2013). Flipping the classroom to improve student performance and satisfaction. *Journal of Nursing Education, 44*(10), 597–599.

Moscato, S. R., Miller, J., Logsdon, K., Weinberg, S., & Chorpenning, L. (2007). Dedicated education unit: An innovative clinical partner model. *Nursing Outlook, 55*, 31–37.

National Council of State Boards of Nursing. (2009). *Report of findings from the effect of high-fidelity simulation on nursing students' knowledge and performance: A pilot study.* NCSBN Research Brief, 40. Chicago, IL: Author.

National League for Nursing Think Tank on Transforming Clinical Nursing Education. (2008). *Final report of the 2008 NLN think tank on transforming clinical nursing education.* Retrieved from http://www.nln.org/facultydevelopment/pdf/think_tank.pdf

Nehring, W. M. (2008). U.S. boards of nursing and the use of high-fidelity patient simulators in nursing education. *Journal of Professional Nursing, 24*(2), 109–117.

Neill, M. A. (2011). Graduate-entry nursing students' experiences of an accelerated nursing degree-a literature review. *Nurse Education in Practice, 11*, 81–85.

Newman, D. (2008). Conceptual models of nursing and baccalaureate nursing education [Editorial]. *Journal of Nursing Education, 47*(5), 199–200.

Nielsen, A. E., Noone, J., Voss, H., & Mathews, L. R. (2013). Preparing nursing students for the future: An innovative approach to clinical education. *Nurse Education in Practice,13*(4), 301–309.

Nokes, K., Nickitas, D. M., Keida, R., & Neville, S. (2005). Does service-learning increase cultural competency, critical thinking, and civic engagement? *Journal of Nursing Education, 44*(2), 65–69.

Noone, J. (2009). Teaching to the three apprenticeships: Designing learning activities for professional practice in an undergraduate curriculum. *Journal of Nursing Education, 48*(8), 468–471.

Noone, J., Sideras, S., Gubrud-Howe, P., Voss, H., & Mathews, L. R. (2012). Influence of a poverty simulation on nursing student attitudes toward poverty. *Journal of Nursing Education, 51*(11), 617–622.

O'Brien-Larivee, C. O. (2011). A service-learning experience to teach baccalaureate nursing students about health policy. *Journal of Nursing Education, 50*(6), 332–336.

Olson-Sitki, K., Wendler, M. C., & Forbes, G. (2012). Evaluating the impact of a nurse residency program for newly graduated registered nurses. *Journal for Nurses in Staff Development, 28*(4), 156–162.

Paul, P., Olson, J., Jackman, D., Gauthier, D., Gibson, B., Kabotoff, W., . . . Hungler, K. (2011). Perceptions of extrinsic factors that contribute to a nursing internship experience. *Nurse Education Today, 31*, 763–767.

Penprase, B., & Koczara, S. (2009). Understanding the experiences of accelerated second-degree nursing students and graduates: A review of the literature. *The Journal of Continuing Education in Nursing, 40*(2), 74–78.

Rafferty, M., & Lindell, D. (2011). How nurse managers rate the clinical competencies of accelerated (second-degree) nursing graduates. *Journal of Nursing Education, 50*(6), 355–357.

Raines, C., & Taglaireni, M. (2008). Career pathways in nursing: Entry points and academic progression. *The Online Journal of Issues in Nursing: A Scholarly Journal of the American Nurses Association, 13*(3). Retrieved from https://nursingworld.org

Raines, D. A. (2007). Accelerated second-degree program evaluation at graduation and 1 year later. *Nurse Educator, 32*(4), 183–186.

Raines, D. A. (2009). Competence of accelerated second degree students after studying in a collaborative model of nursing practice education. *International Journal of Nursing Education Scholarship, 6*(1), 1–12.

Raines, D. A. (2010). Nursing practice competency of accelerated bachelor of science in nursing program students. *Journal of Professional Nursing, 26*(3), 162–167.

Raines, D. A. (2013). Five years later: Are accelerated, second-degree program graduates still in the workforce? *International Journal of Nursing Education Scholarship, 10*(1), 1–6.

Raines, D. A., & Sipes, A. (2007). One year later: Reflections and work activities of accelerated second-degree bachelor of science in nursing graduates. *Journal of Professional Nursing, 23*(6), 329–334.

Reese, C. E., Jeffries, P. R., & Engum, S. A. (2010). Using simulations to develop nursing and medical student collaboration. *Nursing Education Perspectives, 31*(1), 33–37.

Reid, J. M. (1987). The learning style preferences of ESL students. *TESOL Quarterly, 21*(1), 87–111.

Riesen, E., Morley, M., Clendinneng, D., Ogilvie, S., & Murray, M. A. (2012). Improving interprofessional competence in undergraduate students using a novel blended approach. *Journal of Interprofessional Nursing, 26*, 312–318. doi:10.3109/13561820.2012.660286

Salfi, J., Solomon, P., Allen, D., Mohaupt, J., & Patterson, C. (2012). Overcoming all obstacles: A framework for embedding interprofessional education into a large, multisite Bachelor of Science Nursing program. *Journal of Nursing Education, 51*(2), 106–110.

Scherer, Y. K., Myer, J., O'Connor, T. D., & Haskins, M. (2013). Interprofessional simulation to foster collaboration between nursing and medical students. *Clinical-Simulation in Nursing, 9,* e497–e505. Retrieved from http://dx.doi.org/10.1016/j.ecns.2013.03.001

Sharpnack, P. A., & Madigan, E. A. (2012). Using low-fidelity simulation with sophomore nursing students in a baccalaureate nursing program. *Nursing Education Perspectives, 33*(4), 264–268.

Shiyanbola, O. O., Lammers, C., Randall, B., & Richards, A. (2012). Evaluation of a student-led Interprofessional innovative health promotion model for an underserved population with diabetes: A pilot project. *Journal of Interprofessional Care,26,* 376–382.

Simpson, V. L. (2012). Making it meaningful: Teaching public health nursing through academic-community partnerships in a baccalaureate curriculum. *Nursing Education Perspectives,33,* 260–263.

Sinclair, B., & Ferguson, K. (2009). Integrating simulated teaching/learning strategies in undergraduate nursing education. *International Journal of Nursing Education Scholarship, 6*(1), 1–11.

Skiba, D. J. (2007). Emerging technologies center. Faculty 2.0: Flipping the novice to expert continuum. *Nursing Education Perspectives, 28*(6), 342–344.

Skiba, D. J. (2009). Nursing education 2.0: A second look at Second Life. *Nursing Education Perspectives, 30,* 129–131.

Spector, N., & Echternacht, M. (2010). NCSBN focus: 2009 Update on the National Council of State Boards of Nursing's regulatory model for transitioning new nurses to practice. *JONA's Healthcare Law, Ethics, and Regulation, 12*(1), 12–14. Retrieved from http://dx.doi.org.liboff.ohsu.edu/10.1097/NHL.0b013e3181d294c1

Spencer, J. (2008). Increasing RN-BSN enrollments: Facilitating articulation through curriculum reform. *The Journal of Continuing Education in Nursing, 39*(7), 307–313.

Swaner, L. E., & Brownell, J. E. (2008). *Outcomes of high impact practices for underserved students: A review of the literature.* Retrieved from http://www.aacu.org/inclusive_excellence/documents/DRAFTProjectUSALiteratureReview.pdf

Talbert, J. (2009). Distance education: One solution to the nursing shortage? *Clinical Journal of Oncology Nursing, 13*(3), 269–270.

Tanner, C. A. (2006). Thinking like a nurse: A research-based model of clinical judgment in nursing. *Journal of Nursing Education, 45*(6), 204–210.

Tanner, C. A. (2007). The curriculum revolution revisited [Editorial]. *Journal of Nursing Education, 46*(2), 51–52.

Teeley, K. H. (2007). Designing hybrid web-based courses for accelerated nursing students. *Journal of Nursing Education, 46*(9), 417–422.

U.S. Department of Health and Human Services. (2011). Healthy People 2020. Washington, DC: U.S. Government Printing Office. Retrieved from http://www.healthypeople.gov/2020/default.aspx

U.S. Department of Health and Human Services, Health Resources and Services Administration. (2010). *The registered nurse population: Initial findings from the 2008 National Sample Survey of Registered Nurses.* Retrieved from http://bhpr.hrsa.gov/healthworkforce/rnsurvey/initialfindings2008.pdf

Utley, Q., Phillips, B., & Turner, K. (2007). Avoiding socialization pitfalls in accelerated second-degree nursing education: The returning-to-school syndrome model. *Journal of Nursing Education, 46*(9), 423–426.

Walker, J. T., Martin, T. M., Haynie, L., Norwood, A., White, J., & Grant, L. (2007). Preferences for teaching methods in a baccalaureate nursing program: How second-degree and traditional students differ. *Nursing Education Perspectives, 28*(5), 246–250.

Ward, J., Cody, J., Schaal, M., & Hojat, M. (2012). The empathy enigma: An empirical study of decline in empathy among undergraduate nursing students. *Journal of Professional Nursing, 28*(1), 34–40.

Warda, M. R. (2008). Curriculum revolution: Implications for Hispanic nursing students. *Hispanic Health Care International, 6*(4), 192–199.

Weathers, S. M., & Hunt Raleigh, E. D. (2013). 1-year retention rates and performance ratings: Comparing associate degree, baccalaureate, and accelerated baccalaureate degree nurses. *Journal of Nursing Administration, 43*(9), 468–474.

Webber, P. B. (2002). A curriculum framework for nursing. *Journal of Nursing Education, 41*(1), 15–24.

Weimer, M. (2002). *Learner-centered teaching.* San Francisco, CA: Jossey-Bass.

Williams, B. (2001). Developing critical reflection for professional practice through problem-based learning. *Journal of Advanced Nursing, 34*(1), 27–34.

Williams, D. A., Berger, J. B., & McClendon, S. A. (2005). *Toward a model of inclusive excellence and change in postsecondary education.* Washington, DC: AAC&U. Retrieved from http://www.aacu.org/inclusive_excellence/documents/Williams_et_al.pdf

World Health Organization. (2010). WHO *framework for action on interprofessional education and collaborative practice.* Geneva, Switzerland: WHO Press.

Wright, J. A. (2012). Descriptions from accelerated baccalaureate nurses: Determining curriculum and clinical strategies that work best to prepare novice nurses. *International Journal of Nursing Education Scholarship, 9*(1), 1–12.

Yuan, H., Williams, B., & Fan, L. (2007). A systematic review of selected evidence on developing nursing students' critical thinking through problem-based learning. *Nurse Education Today, 28,* 657–663.

Curriculum Planning for Master's Nursing Programs

Sarah B. Keating

Upon completion of Chapter 12, the reader will be able to:

1. Discuss the process of curriculum development for master's programs in nursing including the:
   a. RN to master of science in nursing (MSN) programs
   b. Entry-level MSN
   c. Clinical nurse leader (CNL)
   d. Advanced practice programs
   e. Functional roles, for example, case management, nursing administration/leadership, and nurse educator
   f. Pathways to the doctorate
2. Review recommendations from accrediting, professional specialty and educational organizations, and certification agencies for master's degrees in nursing.
3. Analyze issues surrounding graduate-level nursing at the master's level:
   a. Entry into practice
   b. Terminal degrees and advanced practice
   c. Postmaster's certificates
   d. Certification, licensure, and regulation

OVERVIEW

In the 20th century, as nursing education matured in the academic world and the profession grappled with the issue of defining itself as a discipline, graduate education in nursing evolved. Nursing leaders recognized the need for additional education to be prepared for faculty and administrator roles. Since there was a dearth of graduate nursing programs, nurses often sought degrees in other disciplines such as education, business, and health care administration. Nurses in practice focused their services on clinical specialties such as pediatrics, obstetrics, psychiatric/mental health, medical/surgical nursing, and intensive care; and they too, felt the need for additional specialty training; many seeking nondegree certification. In community settings, it was recognized that public health nurses needed knowledge in epidemiology and the public health sciences, and the specialty roles of nurse midwives and nurse anesthetists required advanced educational preparation and clinical practice. Many of these programs were first offered in baccalaureate programs or as certificate programs to expand on knowledge and skills from basic nursing programs; however, all eventually moved into the graduate level.

In the 1970s, schools of nursing in higher degree institutions developed master's degree programs that focused on the preparation of nursing faculty, administrators, and some of the classic specialties such as pediatrics, maternity, community health, and psychiatric/mental health nursing. These latter specialties became clinical specialties and as they were developing, the advent of the nursing role in primary care began with the introduction of nurse practitioners. With acute care rising in complexity, it became apparent that nurses with blended specialty role preparation were indicated such as the acute care nurse practitioner. More recently, with the implementation of the Affordable Care Act (2014) and the Institute of Medicine's (IOM's) (2014) *The Future of Nursing*, the demand for advanced practice nurses has increased exponentially.

See Chapter 1 for a history of graduate nursing education to gain an appreciation for how nursing evolved in its role in health care to match the needs of the health care system with its growing demands for well-educated providers of care. Out of all of these changes and demands came master's degrees that focused on the specialties, primary care, management/administration, and education. A review of the master's level nursing programs in the United States accredited by the Accreditation Commission for Education in Nursing (2014) and the Commission on Collegiate Nursing Education (2014) found approximately 481 accredited master's nursing programs in the United States in 2013.

Chapter 12 breaks the various master's level programs in nursing into groups from the RN to MSN, entry-level master's, advanced generalist, and finally, to the advanced practice specialty and functional roles that are available in today's graduate programs. Each group is reviewed and its role in graduate nursing and the profession is discussed. Some of the major issues related to master's level nursing education are discussed throughout.

RN TO MSN PROGRAMS

With the call for higher education for nurses by the IOM's recommendations on *The Future of Nursing* (2014) to meet the needs of the U.S. health care system, there is renewed interest in RN to MSN programs. The shortage of nursing faculty adds to this need for nurses with clinical work experience to gain higher education to assume faculty roles. According to the American Association of Colleges of Nursing (AACN) (2014f) and the American Association of Community Colleges (2014), there are more than 173 RN to MSN programs available across the United States and several more in the planning stages.

There are several permutations of curricula for accelerating RNs who have a diploma or associate degree to the master's degree. One format awards the baccalaureate along the way as the RN completes courses equivalent to the upper division level bachelor of science in nursing (BSN). The other format is to not award the BSN but, rather, have the RN complete both upper division baccalaureate and master's level courses and receive the MSN upon completion of the program. Sometimes, both the BSN and MSN are awarded upon completion of the program. Factors that determine the type of program of study include regional accreditation issues, parent institution standards, and the faculty's philosophy. For example, awarding the BSN along the way of the program gives students a baccalaureate whose circumstances prohibit them from completing the master's portion of the program.

The typical patterns for the curricula consist of 1 year accelerated study to complete the baccalaureate upper division level equivalent courses. Following completion of these courses, students enter graduate level courses and depending on the program, may take another 1 ½ to 3 years of master's level courses depending on the type of master's degree, with advanced practice degrees spending more clinical hours and theory courses specific to that branch of advanced practice. Some courses are developed to match the experience of the RNs to the level of education indicated and double count toward both the higher level of the baccalaureate and the introductory level master's courses. Since the large majority of RN students are working, the usual platforms for delivery of the programs are web-based, online, evenings, and/or weekend classes to accommodate their needs.

There are few if any, studies to compare RN to MSN graduates to post-BSN and entry-level master's programs, thus research is called for. The type of master's program (advanced practice or functional role) and the platform for delivery of the program (online, nontraditional, or traditional) should be studied for their effectiveness and student, faculty, and employer satisfaction.

ENTRY-LEVEL (GENERIC) MASTER'S DEGREE PROGRAMS IN NURSING

When planning an entry-level master's program, it is wise to consult with the regional accrediting body and the State Board of Nursing to identify any possible barriers to offering the degree. For example, some regional or state accrediting bodies and Boards of Nursing may require a baccalaureate in nursing prior to earning a master's degree in the same discipline, even if the person has a baccalaureate in another discipline. There are two major pathways or programs of study for nonnursing college graduates to reach licensure (RN) requirements and a graduate degree in nursing. They are described as follows.

The first program provides basic nursing knowledge and skills courses specifically designed for college graduates and taught at the post-baccalaureate level. Included in the program or required as prerequisites are the usual sciences, social sciences, and liberal arts courses. Examples of classic prerequisites for any entry-level nursing program (associate degree, baccalaureate, and master's) are anatomy, chemistry, english, genetics, human development, mathematics/statistics, microbiology, nutrition, physiology, psychology, sociology, and speech/communications. Students in the entry-level master's complete nursing theory and clinical courses at the upper division level, advanced nursing theory and clinical courses at the graduate level, and a capstone experience that can be a thesis, project, and/ or comprehensive examination. Schools of nursing differ in their preparation of these graduates by offering either an advanced generalist master's degree for entry into practice or a specialist track to prepare graduates for advanced levels of nursing practice.

The other entry-level curriculum requires students to complete courses equivalent to or the same as existing courses in baccalaureate level nursing programs. They are not necessarily specifically revised for college graduates. As with the first program, students either must have the prerequisite sciences and liberal arts courses or complete them in the program. After completion of the baccalaureate-level courses, students enter into the master's program to complete either an advanced generalist role such as the CNL, or a specialty, such as case management, clinical specialist, nurse anesthetist, nurse educator, nurse midwife, or nurse practitioner. The track record for the graduates of entry-level master's programs is excellent. Students in the programs bring life experience, a previously earned higher degree, and most programs require at least a 3.0 GPA in the undergraduate program for admission. NCLEX pass rates exceed 90% (author) for entry-level MSN graduates.

According to the AACN (2014a), there were 68 entry-level (generic) master's programs in the United States. Descriptions of the programs and the student and graduate characteristics may be found in the accelerated BSN and MSN programs (www.aacn.nche.edu/publications/issue-bulletin-accelerated-programs). AACN (2014c) conducted a survey of member schools that prepare entry-level baccalaureate and master's degree nurses. One of the purposes of the survey was to identify the employment rates for graduates at the time of graduation and 4 to 6 months later. While the regions of the country varied, with the West lagging somewhat behind the rest of the country, it was found that entry-level master's graduates enjoyed a higher mean rate of employment compared to entry-level baccalaureate graduates at the time of graduation (56% and 74%) and 4 to 6 months later (42%–79%).

There are several recent articles in the literature relative to entry-level master's students' experiences in their educational programs and their performance following graduation that are helpful to programs planning to initiate an entry level master's or revising the existing one. McNiesch (2011) interviewed 19 entry-level master's students for their lived experiences during their accelerated educational program. She found that the students were highly motivated and appreciative of the high stakes involved in delivering safe patient care. Her findings resulted in recommendations for types of faculty support for these students as they develop clinical competence and confidence. Klich-Heartt (2010) summarizes the literature on the socialization of entry-level MSN students into the professional nursing role. According to her review of the literature, graduates of these programs take about a year to become comfortable in the role of staff nurse; however their overall scholastic grades and motivation are higher than nurses prepared at the undergraduate levels. She suggests that nursing administrators need to ensure that the accelerated programs' graduates have support for orientation and socialization into the professional role in health care agencies.

Ziehm, Cunningham, Fontaine, and Scherzer (2011) conducted a follow-up study of graduates of an entry-level MSN program and their managers in their employment settings. They found that as expected, graduates with more than 1 year of experience reported more confidence in their role than those with less than 1 year. There was a high level of agreement when comparing the graduates' self-assessment and their managers' perceptions of job performance that was very positive. Several of the positive characteristics included the graduates' role as patient advocates, their resourcefulness and strong social skills, and that they were more savvy in their professional relationships. These studies verify the success of entry-level master's programs in preparing college graduates for the nursing workforce at higher levels of education to meet the demands of the system and the health care needs of the population.

THE CLINICAL NURSE LEADER

The CNL program was developed by the AACN in response to the need for health care providers to manage clients or groups of clients at the point of care. It applies to all settings of health care. The program is at the master's level and lends itself very well to entry-level master's programs as well as post-baccalaureate in nursing programs. An overview of the development of the role, its characteristics, and place in the United States and international health care systems is described by Baernholdt and Cottingham (2010).

AACN (2007) provides the following description of the role of the CNL: "The CNL is a leader in the healthcare delivery system in all settings in which healthcare is delivered. CNL practice will vary across settings. The CNL is not one of administration or management. The CNL assumes accountability for patient-care outcomes through the assimilation and application of evidence-based information to design, implement, and evaluate patient-care processes and models of care delivery. The CNL is a provider and manager of care at the point of care to individuals and cohorts of patients anywhere healthcare is delivered. Fundamental aspects of CNL practice include:

- Clinical leadership for patient-care practices and delivery, including the design, coordination, and evaluation of care for individuals, families, groups, and populations; participation in identification and collection of care outcomes
- Accountability for evaluation and improvement of point-of-care outcomes, including the synthesis of data and other evidence to evaluate and achieve optimal outcomes
- Risk anticipation for individuals and cohorts of patients
- Lateral integration of care for individuals and cohorts of patients
- Design and implementation of evidence-based practice(s)
- Team leadership, management and collaboration with other health professional team members
- Information management or the use of information systems and technologies to improve healthcare outcomes

• Stewardship and leveraging of human, environmental, and material resources
• Advocacy for patients, communities, and the health professional team" (pp. 4–5)

In October 2013, there were 107 accredited nursing programs that provide the CNL major at the master's level (AACN, 2014b, 2014c, 2014d). The AACN (2014e) document on the *Competencies and Curricular Expectations for CNL Education and Practice* provides specific information for curricular planning for programs wishing to offer this degree. The experience of faculty who developed a curriculum in Alabama to prepare CNLs is described by Jukkala, Greenwood, Motes, and Block (2013). Especially useful are their ideas on preparing the community, faculty, and potential preceptors who may not be familiar with the role.

Upon graduation, graduates of CNL programs are eligible to sit for national certification through the Commission on Nurse Certification (2014). According to the AACN, as reported by Tan (2011), the updated version of the certification is based on a survey of CNL prepared nurses and their competencies in the practice setting. The competencies include horizontal leadership, interdisciplinary communication and collaboration skills, health care advocacy, integration of the CNL role, lateral integration of care services, illness and disease management, knowledge management, health promotion and disease prevention management, evidence-based practice, advanced clinical assessment, team coordination, health care finance and economics, health care systems, health care policy, quality improvement, health care informatics, and ethics. Based on follow-up studies on the effect that the CNL role has on improving care, it is anticipated that more nurses will be prepared for this advanced generalist role in the near future.

ADVANCED PRACTICE MASTER'S DEGREE PROGRAMS IN NURSING

The classic advanced practice roles encompass the clinical specialist, nurse anesthetist, nurse midwife, and nurse practitioner. As discussed in Chapter 1 on the history of master's education, the advanced practice roles emerged in the 1960s and 1970s. Nurse anesthetists (certified registered nurse aesthetists [CRNAs]) and nurse midwives predated these programs by many years (centuries for midwives and 150+ years for CRNAs); however, their move into higher education/graduate education occurred about the same time period as did the clinical specialist and nurse practitioner roles. A few advanced practice nurses still have a certificate to practice depending upon state licensure laws, although most states now require the master's degree for entry into advanced practice. With the advent of the doctor of nursing practice (DNP) degree, many of these nurses will continue their education to earn a DNP. See Chapter 13 for discussion of the DNP. The AACN (2010d) issued a statement that the DNP should be the entry level for advanced practice in nursing by 2015, which has implications for the future when many master's programs for advanced practice will be phased out and moved into the DNP.

All master's degree programs that prepare advanced practice nurses require a baccalaureate in nursing or in rare cases, its equivalent, and some have additional prerequisites; for example, CRNA programs often require more than one or two chemistry courses. Both the clinical specialist and nurse practitioner programs have subspecialties. Examples are adult, cardiovascular, family, geriatric, pediatrics, psychiatric/mental health, women's health, and so on. In addition, there are blended roles such as the adult acute care nurse practitioner. Fulton (2005) writes in her editorial that the blended roles require many more hours of course work and practice that surpasses the usual 40+ credits requirements for an advanced practice master's in nursing. In addition, there is some confusion about the definition of these roles and no specific competencies or standards as yet that are specific to the blended role. Rather, graduates are eligible for national certification for both roles.

The 2008 Consensus Report for APRN Regulation (AACN, 2010b) limits the blended role of primary and acute care foci to adult-geriatric and pediatric roles only and specifies that graduates must be nationally certified for both the primary (practitioner) and acute care (clinical specialist) roles. The consensus model was a product of meetings with the leading professional nursing organizations, specialty organizations, accrediting bodies, nursing education organizations, certification agencies, and the National Council of State Boards. It was the intention of the group to clarify advanced practice roles for the profession and the public and to begin an initiative for consistent licensing, certification, and regulation across the various states in the nation. Recently, the National Council of State Boards presented an update on the Consensus Report for APRN Regulation (Cahill, Alexander, & Gross, 2014). It lists the major elements of advanced practice registered nurse (APRN) regulations as:

- Title: Advanced Practice Registered Nurse (APRN)
- Roles of APRNs and recognition of each: Certified Nurse Practitioner (CNP), Clinical Nurse Specialist (CNS), CRNA, Certified Nurse Midwife (CNM)
- Licensure: APRNs hold both an RN and APRN license
- Education: Graduate education is required for APRNs regardless of role
- Certification: Every APRN is required to meet advanced certification requirements
- Independent practice: The APRN shall be granted full authority to practice independently without physician oversight or a written collaborative agreement
- Full prescriptive author. The APRN shall be granted full prescriptive author without physician oversight or a written collaborative agreement (p. 5)

Cahill et al. (2014) list the progress toward meeting the elements of the Consensus Report state by state with some forward progress. As the health care system evolves in the United States, it is expected that the consensus model will continue to move forward in response to increased demands for well-qualified and educated APRNs.

Advanced practice nurses have a key role in the delivery of quality care. To provide some evidence of the impact they have on the health care delivery system, the following reports from the literature verify this statement. Bourbonniere et al. (2009) conducted a review of the literature on the outcomes of patient care and costs in nursing homes that utilized advanced practice nurses (clinical specialist and nurse practitioners). Their findings affirmed that patient outcomes were improved such as reductions in falls, pressure ulcers, incontinence, and improved patient and family satisfaction. In addition, the consultation and education that these nurses offered for staff led to less absenteeism and increased job satisfaction. Cost effectiveness studies demonstrated that advanced practice nurses save the system money in unnecessary hospitalizations for the residents of nursing homes. While reimbursement for advanced practice nurses is based on medical services, indirect costs such as referrals and staff and patient education are not billable. The panel that studied the effects of advanced practice nurses in nursing homes concluded that there is need for increased services of this kind in these facilities, that new financial systems need to be set for their services, that it is essential that geriatric content be included in nursing curricula, and that geriatric specialties in the advanced roles would be beneficial.

McCorkle (2006) reported on the use of advanced practice nurses to support cancer patients and their caregivers in home care agencies. After refining several instruments to measure symptom distress and enforced social dependency, McCorkle and others conducted several studies to observe the effects of advanced practice nursing interventions on dying patients and their caregivers, many of whom were spouses. The researchers compared patients and their caregivers who received the services of advanced practice nurses to those who received the usual types of care. They found that providing support throughout the dying process for both the patient and the caregiver resulted in lessening of symptoms for the patients and less psychological stress for the caregivers during and after the patient's death. An interesting finding was that caregivers with pre-existing medical conditions when the patient was diagnosed had more psychological difficulties than those who were relatively healthy. It was McCorkel's conclusion that using advanced practice nurses to assess and provide interventions during these episodes of illness and dying results in better outcomes for the patients and their caregivers.

Delgado-Passler and McCaffrey (2006) reviewed the literature for studies to compare the use of RNs to advanced practice nurses for follow-up of heart failure patients. Although, the number of studies was limited, they found that advanced practice nurses were more effective in managing posthospitalized heart failure patients owing to their advanced knowledge in care management and, with the physician, could individualize discharge and follow-up at home, which resulted in fewer readmissions to the hospital. This in turn resulted in cost savings.

Parrish and Peden (2009) reviewed the literature for studies that reported on depressed clients' outcomes when cared for by advanced practice psychiatric nurses (APPNs). They found 10 studies that met their criteria for the review. The studies compared the outcomes of APPNs care to other psychiatric/mental health professionals' care for depressed patients. Overall, the studies found that the most effective treatment for depressed clients is a combination of psychotherapy and medications, which APPNs can provide. In addition, they found that patients were satisfied with the care they received from APPNs. The authors concluded that APPNs are effective providers of care for patients owing to their expertise, and availability of time to spend with the patients, and they can be cost effective, if it is only necessary for one professional to provide care.

In summary, the traditional role for advanced practice continues to play an important role in the delivery of high-quality, safe, and cost-effective care. Nursing continues to find it necessary to illustrate this to not only the health care industry but the public as well. Kleinpell (2007) labels advanced practice nurses in the hospital setting as "invisible" and makes the case for nurse managers and administrators to demonstrate their contributions to the health care system. She offers several recommendations and outlines for gathering the information to promote the role of advanced practice nurses.

COMMUNITY/PUBLIC HEALTH NURSING

Community/public health nursing master's programs prepare nurses for advanced practice roles in community settings. There are some schools of nursing that offer a joint degree awarding both the MSN and the master of public health. Others have community health nursing as a clinical specialty. The American Nurses Credentialing Center (ANCC) (2014) offers a public health nurse advanced certification for graduates of master's in nursing with a specialty in community health nursing or nurses (BSNs) who hold a master's of public health (MPH). Other graduate degrees might be eligible but they must have a baccalaureate in nursing.

Swider et al. (2006) reviewed the core competencies recommended by the Quad Council of Public Health Nursing Organizations, which include the following: analytic assessment skills, basic public health sciences skills, cultural competency skills, communication skills, community dimensions of practice skills, financial planning and management skills, leadership and systems thinking skills, and policy development/program planning skills. The authors compared the competencies to Rush University's curriculum and found that the competencies provide a framework for community/public health nursing practice at an advanced level and recommended that other schools may wish to consider this model as well when planning their programs.

Swider et al. (2009) discuss the DNP as an educational option for master's prepared nurses with community/public health nursing backgrounds. They surveyed community health nursing leaders, and although community health nursing is considered a clinical specialty, it is not always recognized when listing advanced practice nurses. The respondents to the survey raised issues such as their belief that the DNP would not result in salary differentials and they felt that the doctorate in public health is the more accepted degree in their field. They also raised some concerns about nurses in the community and their roles in school health, home care, and hospice. These issues need to be addressed in the near future as the DNP gains recognition in the profession and the health care system.

MASTER'S DEGREES IN NURSING FOR FUNCTIONAL ROLES

There are other roles and specialties for nurses with master's degrees not included in the advanced practice and advanced generalist roles. They include case management, nursing administration, nurse educator, staff development/patient education, and other leadership roles. Nurses prepared for these roles usually have nursing theory, health care policy, and research as core courses along with the courses that focus them into a specific function within the health care system. The following discussion presents a few examples of the programs that prepare nurses for specific roles.

Case Management

The educational preparation for roles in case management in nursing usually requires at least a baccalaureate in nursing, with a master's preferred. Case managers provide coordination of services for aggregates in many health care settings. They work closely with other health care professionals. The role began in the 1970s with its purpose to work with patients to individualize care, avoid duplication of services, enhance the quality of care, and promote cost effectiveness (White & Hall, 2006). White and Hall reviewed the literature to identify journals in the literature that pertain to case management and found three source journals for the specialty, although the topic is mentioned in many other health-related journals. There are approximately 20 schools of nursing that offer case management master's degrees. The ANCC (2014) offers certification, which requires 2,000 hours of clinical practice in case management, RN licensure, practice as an RN for 2 years, and 30 hours of continuing education in case management in the past 3 years.

Nursing Administration

The most common master's degrees in nursing to prepare nurse leaders are the master's in nursing administration or leadership. Some programs offer joint master's degrees with nursing such as business administration (MBA) or health care administration. The graduates of these programs are not prepared for advanced practice roles such as clinical specialists and nurse practitioners, but rather have education in the management of health care systems including staffing, human resources, finances, budgeting, and administration. There are several ways for nurse administrators to receive national certification through the American Organization of Nurse Executives (2014) for executive nursing or as a nurse manager and leader. The latter requires only a baccalaureate in nursing, while the executive certification requires a master's. ANCC (2014) also has a national certification exam for nurse executives. In addition to these roles in management and administration, there are other leadership certifications for infection control nurses, legal nurse consultants, quality control nurses, and risk managers. These certifications occur through specialty organizations and for the most part require or prefer that nurses have a master's degree as well as continuing education and experience for the specific role.

Nurse Educator

The role of the nurse educator in health care agencies includes staff development and patient education. There are programs in schools of nursing that specifically prepare nurses for this role at the master's level. The National Nursing Staff Development Organization (2010) recommends that staff developers become credentialed by ANCC for the nursing clinical specialty in which they are prepared.

With the recent growth of nursing education programs to help relieve the shortage of nursing faculty, many of the programs offer a track for nurse educators in schools of nursing and some offer postmaster's certificates in nursing education. According to the AACN (2010 a, 2010c) report on enrollments, 49,948 qualified applicants to nursing schools were turned away in 2008 to 2009 and two thirds of the schools reported that faculty shortages contributed to the turndowns. Owing to the shortage, there has been a surge of master's programs that prepare nurses for faculty roles. In addition, there are many postmaster's certificate programs in education.

It is recommended that faculty have at least the same degree level for the type of program in which they teach and it is highly recommended that they have one degree higher. Therefore, faculty teaching in associate degree programs should have at the very least a baccalaureate, but most boards of nursing require the master's degree for program approval, while those teaching in baccalaureate and higher degree programs should have a doctorate. However, with the shortage in nursing, it is not uncommon for master's prepared nurses to teach clinical courses in specialties that match their expertise, and in some states, boards of nursing allow nurses with baccalaureates in nursing to teach under the supervision of an experienced educator.

There is continuing debate about whether nursing faculty need to have special courses in education since they are specialists in their fields. There is no question that there is a separate body of knowledge related to curriculum development, instructional design and strategies, instructional technology, and program and student evaluation. Without this knowledge, many instructors in nursing do not have the background in learning theories that support best practices in education for meeting the needs of learners, nor do they have the curriculum planning and evaluation background to connect the program to the actual implementation (teaching) of the program. Such knowledge ensures the quality of the program so that learning experiences are linked to the mission and goals of the program. The same is true for evaluation for program review to measure outcomes and student evaluation to measure students' progress in the program. At the same time, it is equally important that nursing faculty have the content knowledge and theory on the material that they are teaching. To further support these statements the National League for Nursing (2010) offers national certification for nurse educators. Eligibility qualifications require a master's or doctorate in nursing and courses in Curriculum Development and Evaluation; Instructional Design; Principles of Adult Learning; Assessment/Measurement and Evaluation; Principles of Teaching and Learning, and Instructional Technology.

SUMMARY

Chapter 12 reviewed common master's degree programs in nursing and the differences among the majors available in nursing at the master's degree level. Roles for master's degree prepared nurses were discussed and postgraduate certification possibilities were reviewed. Some issues were raised such as the advent of the DNP and its impact on advanced practice master's programs, entry into practice at the master's level, expectations of educational preparation for nursing faculty, and the place for the advanced generalist master's degree in the health care system.

DISCUSSION QUESTIONS

1. Debate the pros and cons of entry into practice at the master's level versus the second baccalaureate for college graduates.

2. How should nursing differentiate between advanced practice roles and advanced knowledge roles such as nurse administrators, case managers, risk managers, and so on?

3. Is it important for nurse educators in the practice setting and in schools of nursing to have graduate degrees and what levels of advanced education are necessary? Why or why not?

LEARNING ACTIVITIES

STUDENT LEARNING ACTIVITIES

1. Review the literature and websites for nursing education to identify how many possible majors there are for master's degrees in nursing. Compare these majors to the job market for these specialties in your region. Discuss the pros and cons for the continuation or discontinuation of some of the programs.

2. Go to the websites of various credentialing and certification organizations for nursing and identify how many require at least a master's degree in nursing. Discuss why or why not certification for advanced roles should continue.

NURSE EDUCATOR/FACULTY DEVELOPMENT ACTIVITIES

1. Review the latest follow-up survey of the graduates of your master's program for data on the employment of the graduates in settings where they use the focus of their graduate degree. Determine if your program prepares graduates for the needs of the health care system and why or why not. Consider the effect of your findings on curriculum revision or, possibly, discontinuance of a program or development of new programs.

2. Discuss among yourselves your beliefs about master's education for advanced practice or roles in leadership and if the master's degree serves your graduates as a terminal degree and/or pathway to doctoral studies.

REFERENCES

Accreditation Commission for Education in Nursing. (2014). *Accredited programs.* Retrieved from http://acenursing.org

Affordable Care Act. (2014). Retrieved from http://www.hhs.gov/healthcare/facts/timeline

American Association of Colleges of Nursing. (2007). *White paper on the education and role of the clinical nurse leader.* Washington, DC: Author.

American Association of Colleges of Nursing. (2010a). *2007-2008 enrollment and graduations in baccalaureate and graduate programs in nursing.* Washington, DC: Author.

American Association of Colleges of Nursing. (2010b). *Consensus model for* APRN *regulation: licensure, accreditation, certification, & education.* Retrieved from http://www.aacn.nche.edu/education/pdf/APRNReport.pdf

American Association of Colleges of Nursing. (2010c). *Nursing faculty shortage.* Retrieved from http://www.aacn.nche.edu/Media/factsheets/FacultyShortage.htm

American Association of Colleges of Nursing. (2010d). *Position statement on the practice doctorate in nursing.* Retrieved from http://www.aacn.nche.edu/DNP/DNPPosition-Statement.htm

American Association of Colleges of Nursing. (2014a). *Accelerated programs. The fast track to careers in nursing.* Retrieved from https://www.aacn.nche.edu/publications/issue-bulletin-accelerated-programs

American Association of Colleges of Nursing. (2014b). *Accredited CNL programs.* Retrieved from http://www.aacn.nche.edu/cnl/about/cnl-programs

American Association of Colleges of Nursing. (2014c). *Clinical nurse leader master's degree programs.* Retrieved from http://www.aacn.nche.edu/CNL/CNLWebLinks.htm

American Association of Colleges of Nursing. (2014d). Commission on Nurse Certification. Retrieved from: http://www.aacn.nche.edu/cnl/cnc

American Association of Colleges of Nursing. (2014e). *Competencies and curricular expectations for clinical nurse leader education and practice.* Retrieved from http://www.aacn.nche.edu/cnl/CNL-Competencies-October-2013.pdf

American Association of Colleges of Nursing. (2014f). *Degree completion programs for registered nurses:* RN *to master's degree and* RN *to baccalaureate programs.* Retrieved from http://www.aacn.nche.edu/media-relations/fact-sheets/degree-completion-programs

American Association of Community Colleges. (2014). *RN to MSN program information.* Retrieved from http://www.aacc.nche.edu/Resources/aaccprograms/health/cap/Pages/rn-msn.aspx

American Nurses Credentialing Center. (2014). Retrieved from http://www.nursecreden-tialing.org/default.aspx

American Organization of Nurse Executives. (2014). *Credentialing center.* Retrieved from the home page of http://www.aone.org

Baernholdt, M., & Cottingham, S. (2010). The clinical nurse leader—new nursing role with global implications. *International Nursing Review, 58,* 74–78.

Bourbonniere, M., Mezey, M., Mitty, E., Burger, S., Bonner, A., Bowers, B., . . . Nicholson NR, Jr. (2009). Expanding the knowledge base of resident and facility outcomes of care delivered by advanced practice nurses in long-term care: Expert panel recommendations. *Policy, Politics, & Nursing Practice, 10*(1), 64–70.

Cahill, M., Alexander, M., & Gross, L. (2014). The 2014 NCBSN report on APRN regulation. *Journal of Nursing Regulation, 4*(3), 3–12.

Commission on Collegiate Nursing Education. (2014). *Accredited programs.* Retrieved from http://ccne.desertrose.net/reports/accprog.asp

Delgado-Passler, P., & McCaffrey, R. (2006). The influences of postdischarge management by nurse practitioners on hospital readmission for heart failure. *Journal of the American Academy of Nurse Practitioners, 18*(4), 154–160.

Fulton, J. S. (2005). Calling blended role programs to account. *Clinical Nurse Specialist: The Journal for Advanced Nursing Practice, 15*(5), 221–222.

Institute of Medicine. (2014). *The future of nursing: Leading change advancing health.* Retrieved from http://www.iom.edu/Reports/2010/The-future-of-nursing-leading-change-advancing-health.aspx

Jukkala, A., Greenwood, R., Motes, T., & Block, V. (2013). Creating innovative clinical nurse practicum experiences through academic and practice partnerships. *Nursing Education Perspectives, 34*(3), 186–191.

Kleinpell, R. (2007). APNs: Invisible champions? *Nursing Management, 38*(5), 18–22.

Klich-Heartt, E. I. (2010). Special needs of entry-level master's-prepared nurses from accelerated programs. *Nurse Leader, 8*(5), 52–54.

McCorkle, R. (2006). Leadership & professional development. A program of research on patient and family caregiver outcomes: three phases of evolution. *Oncology Nursing Forum, 33*(1), 25–31.

McNiesch, S. G. (2011). The lived experience of students in an *accelerated nursing program:* Intersecting factors that influence experiential learning. *Journal of Nursing Education, 50*(4), 197–203.

National League for Nursing. (2010). *Certification for nurse educators.* Retrieved from http://www.nln.org/facultycertification/index.htm

National Nursing Staff Development Organization. (2010). *Become a staff educator.* Retrieved from https://www.nnsdo.org

Parrish, E., & Peden, A. (2009). Clinical outcomes of depressed clients: A review of current literature. *Issues in Mental Health Nursing, 30*(1), 51–60.

Swider, S., Levin, P., Ailey, S., Breakwell, S., Cowell, J., McNaughton, D., & O'rourke, M. (2006). Matching a graduate curriculum in public/community health nursing to practice competencies: The Rush university experience. *Public Health Nursing, 23*(2), 190–195.

Swider, S., Levin, P., Cowell, J., Breakwell, S., Holland, P., & Wallinder, J. (2009). Community/public health nursing practice leaders' views of the doctorate of nursing practice. *Public Health Nursing, 26*(5), 405–411.

Tan, R. J. B. (2011). CNL *clinical nurse leader. Job analysis summary report.* Commission on Nurse Certification. Washington, DC: American Association of Colleges of Nursing.

White, P., & Hall, M. E. (2006). Managing the literature of case management nursing. *Journal of the Medical Library Associaiton, 94*(2), 99–106.

Ziehm, S. R., Uibel, I. C., Fontaine, D. K., & Scherzer, T. (2011). *Success indicators for accelerated master's entry nursing program:* Staff RN performance. *Journal of Nursing Education, 50*(7), 395–403.

The Doctor of Nursing Practice (DNP)

Sarah B. Keating

OBJECTIVES

Upon completion of Chapter 13, the reader will be able to:

1. Differentiate between applied practice/professional doctorates and research-focused degrees
2. Describe the role(s) of the doctor of nursing practice (DNP) in practice, the health care system, and education
3. Analyze the educational preparation necessary for the DNP
4. Review program evaluation and accreditation requirements for DNP programs

OVERVIEW

The movement toward a doctorate in nursing for advanced practice and leadership roles has grown tremendously over the past decade. According to the American Association of Colleges of Nursing (AACN), the DNP is the highest level of advanced nursing practice (AACN, DNP Fact Sheet, 2014a). AACN (2013b), in its annual report, listed a total of 217 existing DNP programs with another 97 planning to open. There were 40 states in the nation and the District of Columbia with DNP programs reported by AACN. In addition, nine states each have one clinical doctorate program accredited by the Accreditation Commission for Education in Nursing (ACEN, 2014).

Chapter 13 reviews the DNP, the nature of the professional doctorate and differences from research-focused degrees; its role in practice, health care, and education; the essentials of a curriculum for the degree as recommended by AACN; and the standards for accreditation by the ACEN and the Commission on Collegiate Nursing Education (CCNE).

DIFFERENCES BETWEEN PROFESSIONAL AND RESEARCH-BASED DOCTORATES

Melnyk (2013) succinctly describes both the PhD and the DNP degree programs and their specific purposes and differences with implication for both practice and research. While nursing has a history for developing various titles for its doctoral programs, academe recognizes two types of degrees. The first is the research-focused PhD program or in the case of nursing, the PhD, doctor of nursing science (DNS). Research-focused doctorates emphasize nursing theory and research and educate nurses who are prepared to conduct research and foster the development of new knowledge in health care and nursing. Often, nurse educators in higher education prefer the research-focused degree for faculty who wish to teach in tenure-track positions. The rationale for this is that research-focused institutions prefer faculty prepared to develop new knowledge and theories in their respective disciplines. Academe in these institutions and other colleges or universities with productive research records award tenure to faculty members who demonstrate research productivity through publications, grants, and other scholarly works that advance knowledge in their disciplines. This results in keeping the curriculum up-to-date and prepares graduates who are abreast of changes in their disciplines and have the potential for further research.

The professional doctorate degree, including the DNP, prepares graduates for application of research to practice; another way to say it is to translate research into evidence-based practice. A few examples from other disciplines that have professional doctorates are the doctor of business administration (DBA); doctor of dental surgery (DDS); doctor of law (LLD); doctor of medicine (MD); doctor of pharmacology (PharmD); doctor of physical therapy (DPT); and doctor of psychology (PsyD). The doctor of education (EdD) is a recognized doctorate that in the past included research and dissertation requirements, although the current trend is for these types of degrees to carry the PhD in education title (doctor of philosophy). The EdD has become an applied professional degree that includes application of research and theories in education to evidence-based practice.

Nursing education programs are sometimes reluctant to hire DNPs into tenure-track positions owing to the DNP focus on applied research and translational science as compared to research for discovering new knowledge. However, the profession and educators recognize the role of DNP graduates for providing instruction and clinical supervision in undergraduate and graduate nursing programs owing to their expertise in evidence-based clinical practice and in translational science. Many DNP graduates demonstrate extensive research in practice that contributes to the science of nursing; therefore, they are eligible for tenure-track positions. DNP graduates who expect to teach in schools of nursing should compare tenure-track policies in potential employing institutions to other types of positions such as clinical faculty that are not research-focused, but still offer academic ranks from instructor to professor and the potential for job stability over time. For both the research-focused degrees (PhD, DNS) and the DNP, AACN (2010) strongly recommends taking courses in education if graduates intend to teach. The National League for Nursing (NLN) (2014) has a vision statement on doctoral preparation for nurse educators that emphasizes the need for evidence-based practice in education and the preparation of educators for teaching, assuming leadership in academe and health care systems, and conducting and translating research in nursing education. It lists recommendations to prepare nurse educators for the nursing profession, doctoral programs, and administrators of nursing education programs.

THE ROLE OF THE DNP IN PRACTICE

When the notion of a professional/applied practice doctoral degree in nursing was first introduced in the late 1990s and early 2000s, there was much controversy from the profession and outside of the profession about the role of nurses with doctorates. Among the issues raised by nursing when the programs were fairly new were the many different nursing doctoral degree programs and titles that confuse the public and nursing such as, DNS, EdD, ND, PhD, and so on. Objections to the use of the title "doctor" were raised for fear the public would assume that the provider was a medical doctor. The Unified Statements by the organization representing nurse practitioners and faculty for nurse practitioner programs clearly state that nurses who earn the DNP have a right to title themselves as doctor, as no one profession has exclusive rights to this title (Nurse Practitioner Roundtable, 2014). Dennison, Payne, and Farrell (2012) point out that the doctorate is an academic degree and therefore the graduate is authorized to use the title of doctor, and they add that nurses with doctorates collaborate with other professionals and patients by identifying their role as nurses. Another source for promulgating the use of the title "doctor" was identified by Smolowitz (2011) in her interview of O'Dell, who with his associates founded the website Doctor of Nursing Practice (www.doctorsofnursingpractice.org; 2014). O'Dell discusses the continuing debate about the use of the title and the usefulness of the website for discussion of the issue by not only nurses but other disciplines as well. In addition, the website is a platform for discussions among DNP graduates and educators on issues surrounding the degree as well as current changes in nursing practice, the profession, and the health care system.

There are several major roles for DNP-prepared nurses in the health care system. One role is in advanced practice including those nurses who are clinical specialists, nurse anesthetists, nurse midwives, and nurse practitioners; however, this is not limited to these roles and could include others, for example, advanced practice community/public health nurses. Another essential role for DNPs is to apply research to bring about change in evidence-based nursing practice and health care. A major role is for systems leadership in public policy to improve health care. While the focus of the DNP is not to prepare nurse educators, graduates of DNP programs are involved in the clinical education of nurses and the AACN and NLN recommend that DNP graduates (as well as PhD graduates), who wish to have faculty roles, complete education courses to prepare for the teaching role (AACN, 2013a; NLN, 2104).

Grey (2013) discusses the issues related to DNP practice and education that summarizes articles on the DNP in a special issue of the *Journal of Nursing Education*. She states that the original intention of DNP education was to prepare nurses for advanced practice roles with a focus on population-based practice, that is, a professional practice degree. However, many of the existing MSN to DNP programs provide advanced practice education or advanced leadership strategies such as administration, health care policy, and for a few, education. As additional bachelor of science in nursing (BSN) to DNP programs graduate students, it is assumed that the graduates will enter into the previously master's-prepared traditional roles of nurse practitioners, clinical specialists, nurse midwives, and nurse anesthetists. However, since the programs are relatively young, there is not sufficient evidence to demonstrate if this is true and studies to determine graduates' employment placements are indicated.

Several articles in the literature describe some of the roles of DNPs in practice. Ferguson and Forest (2012), as graduates of a postmaster's DNP program, describe how they as nurse practitioners applied the additional knowledge and skills gained from the DNP program to their practice. Included in additional knowledge and skills was a focus on population-based services, evaluation, and interpretation of evidence for translation into practice, all of which result in improved clinical services. They believe that as a result of their education, their clinical services (one is in acute care and the other in primary care) have gained in breadth and depth for the benefit of the populations they serve.

Dunbar-Jacob, Nativio, and Khalil (2013) reported on the types of positions graduates of DNP programs in Pennsylvania held in 2012. While the DNP is fairly new to the profession of nursing, some of the programs in Pennsylvania were started as early as 2006 and thus provide a possible sample of the outcomes from DNP programs. Of the 589 graduates of Pennsylvania DNP programs, the authors reported that about two thirds of the graduates were educated in administrative/leadership DNP programs and the other third graduated from advanced practice (nurse practitioner, clinical specialist, etc.) programs. Only 163 of the 589 had postgraduation placement data available, and of those, the majority practiced in acute care, with the remaining in academe. Clearly, additional national research is indicated to learn where DNP graduates are practicing, differences between postmaster's and BSN to DNP graduates' areas of practice, and if the programs are having an impact on increasing advanced practice nurses in the workforce as well as changing health care policy and practices.

EDUCATIONAL PREPARATION FOR THE DNP

DNP programs continue to grow across the country and according to the 2013 Annual Report of the AACN there was a total enrollment in member AACN, DNP programs of 11,575 students (AACN, 2013a). Most DNP curricula are based upon *The Essentials of Doctoral Education for Advanced Nursing Practice* (2006). These eight *Essentials* include (1) Scientific Underpinnings for Practice, (2) Organizational and Systems Leadership for Quality Improvement and Systems Thinking, (3) Clinical Scholarship and Analytical Methods for Evidence-Based Practice, (4) Information Systems/Technology and Patient Care Technology for the Improvement and Transformation of Health Care, (5) Health Care Policy for Advocacy in Health Care, (6) Interprofessional Collaboration for Improving Patient and Population Health Outcomes, (7) Clinical Prevention and Population Health for

Improving the Nation's Health, and (8) Advanced Nursing Practice. Each of these *Essentials* is described in detail by AACN and specific learning objectives are listed for each. AACN discusses the incorporation of specialty competencies for programs that prepare DNPs for advanced practice roles such as clinical specialists, nurse practitioners, nurse midwives, nurse anesthetists, and others. The National Organization for Nurse Practitioner Faculties (2014) lists specific competencies expected for the nursing practice doctorate and nurse practitioners. Program developers are directed to specialty organizations for the lists of competencies required for national certification in advanced nursing roles.

There are two major types of DNP programs. The first is the postmaster's DNP program that admits nurses with master's degrees who are nationally certified for advanced practice including nurse anesthetists, midwives, practitioners, and clinical specialists. Additionally, nursing administrators, managers, and other nurse leaders with or without national certification enroll in DNP programs to gain additional education and experiences for leadership roles in the health care system. These include administration, informatics, health care systems analysis, development of policies, and other leadership roles. Many of these programs were first initiated to meet the needs of master's-prepared nurses wishing to earn a doctorate to advance their practice, act as change agents in the health care system, increase interprofessional collaboration, and gain professional credibility in a system with most of the major disciplines prepared at the doctoral level, for example, medical doctors (MDs), pharmacology (PharmD), physical therapy (DPT), psychology (PsyD), and so on. While it is expected that advanced practice nurses currently in practice who do not have the DNP will be "grandparented in" for licensure to practice in the states in which they are licensed and recognized, it is anticipated that many will wish to have the DNP credential. This is validated by the AACN report of *Enrollments and Graduations in Baccalaureate and Graduate Programs,* which reported that 1,742 students were enrolled in postmaster's DNP programs (AACN, 2013a).

The other type of DNP educational program is to move the baccalaureate/BSN prepared nursing generalist into a DNP program. These programs prepare BSNs for advanced practice roles similar to the programs for advanced practice nurses at the master's level, for example, certified registered nurse anesthetists (CRNAs), clinical specialists, nurse midwives, and nurse practitioners. Additional course work related to health care systems management and leadership at the doctorate level is included. In addition to the traditional advanced practice courses and roles, some BSN to DNP programs offer other options for roles in informatics and technology, health care management, and/or administration roles. Supervised clinical experiences are included in the programs to meet professional accreditation and/or certification standards and account for at least 1,000 hours of practice. Students have courses that include the content of the eight *Essentials* recommended by AACN (2006) as well as completion of the specialty role in which they are enrolled. Graduates are eligible for national certification depending upon the program of study's specialization and meeting of eligibility requirements for certification.

Dennison et al. (2012) reviewed the history of DNP programs by tracing them from research-focused doctoral degrees to the nursing practice doctorate (DNP). The authors focused on the advanced practice roles of the DNP and linked them to the AACN *Essentials* (AACN, 2006). The article provides a model for curriculum planners for both the postmaster's and the BSN to DNP programs with a table that ties the AACN *Essentials* to program competencies. The authors surveyed advanced practice specialty organizations for their positions on the DNP as entry into practice. While the organizations vary from requiring that all educational programs have the DNP as entry to advanced practice by 2022 to requiring the master's but recognizing the doctorate for the future, there is consensus among the organizations that the doctorate includes competencies for advanced practice.

Grey (2013) reiterated the original intent for the DNP program to prepare nurses for advanced practice. Based on a review of the conference held by the Committee on Institutional Collaboration that was sponsored by nursing school deans, she identified similarities (consensus) and differences (controversies) across programs. Based on her observations and a review of the literature, Grey calls for consistency among DNP programs' curricula; that the "product" be defined according to the roles that graduates are prepared for; that the BSN to DNP and the postmaster's to DNP graduates be similar; that education include interprofessional collaboration and not just intraprofessional collaboration; and that nurse educators determine the curriculum, not other disciplines with outside interests.

Frantz (2013) provides an overview of the resources that schools of nursing need when planning, implementing, and sustaining a DNP program. Included on her list are the necessary faculty members and their qualifications; resources such as classrooms and simulation facilities; the infrastructure for delivering courses online and on campus; potential collaboration between the PhD and DNP programs' course faculty and, possibly, other academic institutions; faculty and student practice opportunities; health care agencies' resources for clinical experiences (both advanced practice and administrative); and administrative and staff support specific to the DNP program.

Honig and Smolowitz (2009) describe the initiation of a clinical doctorate program at Columbia University that emphasized advanced practice. First, the authors explained how faculty members for the DNP program were recruited and prepared by enrolling advanced practice nurses from various specialties and clinical experiences in the first cohort of scholars to earn the doctorate. They continue with a description of the processes the school underwent such as university and state approvals, how the curriculum tied to the AACN *Essentials*, how the scholarly project related to the final practicum, and the formative program evaluation they underwent to ensure the quality of the program.

A topic of concern that arises at many national DNP nursing faculty meetings is students' scholarly writing abilities. Shirey (2013) describes one school of nursing's strategy to promote students' scholarly writing skills. It is a developmental approach that occurs throughout the program and is learner-focused. It consists of a five-step process that starts with an assessment of scholarly writing skills and culminates in a faculty-mentored, publishable, scholarly written capstone project. Writing skills assessment and development are integrated throughout the program in various courses. The process is described as the "SMART" model, that is, strategies, methods, assessment of outcomes, related to teaching/learning.

Yet another skill essential for graduates of DNP programs is that of interprofessional leadership. Montgomery and O'Grady (2010) describe an integrated approach to acquiring these skills at the University of Maryland postmaster's DNP program. All students, whether in advanced practice, informatics, education, or administration, participate in two courses to develop evidence-based leadership skills. With faculty support, students self-assess leadership skills and develop a multidimensional and interactive "mind map" that culminates in the application of leadership skills to address an issue in the health care system. While these latter articles pertain to the implementation of the curriculum, they are useful to program developers as the program of study is developed.

PROGRAM EVALUATION AND ACCREDITATION

Program evaluation and accreditation are essential to the quality of DNP programs. Each school of nursing that has a DNP program usually has a master plan of evaluation for all programs and the DNP is included. DNP programs, in addition to the usual layers of approval within the home institution, are subject to the institution's governing board's approval, and if they are preparing entry-level advanced practice nurses, depending upon state regulations, they must undergo program approval by their state board of nursing. Program evaluation provides the data for assessing the effectiveness and quality of the program. Developing evaluation plans that incorporate all of the parameters of the program for assessment are important but it is also essential that plans are in place to implement the assessment. The methods for collecting and analyzing the data, the persons responsible, and when and how the findings from the analysis are used for program improvements are key factors to include.

Specific to DNP program accreditation are the roles of the ACEN (2013) and the CCNE (2014). The *Standards for Accreditation of Clinical Doctorate Programs* by the ACEN (2013) can be found at www.acenursing.net/manuals/SC2013.pdf. There are six standards:

1. Mission and Administrative Capacity
2. Faculty and Staff
3. Students
4. Curriculum
5. Resources
6. Outcomes

Details concerning these standards are found at the ACEN website.

CCNE (2009) determined that it would accredit doctoral degrees that reflected the terminal practice degree in the profession, not research-focused degrees. This is in line with other professional or applied practice doctoral degrees in other disciplines. To be eligible for CCNE accreditation, programs are required to base their curricula on the AACN *Essentials of Doctoral Education for Advanced Practice* (2006). In addition, programs must have students enrolled for at least 1 year before hosting an on-site evaluation with a self-study submitted prior to the visit (CCNE, 2014). Action on accreditation takes place after a site visit and during the next scheduled CCNE Board of Commissioners meeting. This usually means that students enrolled in the program will graduate from a CCNE accredited program.

Since the DNP is a relatively new degree, most programs must also have regional accreditation, as a new degree is considered a substantive change. See Chapters 16 and 17 for more details on program evaluation and accreditation.

SUMMARY

Chapter 13 reviewed the growth of DNP programs in the nation and the role of DNPs in the health care system including evidence-based advanced practice and leadership in the health care system and health policy. Many of the issues pertaining to the roles of DNP graduates in practice, the health care system, and education and the type of educational preparation necessary for these roles were discussed. References for guidelines on the development of DNP curricula and suggestions for accreditation of programs were listed.

DISCUSSION QUESTIONS

1. To what extent do you believe the DNP as the terminal degree for advanced practice resulted in consensus within the nursing profession?
2. Debate research-focused degrees as contrasted to professional degrees and how research activities differ or are the same. What effect do you believe this debate has on the profession of nursing as a discipline?

LEARNING ACTIVITIES

STUDENT LEARNING ACTIVITY

Review the latest research and literature (the past 2 years) to identify the state of debate on the DNP and its role in research and academe.

NURSE EDUCATOR/FACULTY DEVELOPMENT ACTIVITY

If your school of nursing has a DNP program, analyze its curriculum for its congruence with the AACN *Essentials* document. If your school does not have a DNP program, find a school that does and review its program of study to compare to the *Essentials*.

REFERENCES

Accreditation Commission for Education in Nursing. (2013). *ACEN 2013 standards and criteria clinical doctorate.* Retrieved from www.acenursing.net/manuals/SC2013.pdf

Accreditation Commission for Education in Nursing. (2014). *Search accredited programs.* Retrieved from www.acenursing.us/accreditedprograms/programsearch.asp

American Association of Colleges of Nursing. (2006). *The essentials of doctoral education for advanced nursing practice.* Retrieved from www.aacn.nche.edu/publications/position/DNPEssentials.pdf

American Association of Colleges of Nursing. (2013a). 2012-2013. *Enrollments and graduations in baccalaureate and graduate programs in nursing.* Retrieved from www.aacn.nche.edu/downloads/ids/2013/EG12.pdf

American Association of Colleges of Nursing. (2013b). *Annual report.* Retrieved from www.aacn.nche.edu/aacn-publications/annual-reports/AnnualReport13.pdf

American Association of Colleges of Nursing. (2014a). DNP *fact sheet.* Retrieved from www.aacn.nche.edu/media-relations/fact-sheets/dnp

American Association of Colleges of Nursing. (2014b). *Doctor of nursing practice. DNP Programs. Frequently asked questions.* Retrieved from www.aacn.nche.edu/dnp/FAQ.pdf

Commission on Collegiate Nursing Education. (2009). *Achieving excellence in nursing education: The first 10 years of CCNE.* Washington, DC: Author.

Commission on Collegiate Nursing Education. (2014). *DNP: Program accreditation information.* Retrieved from www.aacn.nche.edu/Accreditation/DNPaccred.htm

Dennison, R. D., Payne, C., & Farrell, K. (2012). The doctorate in nursing practice: Moving advanced practice in nursing even closer to excellence. *Nursing Clinics of North America, 47,* 225–240.

Doctor of Nursing Practice. (2014). *Website.* Retrieved from www.doctorsofnursingpractice.org

Dunbar-Jacob, J., Nativio, D. G., & Khalil, H. (2013). Impact of doctor of nursing practice education in shaping health care systems for the future. *Journal of Nursing Education, 52*(8), 423–427.

Ferguson, L. A., & Forest, S. (2012). The practice doctorate in nursing: Perspective on how the DNP changes practice and improves clinical care. *Pelican News,* 11.

Frantz, R. A. (2013). Resource requirements for a quality doctor of nursing practice program. *Journal of Nursing Education, 52*(8), 449–452.

Grey, M. (2013). The doctor of nursing practice: Defining the next steps. *Journal of Nursing Education, 52*(8), 462–465.

Honig, J., & Smolowitz, J. (2009). Clinical doctorate at Columbia University school of nursing: Lessons learned. *Clinical Scholars Review, 2*(2), 51–59.

Melnyk, B. M. (2013). Distinguishing the preparation and roles of doctor of philosophy and doctor of nursing practice graduates: National implications for academic curricula and health care systems. *Journal of Nursing Education, 52*(8), 442–448.

Montgomery, K. L., & O'Grady, T. P. (2010). Innovation and learning: Creating the DNP nurse leader. *Nurse Leader, 8,* 44–47.

National League for Nursing. (2014). *A vision for doctoral preparation for nurse educators.* Retrieved from www.nln.org/aboutnln/livingdocuments/pdf/nlnvision_6.pdf

National Organization of Nurse Practitioner Faculties. (2014). *NONPF recommendations for the nursing practice doctorate and nurse practitioner preparation.* Retrieved from ww.nonpf.org/?page=16

Nurse Practitioner Roundtable. (2014). *Nurse practitioner DNP education, certification and titling: A unified statement.* Washington, DC: Author. Retrieved from www.nonpf.com/associations/10789/files/DNPUnifiedStatement0608.pdf

Shirey, M. R. (2013). Building scholarly writing capacity in the doctor of nursing practice program. *Journal of Professional Nursing, 29,* 137–147.

Smolowitz, J. (2011). Doctors of nursing practice on the web: An interview with David D. O'Dell, DNP, FNP-BC. *Clinical Scholars Review, 4*(1), 62–64.

Curriculum Planning for PhD and Other Research-Focused Doctoral Nursing Programs

Nancy A. Stotts

OBJECTIVES

Upon completion of Chapter 14, the reader will be able to:

1. Describe the purpose of the research-focused doctorate in nursing
2. Analyze the components of the research-focused doctoral programs as recommended by the American Association of Colleges of Nursing (AACN)
3. Propose strategies to evaluate the quality of research-focused doctoral programs
4. Identify common issues faced by research-focused doctoral programs

OVERVIEW

Nurse scientists are the major product of research-focused doctoral programs, including the doctor of philosophy (PhD) and doctor of nursing science (DNS) programs. These programs are designed to enhance the health of the population by preparing graduates to conduct, disseminate, and translate research. They extend knowledge of the discipline through research (AACN, 2010). The purpose of the research-focused doctoral programs in nursing, the curriculum, and evaluation of its quality are addressed, and issues common to research-focused programs are discussed.

THE ROLE OF THE RESEARCH-FOCUSED DOCTORAL PROGRAM IN NURSING

Research-focused doctoral programs prepare students to pursue intellectual inquiry and conduct independent research that results in extension of knowledge (AACN, 2010; Melnyk, 2013). From a theoretical perspective, PhD programs are theory based and focus on testing theory, while DNS programs are oriented more toward clinical practice research (Keithley et al., 2003; Robb, 2005). However, AACN does not differentiate the PhD from DNS program and it is often difficult to tell the difference in the programs based on their curricula. Clearly the commonality in the program designations is the focus on original research that has potential to contribute to the body of knowledge in the discipline. The PhD in the scientific world is the entry-level preparation needed to develop an independent program of research (AACN, 2010). Graduates are scholars (Melnyk, 2013; Walker, Golde, Jones, Bueschel, & Hutchings, 2008), although the nature of the knowledge and how it contributes to the field is unique to each candidate and may reflect the explicit foci within the various schools.

In reality, the designation as a PhD or DNS program often is determined by the school's specific mission and philosophy as well as by institutional criteria for research doctoral program approval. While holding the highest academic degree in the field, nurses from research-focused institutions are prepared and expected to be leaders in nursing as demonstrated by their role in knowledge generation and dissemination, professional organizations, and policy. In fact, graduates of research doctoral programs have been called the stewards of the discipline, those entrusted with preserving the past as the basis for the future of the discipline (AACN, 2010; Walker et al., 2008).

In the United States, there are 125 research-focused programs that offer a nursing PhD/DNS. In 2012, the year of the most recent AACN data, 4,909 students were enrolled and 601 students graduated. Forty-two states have research-focused doctoral program in nursing; eight states and two territories have none. The number of research-focused program as well as enrollment is stable and growing slowly. Neither the number of programs nor enrollment has increased as rapidly as that of the doctor of nursing practice (DNP) programs (AACN, 2012a). Of the enrollees, 75% are White, indicating that one in four is non-White (AACN, 2012a). Race/ethnicity of enrolled students varies greatly by state (range 4–100% White) (AACN, 2012b). Male students comprise 6.8% of the research-focused doctoral program student body (AACN, 2012a).

There remains a shortage of faculty, illustrated by the fact that 7.6% of full-time budgeted nursing faculty positions are vacant in the United States. Vacancies range from 1 to 20 and the average is 1.8 per school. In addition 6.6% of schools report no full-time vacancies but need additional faculty (Fang, 2013). Slightly fewer part-time (6.8%) than full-time faculty positions are available, with a mean of 1.1 part-time vacancies per school and a range of 1 to 38 vacancies per school. In the schools that responded to an AACN survey, hiring for 2012 through 2013 was precluded by lack of funds for salaries (64.1%), unwillingness of administration to commit to full-time positions (51.5%), inability to recruit due to marketplace competition (35.9%), and lack of qualified applicants (26/2%) (Fang, 2013). The most critical faculty recruitment related issues are limited number of doctorally prepared faculty (32.9%), noncompetative salaries (27.6%), and having faculty with the right specialty mix (19%) (Fang, 2013).

Lack of faculty impacts student enrollment; students are not being accepted into programs due to lack of faculty (AACN, 2012a). In addition, the faculty in nursing education is aging. Across the various levels of nursing programs, the mean age of professors is 61.0 years, associate professors is 57.5 years, and assistant professors is 51.8 years (AACN, 2012a). Clearly a cadre of new faculty is needed to replace the aging and soon to be retiring faculty (AACN, 2012a; Meleis, 2005; Meleis & Dracup, 2005).

Most graduates from research-focused programs work in academia where scholarly activity/research, service to the university and profession, professional competence, and teaching are core criteria for tenure and promotion. Recognizing responsibilities across these various areas, there is no question that research is the focus of research-intensive doctoral education. Pedagogical preparation requires additional course work and practice that focuses on teaching to develop skills and knowledge commensurate with role expectations (AACN, 2010). Similarly, preparation in health policy may require additional coursework and practice.

PhD/DNS graduates work in research-intensive or teaching-intensive universities. In the research-intensive university, the most highly rewarded activity is research and scholarship. New PhD/DNS faculty members are expected to develop a program of research that is externally funded, publish in peer-reviewed journals, develop a national and, eventually, international reputation as a scholar, provide scientific critique and review for journal articles and grants, and influence policy (AACN, 2010; Billings, 2008; Cleary, Hunt, & Jackson, 2011). The expectation is that they will mentor and teach PhD/DNS students who subsequently will become faculty who are research scientists. Leadership in the profession, a national reputation (and eventually international), and service to their institution are markers of a successful faculty member at a research-intensive university.

In teaching-intensive programs, PhD/DNS faculty members teach and mentor pre-licensure students as well as graduate students. Scholarly activity is required but may be more broadly defined than in the research-intensive university and may include writing textbooks, conducting externally funded quality assurance or education-focused studies, and publishing clinically focused papers. Committee service in the university and leadership in professional organizations and the community are also usual expectations in these schools.

Some graduates work in industry, government, and policy. While their roles vary, they are hired for their expertise and leadership capacity, much of which is the product of their doctoral education. In industry, they may work in clinical research and direct or monitor research studies. In government, they may assume a role in the National Institute of Nursing Research as well as various other agencies (e.g., Veteran's Administration or a branch of the military). Doctorally prepared nurses may work in policy to affect public, industry, or government opinion on health-related issues (e.g., smoking).

Postdoctoral work often follows graduation from a research-focused doctoral program (AACN, 2010; Nolan et al., 2008). Postdoctoral study focuses on increasing depth in research expertise to help develop a robust program of research. Activities during postdoctoral study may include learning a new method, extending expertise in substantive content, publication of papers from the dissertation, and writing research grants to fund future research. Those who have completed a postdoctoral program are better prepared to enter academia and successfully complete the research related milestones of obtaining external funding and publishing in peer-reviewed journals than PhD/DNS-prepared nurses who have not gone on for further preparation (National Research Council, 2005).

THE CURRICULUM

The curriculum of each research-focused doctoral program is unique and is based on the school's mission and philosophy as interpreted and implemented by the faculty. Usual core coursework includes the history and philosophy of nursing science, theories that guide the discipline and practice, research methods, advanced statistics, substantive nursing in a specific area of expertise, and role-related content (e.g., pedagogy). Depending on the program, required content may include mentoring, leadership, interdisciplinary research teamwork, and health policy. Cognates from supporting disciplines, such as sociology or physiology, often are required. The faculty, their program of research, funding success, and area of expertise are recognized as pivotal as are the resources available such as an office of research (Bevil, Cohen, Sherlock, Yoon, & Yucha, 2012). The variability in the curriculum among programs is seen in the requirements in research-focused doctoral programs. Surveys of research-focused doctoral programs show that a research practicum was required by 77.1%, attendance at a professional meeting by 36.8%, presentation at a professional meeting by 21.1%, and submitting a paper for publication by 31.6%. Dissertation format also was quite variable where traditional format was utilized by the majority of schools (61.4%), while the publication of at least one paper was required by a few schools (6.9%); and some schools (30.7%) allowed either approach (Minnick, Norman, & Donaghey, 2013).

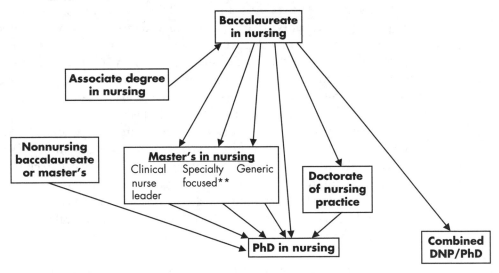

AACN (2010) identified pathways to the research-focused doctoral degree, designated here as the PhD. The pathways are diagrammed above.
1. Baccalaureate in nursing (BSN) to master's in nursing (MSN) to PhD
2. BSN to PhD
3. BSN to doctoral of nursing practice (DPN) combined with PhD
4. BSN to DNP to PhD
5. BSN to MS (specialty practice) to PhD
6. Generic MSN to PhD
7. Associate degree in nursing (ADN) to BSN to PhD
8. Nonnursing BSN or MS to PhD
**The MS in specialty practice is being phased out and replaced with the DNP.

FIGURE 14.1   Pathways to research-intensive doctoral programs in nursing.

With the focus of doubling the number of doctorally prepared nurses by 2020 (IOM, 2010), there is concern about capacity issues and whether the goal of increasing the number of graduates will threaten the quality of their educations (Gill & Burnard, 2012; Henly, 2013). To address the capacity issue, AACN (2010) proposed articulation and facilitation of multiple entry points to the research-focused doctoral program. Figure 14.1 diagrams the proposed pathways. Implementation of the schemata requires changes in traditional perspectives and discussion about the value of requiring clinical practice as the basis for the research doctorate.

From a process perspective, most programs require coursework and then a formal evaluation of substantive knowledge prior to students undertaking their original research projects. All programs have a process by which the research topic is approved by the faculty and the quality of the dissertation research evaluated.

PROGRAM EVALUATION

The quality of research-focused doctoral nursing programs is established and maintained by the individual programs. There is no professional accreditation for research-focused doctoral programs. However, quality indicators are provided by AACN (2010) to guide the evaluation of these programs. Evaluation criteria are divided into categories of faculty and administration, students, resources and infrastructure, and evaluation plan. Table 14.1 provides examples of quality indicators

TABLE 14.1 EXAMPLES OF QUALITY INDICATORS IN RESEARCH-FOCUSED DOCTORAL PROGRAMS IN NURSING

Faculty

Make scholarly contribution to the discipline with peer-reviewed publications
Present research or theory at national/international meetings
Participate in National Institutes of Health panels
Maintain program of research and extramural funding
Collaborate on interdisciplinary research teams

Students

Selected from a pool of highly qualified diverse applicants
Goals and objectives are congruent with faculty research
Dissertation is guided by faculty mentor with expertise in the field
Publish papers and provide podium presentations and posters at national meetings
Scholarship and leadership of graduates are recognized in awards, honors, external funding within 3–5 years

Resources and Infrastructure

Office of research exists
Sufficient space is available for faculty research needs, doctoral student study, and seminars
Internal research funds are awarded
University environment fosters interdisciplinary research and collaboration

Evaluation

Evaluation is comprehensive, systematic, and ongoing
Process and outcome data are obtained related to indicators of quality
Engages students, graduates, faculty, employers, and stakeholders
Assesses financial and institutional resources

cited in the AACN (2010) document. Programs often supplement these measures with their own indicators. For example, for a state supported program, one rubric might be the proportion of state residents in the student body and/or the number of international students enrolled.

However, to date, little comparative data exist about quality of programs other than objective measures of enrollment, race/ethnicity and gender of students, length of program, number of grants, and the amount of funding awarded from federal and private grants to nursing faculty.

At times, the parent institution in which the program or school is located has internal processes for ensuring quality of their programs. For example, within the University of California 10-campus system, an external review is conducted every 5 years for PhD programs to ensure program quality. Reviewers from similar doctoral programs within the discipline use a set of established criteria to evaluate the program. A self-study as well as in-person meetings with the program and school's administration, faculty, predoctoral students, postdoctoral students, and graduates are conducted. At the end of the visit, the reviewers write a report to the campus-wide committee responsible for graduate education. Program directors are then charged to address the items identified in the review. Overall it is a positive process and helps maintain parity both of the nursing program nationally and the doctoral programs within the larger University of California system.

COMMON ISSUES FACED BY RESEARCH-FOCUSED DOCTORAL PROGRAMS

Internal and external forces create issues for research-intensive programs. Shrinking funding for higher education is a major external issue in academia. Tuition is rising and fewer grants are available to students. Less money is available to both public and private schools due to the downturn in the economy and the reconceptualization of priorities.

There is a change in many schools about how faculty members are funded. Increasingly the expectation is that faculty will bring in their own salary from grants, as well as fund the salary and tuition of their PhD/DNS students. While requiring grants to provide research assistant salaries for doctoral/postdoctoral students is a long-standing norm in the basic sciences, only recently has it become explicit in nursing. To make matters more challenging, the budget for the National Institutes of Health is stretched and there is increasing competition for those funds as well as private foundation grants. The number of research-focused graduates seeking funding has increased (AACN, 2012a) without similar increases in available support for new grants (National Institutes of Nursing Research, 2011).

Increasingly, nursing programs have looked to collaboration with industry as another source of revenue for their studies; this has raised questions of conflict of interest. New faculty members are advised to be cautious when obtaining funding from commercial vendors to avoid even the perception of bias or tainted scientific objectivity (Nolan et al., 2008). A new business model for research-focused doctoral programs is emerging and how the model is shaped will have a profound effect on the number and nature of future research-focused nursing doctoral programs.

Clear differentiation of the product of research- and practice-focused doctoral programs is needed as the DNP is accepted as the nursing parallel of the doctor of medicine (MD) or doctor dental science (DDS). It will be important for the discipline and the profession that nursing speak as a single voice as to the nature of education and then ensure implementation of the uniqueness of each program to avoid divisiveness, such as that which existed with the issue of entry into practice (Meleis & Dracup, 2005). Although the National Institutes of Health (NIH) does not specify the type of doctoral degree required for the Principal Investigator awarded NIH grants, the expectation is that the research training commensurate with large grant funding will be obtained primarily by graduates of research-focused doctoral programs. This is a perfect time to re-think, clarify, change, and reaffirm the pivotal tasks of the various levels of nursing education, including research-focused doctoral programs (Benner, Sutphen, Leonard, & Day, 2009; Institute of Medicine [IOM], 2010).

Several issues could be rolled into such a reevaluation, change, and reaffirmation package. The issue of pedagogy (i.e., how to teach, the role of active learning, distance approaches to learning) needs increased attention. The nature of the students also needs to be addressed. At the moment, the normative expectation is that the doctoral preparation is built on the foundation of expertise attained in a master's program (AACN, 2010). Widespread implementation of AACN's multiple pathways to the PhD (Figure 14.1) will require early and ongoing advising to help students identify and qualify for their chosen pathway.

While not unique to research-focused programs, a related issue is how to recruit, educate, and graduate racial/ethnic minority nurses (Nnedu, 2009). More are needed if nurse scientists are going to reflect the characteristics of the population they serve, which is the goal of AACN and its member schools (2010). Progress has been made in the area; however, more is needed as AACN continues to address this issue (2010).

Finally, while there is growing appreciation of the need for interdisciplinary education, there needs to be clearer delineation of how interdisciplinary education can be mounted in research-focused programs. Discussion needs to center on a variety of issues beyond the practical issues of cross-discipline teaching and scheduling. Topics that might be addressed include the ethics that underlie work produced by multiple persons and how interdisciplinary work informs the science differently than a single discipline perspective. Much progress has been made in enhancing interdisciplinary learning, but most has been on an individual basis. Nursing has much to give and gain from interdisciplinary education. It would behoove us to better define our expectations in research-focused doctoral programs.

SUMMARY

Research-focused doctoral programs produce scientists. Most work in academia after graduation balances research with the other dimensions of their work (teaching, service). The curriculum varies by program but has identified threads that are comparable with research-focused preparation in other disciplines. Ongoing evaluation is an important component of these programs. While the number of programs and enrollment is stable and slowly increasing, research-focused doctoral programs face ongoing issues having to do with funding, strategies to recruit applicants that reflect the population served, and determining how to actualize interdisciplinary education so that it best contributes to the development of science and health of the nation.

DISCUSSION QUESTIONS

1. Propose how interdisciplinary research might be supported and developed as part of a PhD/DNS program.
2. What are the strengths and limitations of having students admitted to a PhD/DNS with a baccalaureate degree in nursing, a master's degree in nursing, and a doctor of nursing practice degree?

LEARNING ACTIVITIES

STUDENT LEARNING ACTIVITIES

Compare and contrast two PhD/DNS programs. What are the similarities and differences in coursework, research training, and available faculty mentorship in your area of expertise?

NURSE EDUCATOR/FACULTY DEVELOPMENT ACTIVITIES

1. Compare one online and one in-person PhD/DNS program. What are the strengths of each? Consider how you can make the best use of these data in your program.
2. If the student population in your program does not reflect the racial-ethnic or gender mix of the general population, what three things might you consider to rectify this disparity?

REFERENCES

American Association of Colleges of Nursing. (2010). *The research focused doctoral program in nursing: Pathways to excellence.* Report from the AACN Task Force on the research-focused doctorate in nursing. Washington, DC: Author.

American Association of Colleges of Nursing. (2012a). *Annual report: Advancing higher education in nursing.* Washington, DC: Author.

American Association of Colleges of Nursing. (2012b). *Race/ethnicity of students enrolled in nursing programs by state 2011.* Washington, DC: Author.

Benner, P., Sutphen, M., Leonard, V., & Day, L. (2009). *Educating Nurses: A call for radical transformation.* San Francisco, CA: Jossey-Bass.

Bevil, C. A., Cohen, M. Z., Sherlock, J. R., Yoon, S. L., & Yucha, C. B. (2012). Research support in doctoral-granting schools of nursing: A decade later. *Journal of Professional Nursing, 29*(2), 74–81.

Billings, D. M. (2008). Managing your career as a nurse educator: Considering an academic appointment. *Journal of Continuing Education in Nursing, 39,* 392–393.

Cleary, M., Hunt, G. E., & Jackson, D. (2011). Demystifying PhDs: A review of doctorate programs to fulfill the needs of the next generation of nursing professionals. *Contemporary Nurse, 29*(2), 273–280.

Fang, D. (2013). Special Survey on vacant faculty positions for academic year 2012-2013. Retrieved January 2, 2014 from www.aacn.nche.edu

Gill, P., & Burnard, P. (2012). Time to end the vagaries of PhD examining? *Nurse Education Today, 32*(5), 477–478.

Henly, S. J. (2013). PhD education in nursing: Changing times, time for reflection. *Nursing Research, 82*(5), 293.

Institute of Medicine. (2010). *The future of nursing: Leading change, advancing health.* Washington, DC: Author.

Keithley, J. K., Gross, D., Johnson, M. E., McCann, J., Faux, S., Shekleton, M., et al. (2003). Why Rush will keep the DNSc. *Journal of Professional Nursing, 19*(4), 223–229.

Meleis, A. I. (2005). Shortage of nurses means shortage of nurse scientists. *Journal of Advanced Nursing, 49*(2), 111.

Meleis, A. I., & Dracup, K. (2005). The case against the DNP: History, timing, substance, and marginalization. *Online Journal of Issues in Nursing, 10*(3), 3.

Melnyk, B. M. (2013). Distinguishing the preparation and roles of doctor of philosophy and doctor of nursing practice graduates: National implications for academic curricula and health care systems. *Journal of Nursing Education, 52*(8), 442–448.

Minnick, A. F., Norman, L. D., & Donaghey, B. (2013). Defining and describing capacity issues in U.S. Doctor of Nursing Practice programs. *Nursing Outlook, 61*(2), 93–101.

National Institutes of Nursing Research. (2011). FY 2011 congressional justification. Retrieved January 30, 2014 from http://www.ninr.nih.gov/aboutninr/budgetandlegislation/fy-2011-cj#.Uuz-NI2A1y0

National Research Council. (2005). *Advancing the national's health needs.* Washington, DC: National Academics Press.

Nnedu, C. C. (2009). Recruiting and retaining minorities in nursing education. *ABNF Journal, 20*(4), 93–96.

Nolan, M. T., Wenzel, J., Han, H. R., Allen, J. K., Paez, K. A., & Mock, V. (2008). Advancing a program of research within a nursing faculty role. *Journal of Professional Nursing, 24*(6), 364–370.

Robb, W. J. (2005). PhD, DNSc, ND: The ABCs of nursing doctoral degrees. *Dimensions of Critical Care Nursing, 24*(2), 89–96.

Walker, G. E., Golde, C. M., Jones, L., Bueschel, A. C., & Hutchings, P. (2008). *The formation of scholars: Rethinking doctoral education for the twenty-first century.* San Francisco, CA: Jossey-Bass.

Curriculum Development and Evaluation in Staff Development

Peggy Guin

Betty Jax

Upon completion of Chapter 15, the reader will be able to:

1. Analyze the role of the staff development educator and advanced practice nurse (APN) in promoting competency in the practice setting
2. Apply learning theories and research to staff development programs
3. Conduct a needs assessment of internal and external frame factors as it relates to staff development programs
4. Apply the components of curriculum development to staff development and programs
5. Realize the importance of budget planning as it applies to staff development
6. Apply program evaluation concepts to staff development
7. Consider the issues and trends in staff development programs

OVERVIEW

This chapter applies the previous information on curriculum development and evaluation in academic settings to staff development programs in health care organizations. The staff development function involves the postlicensure education of nurses in health care organizations to ensure that members of the nursing staff have the most current, evidence-based knowledge and skills for nursing practice. In large health maintenance organizations (HMOs), university medical centers, major county hospitals, and other health care agencies, the staff development function is often centralized with responsibilities for the training and professional development of all personnel from custodial staff and unlicensed health care workers to nurses, physicians, managers, and administrators. For the purposes of this chapter, the terms staff development educator and APN are used. Other terms to describe educators with a staff development role include clinical nurse educator, hospital-based educator, education specialist, and education coordinator. APNs with a staff development component to their role include positions such as clinical nurse specialists (CNSs), nurse clinicians, and clinical nurse leaders (CNLs). These positions may be centralized, departmental, and/or population based; or de-centralized, providing leadership support to a specific nursing unit or area. How APNs are used in this capacity is highly variable and based on the needs of the organization, administrative structure, and its professional practice model.

Activities of staff development educators often include new graduate programs, orientation, competency assessment, cross training, new product and technology training, specialty practice education, research utilization education, leadership development, and continuing education to encourage lifelong learning. Additionally, staff development educators are often involved in providing ongoing education to ensure that health care providers have up-to-date information on standards and guidelines set by government and regulatory agencies such as state health departments, The Joint Commission, and the Centers for Medicare and Medicaid Services (CMS).

In accordance with the mission of a health care organization, additional areas of education may include quality improvement processes, interpersonal relationships, customer service, information technology, and health care economics. Through the provision of initial and ongoing support and education, staff development educators play a key role in the retention of nurses and other health care providers within an organization. APNs have an important role in the initial and ongoing professional development of nurses. As expert clinicians, APNs facilitate the provision of clinically competent care, critical thinking, and the development of good clinical judgment through role modeling, teaching, coaching, and/or mentoring. APNs' abilities to demonstrate the translation of evidence into practice demonstrate and reinforce the importance of nursing interventions and their impact on the achievement of safe, quality, and cost-effective outcomes.

Clinical judgment and collaboration are used to enhance nursing care and its impact on the unique characteristics of the patient in order to devise a plan of care that ensures advocacy. By influencing nurses, other members of the health care team, and organization/systems, the APN meets the needs of diverse groups and enhances quality and cost-effective patient-centered care.

Most health care facilities have a major educational plan for staff development services. Curriculum development in staff development often involves revisions to the plan based on changes in health care delivery, population demographics, emerging health risks and health problems, advances in practice and technology, and program feedback from the recipients of educational programs. The intended impact of staff development is quality patient care by a well-prepared staff with an ultimate outcome of improved health and quality of life in the patient population served by the agency. Information in this chapter includes roles and responsibilities of nurse educators and APNs in the practice setting, adult learning theories appropriate for staff development programs, the emphasis on quality improvement and patient safety as it applies to staff education, a needs assessment of external and internal frame factors relevant to developing or revising staff development programs, adaptation of curriculum components to the practice setting, evaluation strategies, preparing and managing budgets, and issues in nursing education in the practice setting.

QUALIFICATIONS, RESPONSIBILITIES, AND FUNCTIONS OF NURSE EDUCATORS AND ADVANCED PRACTICE NURSES IN STAFF DEVELOPMENT PROGRAMS IN HEALTH CARE AGENCIES

In addition to nursing and health care knowledge, the staff development educator needs knowledge and skills in program and curriculum development, learning theories, instructional design and technology, teaching strategies, program evaluation, and budget management. APNs need advanced assessment skills, expert use of the nursing process, organizational and systems leadership, knowledge about outcome focused patient care programs, and skills in evaluation, translation, and integration of evidence and practice standards into systems of health care delivery.

Excellence in communication is critical to building support for the program, interacting with the public and vendors, and fostering relationships with administrators, advisory boards, staff, academic faculty and students, other agency personnel, patients, families, and the community. While many of these qualifications come with experience, additional education is recommended, preferably at the master's or doctorate level. Additionally, it is preferable for nurses working in staff development and advanced practice roles to be certified in their specialties and/or in continuing nursing education or nursing professional development (NPD). Information on specialty certification can be found at http://www.nursecredentialing.org (American Nurses Credentialing Center [ANCC], 2014). The NPD Role Delineation Study (RDS) summary outlines the practice of NPD based on the results of a ANCC (2012) national study of NPD practice. The study results can be found at http://www.nursecredentialing.org/Certification/NurseSpecialties/Nursing Professional Development/NPD-RelatedLinks/2012-RDS-Survey.pdf

The current standards for NPD were published by the American Nurse's Association (ANA) in 2010. Just as nurses have a responsibility to lifelong learning in order to maintain and increase competence in their practice, so do staff development educators and APNs (ANA, 2010). The Education Standard in the *Scope and Standards of Practice for Nursing Professional Development* requires that in order to maintain current knowledge and competency, all registered nurses must:

1. Participate in ongoing educational activities related to practice knowledge and professional issues
2. Demonstrate a commitment to lifelong learning through self-reflection and inquiry to address learning and personal growth needs
3. Seek experiences that reflect current practice to maintain knowledge, skills, abilities, and judgment in clinical practice or role performance
4. Acquire knowledge and skills appropriate to the role, population, specialty area, practice setting, or situation
5. Seek formal and independent learning experiences to develop and maintain clinical and professional skills and knowledge
6. Identify learning needs based on nursing knowledge, the various roles the nurse may assume, and the changing needs of the population
7. Participate in formal or informal consultations to address issues in nursing practice as an application of education and a knowledge base

8. Share educational findings, experiences, and ideas with peers
9. Contribute to a work environment conducive to the education of health care professionals
10. Maintain professional records that provide evidence of competence and lifelong learning

In addition, the graduate-level prepared specialty nurse and APN should use current health care research findings and other evidence of expanded clinical knowledge, skills, abilities, and judgment to enhance role performance, and to increase knowledge of professional issues (ANA, 2010, pp. 49–50).

The role of the staff development educator and APN is multifaceted and can vary on a daily, sometimes even hourly, basis. Activities of staff development educators often include preparation and support of new graduate programs, orientation, competency assessment, cross training, new product and technology training, specialty practice education, research utilization education, leadership development, and continuing education to encourage lifelong learning. To sustain and build on research and evidence-based practice along the novice to expert continuum (Benner, Kyriakidis, & Stannard, 2011), APNs work with nurses to foster a practice environment that is congruent with clinical inquiry and evidence-based nursing actions. The role of the APN in staff development often varies according to how the role is positioned in the organization. For example, CNSs are often in "central" positions, having expertise within three spheres of influence (patient, nurse and nursing, and organization/systems) around a specific type of patient population. Staff development activities of CNSs therefore are directed at sharing their expertise as it relates to their area of clinical practice. This may be done through didactic teaching, case studies, patient care rounds, module development, patient advocacy, education regarding the evaluation and use of clinical practice guidelines, evidence-based practice, and research.

In contrast, CNLs are expert practitioners in the management and coordination of care for a group of patients on a particular nursing unit or area. They are often involved in unit-level activities that pertain to quality and education. Staff development activities include unit-based orientation, preceptor development, ongoing inservice, and continuing education activities to support clinical and quality initiatives on the unit.

In an ever-changing health care environment with a renewed focus on patient safety and quality outcomes, staff development educators and APNs provide leadership roles in ensuring that nurses and other health care professionals have the knowledge and resources to provide evidence-based care. Through the provision of initial and ongoing support and education, staff development educators and APNs play a key role in the retention of nurses and other health care providers within an organization.

With the renewed focus on patient safety and quality outcomes in health care organizations, the nursing profession is held accountable for nursing-sensitive quality indicators such as skin integrity, hospital acquired infections, and patient falls. The application of research utilization and evidence-based practice in nursing highlights one of the many roles of nurse educators and APNs in the practice setting and their potential to impact patient safety and outcomes. Acting as change agents, the staff development educators and APNs are key to creating a culture of inquiry, promoting research utilization, and preparing nurses and other health care providers to seek out and evaluate the evidence, and ultimately improve the quality of care within their organizations (Krugman, 2003; Strickland & O'Leary-Kelley, 2009).

Also, with regard to patient safety and quality outcomes, nurse educators and APNs are responsible for educating nurses about the "measurement, improvement, and benchmarking of clinical costs, quality, and outcomes specific to nursing" (Gallagher, 2005, p. 39). To this end, nurse educators and APNs must be engaged in data gathering and evaluation activities and, more importantly, in communicating findings and benchmarking information to nursing staff. It is difficult, if not impossible, to change practice and improve outcomes if knowledge about current performance and progress is not shared with the nurses who are actually providing interventions and evaluating patient care at the bedside. Staff development educators and APNs are challenged to implement teaching methodologies that prepare bedside nurses to continually question the effectiveness of their interventions, determine if the evidence supports their practice, and utilize their clinical judgment to impact the outcomes of the care they are providing (Durham & Sherwood, 2008).

The responsibilities and functions of the staff development educator and APN include program planning, implementation, and evaluation. If the educator is the sole person responsible for the educational program, other nursing staff members and/or health care providers are consulted for their content expertise in developing educational sessions and the management staff for infrastructure support. In contrast, a large health care system will have an administrator or director of the staff development program, administrative staff, and educators to implement the program. In either case, all of the components of educational program development, implementation, management, and evaluation apply.

LEARNING THEORIES

Chapter 4 describes in detail classic and postmodernistic learning theories applied to nursing education. For the health agency setting, adult learning theories usually prevail in educational programs, especially for staff development. The five assumptions described by Malcolm Knowles (Knowles, Holton, & Swanson, 1998), an influential leader in the field of adult education, are outlined below:

1. Self-concept; with maturity, self-concept moves from dependent to self-directed
2. Experience; with maturity, a person's life experiences become a resource for learning
3. Readiness to learn; with maturity, readiness to learn becomes linked to the "developmental tasks of social roles"
4. Orientation to learning; with maturity, perspective changes from "postponed application of knowledge to immediacy of application" and learning shifts from subject-centered to problem-centered
5. Motivation to learn; with maturity, motivation to learn becomes internal (Smith, 2002, p. 7)

When developing and implementing staff development courses, adult learning principles must be utilized to engage the learner. Nursing staff must see the relevancy of the learning to their immediate work or life situation. Learning activities must draw from the experiences of the staff and be interactive whenever possible. Case studies, role playing, group discussion with problemsolving, and simulation are effective learning modalities for the adult learner in the classroom setting. Online learning activities must engage the nurse through learning activities such as case examples, pertinent data, videos, and interactive questions.

Access to education resources in real time is critical for the adult learner in the fast-paced hospital and other health care settings. Staff needs to be able to access current and evidence-based information online. Some facilities are able to financially provide an authoritative suite of online, evidence-based learning and clinical information at the point of care. Smaller institutions can provide staff with information on websites that have been vetted for accuracy and relevancy.

NEEDS ASSESSMENT

Curriculum development for staff development programs begins with a needs assessment that examines the frame factors that are external and internal to the organization and have an impact on the curriculum (Johnson, 1977). Chapters 6 and 7 provide a comprehensive discussion of the adaptation of the Johnson model to current curriculum development activities. The discussion to follow applies these same frame factors to a needs assessment for developing and revising curricula for staff development educators.

EXTERNAL FRAME FACTORS

External frame factors to consider are the community (including changes in population demographics), health needs of the population served by the health care agency, the physical, social, and economic environment, the health care system, the nursing workforce, regulations and accreditation requirements for staff development programs, resources for staff education programs, and the need for program development or revision. See Table 15.1 for a summary of the external frame factors to consider.

TABLE 15.1   GUIDELINES FOR ASSESSING EXTERNAL FRAME FACTORS

FRAME FACTOR	QUESTIONS FOR DATA COLLECTION	DESIRED OUTCOME
The Health Care System	What are the major health insurance programs and entitlement programs within the population served by the health care facility, such as HMOs, Medicare, Medicaid, Supplemental Security Income, General Assistance and Veterans Administration (VA) benefits? What impact has the Patient Protection and Affordable Care Act (PPACA), commonly called the Affordable Care Act (ACA), had on access to health care insurance? What are other health care and social service resources in the community such as hospitals, clinics, home care and long-term care agencies, governmental agencies, e.g., VAMC (VA Medical Center), public health services, voluntary health organizations?	Staff development programs include knowledge of impact of health care systems on patient health related conditions, risk factors, and adherence Partnerships between health care agencies provide joint educational programs

(*continued*)

TABLE 15.1	GUIDELINES FOR ASSESSING EXTERNAL FRAME FACTORS (*continued*)	
FRAME FACTOR	QUESTIONS FOR DATA COLLECTION	DESIRED OUTCOME
The Nursing Workforce	What are the numbers of nurses in the region served by the health care facility? Is there a shortage of nurses, and if so, what are the specific areas of severe nursing shortages, such as emergency department, critical care, gerontology, and long-term care?	Staff development programs are tailored to the educational level, job responsibilities and learning needs of the nursing workforce
	Among the nursing staff at the health care facility, what is the level of education and how many are certified?	Creative staff development approaches address the shortage of nurses
	How many are prepared for and certified in advanced practice roles, such as nurse practitioner, CNS, nurse midwife, and nurse anesthetist?	
Regulations and Accreditation	What are the state regulations governing approval of continuing education curricula and course offerings for nurses? What are ANA standards for professional development of staff?	Staff development and continuing education programs offered in the health care facility meet state requirements for approval of continuing education offerings and ANA Standards for Nursing Professional Development programs
Need for Development or Revision of the Program	Has there been a major shift in population demographics? Are there major changes in health risks, morbidity and mortality in the population served by the health care facility?	Staff development programs address changing demographics and emerging health risks, morbidity and mortality
	Do the external and/or internal program evaluation findings reveal areas for improvement?	Program revisions address areas identified for improvement by program from internal and external evaluations
	Are staff education programs culturally, linguistically and educationally appropriate for the intended recipients? Are staff education programs and teaching methods based on the latest research evidence? Are there newer technologies for delivery of effective staff education?	Program revisions are based on current research findings on teaching methods and learning strategies, including effective use of advances in technology in delivering educational programs

Description of the Community

An assessment of the community or geographical area served by the health care agency yields information useful for developing and/or revising staff development programs. Urban and suburban areas may have a number of community characteristics and resources that enrich staff. Technology support systems such as the Internet, email, web-based learning management systems, and videoconferencing offer people access to health education materials that might otherwise not have access. However, lack of access to these technological resources or an inability to utilize them are potential barriers. Other existing health resources, such as hospitals, clinics, public health services, voluntary health organizations, public libraries, and other social service organizations in the community may be tapped for support and collaborative partnerships in providing staff education.

Compared to urban and suburban communities, continuing education and ongoing professional development may be challenging in rural areas. Staff educators in rural areas need to develop creative approaches for overcoming barriers to learning. Examples include making low-cost staff development videos available for rent or purchase, developing web-access and e-mail or list-serve services, and forming partnerships with other communities in the area to purchase distance learning technology or web-based learning management systems and sharing access to resources.

Health Needs of the Populace

Health status reports provide data on current or emerging health risks and health problems as well as existing morbidity and mortality data in a given region or specific patient population. These reports yield information useful for developing and/or revising staff development programs. Health status reports relevant to the population served by health care organizations are usually available in print form from local libraries or online from city, county, state departments of health, or the federal government. The U.S. Department of Health and Human Services publication Healthy People 2020 (2010) is an excellent resource for targeting major health problems in the populace and strategies for promoting health and preventing disease (http://www.healthypeople.gov). More than likely, the health care agency itself has demographic and health status data available on the client population served in recent years, such as the most common diagnoses, diagnoses-related groups (DRGs), injuries and surgeries, thereby providing a basis for determining current needs and projecting trends for the future.

The Health Care System and Nursing Workforce

An assessment of major health care providers in the area, such as managed care systems, health insurance programs, public health services, hospitals, clinics, voluntary health care organizations, other health care facilities, and social services in the area reveal community resources that may be tapped for staff development support as well as potential partners for collaboration. This assessment should include the nursing workforce in the area served by the health care organization, number of nurses employed by the health care organizations, level of education from the licensed practical/vocational nurse to nurses prepared at the doctorate level, numbers of APNs by type (nurse practitioner, CNS, nurse midwife, nurse anesthetist), and critical areas of nursing shortage in the health care organization.

Regulations and Accreditation Requirements

As an integral part of program development or revision, the most current regulations, standards of practice, and accreditation criteria governing staff development are reviewed to ensure that new and revised programs are in compliance. Staff development educators in states with mandatory continuing education for nurses need to review their state regulations for receiving approval for continuing education offerings. The current standards for NPD include continuing education, staff development, and academic education as areas in which nurses may take advantage of professional development opportunities.

Need for Program Development or Revision

Since most staff development departments have a major education plan in place, it is rare that a staff development educator actually develops a new staff education program from the ground up. The need for program revision often arises from the changing demographics and health status in the population served by the health care organization and in response to emerging threats to the health of the community. In addition, feedback from staff, patients, families, health facility managers, and administrators indicate areas of program weakness needing change and improvement. Prior evaluations of staff education programs provide information on the satisfaction of program recipients and the extent to which the program goals of each were achieved.

INTERNAL FRAME FACTORS

Internal frame factors to consider in developing staff education curricula are the mission, philosophy, and goals of the institution; characteristics of the health care setting such as organizational structure, including the decision-making structure, particularly as it applies to staff development; institutional economics, including resources for staff development; the characteristics and learning needs of staff; and potential educators for staff development programs. See Table 15.2 for a summary of the internal frame factors to consider.

TABLE 15.2 GUIDELINES FOR ASSESSING INTERNAL FRAME FACTORS

FRAME FACTOR	QUESTIONS FOR DATA COLLECTION	DESIRED OUTCOMES
Mission, Philosophy, and Goals of the Health Care Organization	Do the mission, philosophy, and goals of the institution speak to staff development and curricula?	The mission, philosophy, and goals of the institution address the professional development of staff
	Are the mission, philosophy and goals of the staff development program congruent with the institutions?	The mission, philosophy, and goals of the staff development programs are congruent with those of the health care organization
Characteristics and Educational Needs of Staff	What are the educational needs of staff?	Educational needs of staff are assessed using multiple sources of information
	What are important characteristics of staff to consider in developing appropriate and effective educational programs?	Characteristics of staff affecting access to education and having impact on learning are taken into consideration in developing educational programs

(*continued*)

TABLE 15.2 GUIDELINES FOR ASSESSING INTERNAL FRAME FACTORS (*continued*)

FRAME FACTOR	QUESTIONS FOR DATA COLLECTION	DESIRED OUTCOMES
Institutional Economics and Resources for Staff Development	What is the present financial health of the institution?	Creative strategies, such as partnering with other experts from nearby health and social service organizations in the community, submitting grants, and recruiting course faculty from among the in-house professional staff, are implemented
	What are the existing and potential resources for staff education programs?	
	What are creative strategies for increasing resources for educational programs?	
	If resources are limited, what are the priority programs that will impact patient outcomes?	Resources are sufficient for developing and implementing needed staff education programs

Mission, Philosophy, and Goals of the Health Care Setting

The health care facility's mission, philosophy, and goals provide the overall framework and direction for the organization. Therefore, the mission, philosophy, and goals of the staff education programs should be closely aligned with those of the parent organization. Staff educators and APNs should have a solid understanding of the organizational structure and decision-making processes as they relate to staff education programs. Final decisions regarding program course offerings for staff education programs, including the commitment of resources to them, are made with consideration for the extent to which the offerings will support the goals of the overall organization. Successful staff education programs are those that prepare health care providers to meet the needs of the community and population served, and the goals and priorities of the health care organization.

Educational Needs Assessment Specific to Staff Development

The characteristics and needs of the learners should be considered in developing and revising staff development curricula. The characteristics of staff members are their levels of education and scope of practice, work experiences, present level of knowledge and skills, particularly in relationship to new or changing job responsibilities, and clinical practice expectations. It is not unusual for staff development educators to have the responsibility for the staff development of nonnursing/ancillary staff, nursing assistants, and various levels of licensed and certified personnel. Therefore, part of the educational needs assessment must include the identification of knowledge and skills that are common to the various types of staff and their differences in learning needs. The educator then develops strategies to enhance the best learning environment for each type of staff member through group work, small classes, individual learning modules, simulation, and/or online learning modalities.

Staff members may have additional needs and skills arising from other demands and situations in their lives. For example, they may have family responsibilities that at times take priority over the employment setting. Some may have multilingual skills and represent various cultural and ethnic groups and thus have additional knowledge to contribute to the care of clients. The availability of staff to attend professional development programs outside of scheduled work shifts may be limited among those with family responsibilities or those who live a long distance from the health care organization. Using advanced technology, such as distance education technology, web-based learning management systems, and other online learning modalities, can ameliorate some of the problems associated with staff access to professional development programs.

There are a number of methods for assessing the educational needs of staff. Educational needs are defined as "any gap between needed and actual knowledge, skills, and behaviors, which can be remedied by an educational intervention" (Burk, 2008). Sources of data include chart audits, quality improvement/benchmarking reports, patient satisfaction surveys, patient safety reports, performance evaluations of staff, input from key stakeholders including administrators and managers from within and outside of nursing, and surveys of individual learners (Abruzzese, 1996; Burk, 2008). Annual surveys of staff utilizing electronic survey tools assist in targeting learning needs. Many hospitals and other health care facilities seek to achieve The Joint Commission, state or national certifications, such as Magnet, Stroke, or Chest Pain Accreditation, Trauma designation, BestFed designation, and centers of excellence such as bariatric surgery and minimally invasive gynecological surgery. These accreditations and certifications require specific staff education. Therefore, a gap analysis between required education and actual knowledge and skills must be conducted to determine education needs for these programs.

Institutional Economics and Resources for Staff Development Programs

An analysis of the institutional economics and financial health of the health care organization provides information on fiscal resources for curriculum development in staff development programs. A lack of resources for staff development is primary among the major issues faced by nursing educators in health care agencies. In lean financial times, the education function is often the first to be downsized. Staff development educators need to develop strong relationships with financial officers and agency administrators to build the case for financial investment in staff development programs. A description of budget planning and budget management appears later in this chapter.

Showing the relationship between educational programs and the achievement of organizational goals is an effective strategy for securing support and material resources for education, particularly if there is program evaluation and/or cost-effectiveness data to support the positive returns on investment in education. Existing resources for staff development programs include classrooms, simulation laboratories and equipment for practicing clinical skills, a medical/nursing/health library, instructional technology for computer-assisted instruction and distance learning, and access to the Intranet. Table 15.2 summarizes the guidelines for assessing the internal frame factors that influence the curriculum.

ANALYSIS OF THE NEEDS ASSESSMENT DATA AND PROGRAM DECISIONS: STAFF DEVELOPMENT

Analyzing the data from the external and internal frame factors assessment often reveals multiple learning needs, more than can be addressed simultaneously. Reasoned choices will need to be made regarding the educational programs to be developed with the mission, philosophy, and goals of the institution serving as the foundation and rationale for decision making.

COMPONENTS OF CURRICULUM DEVELOPMENT IN STAFF DEVELOPMENT PROGRAMS

The same components of curriculum development discussed in Chapter 9 for schools of nursing apply to staff education. The following is a brief discussion of the adaptation of these components to the health care setting. Table 15.3 summarizes the questions for data collection and the desired outcomes that relate to each component for nurse educators to use in these settings when assessing, revising, or developing educational programs.

TABLE 15.3   ADAPTATION OF THE COMPONENTS OF THE CURRICULUM TO STAFF DEVELOPMENT

COMPONENT OF THE CURRICULUM	QUESTIONS FOR DATA COLLECTION	DESIRED OUTCOME
Agency Mission, Vision, and/or Philosophy Statements	To what extent are the mission, vision, and/or philosophy statements visible to the agency's consumers?	The mission, vision, and/or philosophy statements are readily apparent and drive the type of health care services it provides to the community
	To what extent are the mission, vision, and/or philosophy statements of the agency congruent with its educational programs' missions?	All educational programs in the institution have mission, vision, and/or philosophy statements and they are congruent with that of the agency
Purpose or Overall Goal	To what extent does the overall goal or purpose of the agency flow from the mission, vision, and/or philosophy statements?	The agency's overall goal or purpose flows logically from the mission, vision, and/or philosophy statements
	To what extent does the overall goal or purpose of the agency imply the need for educational programs?	The overall goal or purpose of the agency explicitly or implicitly includes educational programs as part of its service
	What is the evidence of an overall goal or purpose for the agency's educational programs and is it congruent with the agency goal or purpose?	All educational programs within the agency have statements relating to their overall purpose and goals that are congruent with the agency's goal or purpose

(continued)

TABLE 15.3	ADAPTATION OF THE COMPONENTS OF THE CURRICULUM TO STAFF DEVELOPMENT (*continued*)	
COMPONENT OF THE CURRICULUM	QUESTIONS FOR DATA COLLECTION	DESIRED OUTCOME
Organizing Framework	To what extent is the framework (if it exists) congruent with the mission, vision, philosophy, and/or overall goal or purpose?	The organizing or conceptual framework is congruent with agency's mission, vision, philosophy, and/or overall purpose or goal
	If the agency or service unit of the agency uses an organizing or conceptual framework for its educational program, to what extent do the programs' curricula reflect that framework?	Educational programs within the agency integrate its organizing or conceptual framework into curriculum plans
Program Objectives	To what extent do the educational programs' objectives flow from the overall goal or purpose of the agency?	Educational programs within the agency have specific goal statements that are congruent with the agency's overall goal or purpose statements
	To what extent are the educational objectives in a format that allows for measurement of the learners' success and evaluation of the teaching session(s)?	Each objective is learner-centered and includes the content of the learning experience, how the learner will achieve the specified behavior, the knowledge or skill desired, at what level of competency, and when
Implementation Plan	To what extent does the agency demonstrate support for its educational programs through staff, resources, facilities, and materials?	There is a central place for educational programs, staff, resources, learning environment facilities with available instructional support, and a listing of all educational offerings
	Is there a dedicated budget for the educational program and under whose control is it?	There is a dedicated budget in place for educational programs and the budget is managed by the leader of the Staff Development Department
	To what extent does each educational program include an overview, objectives, learner characteristics, content outline, teaching and learning methods, setting, and resources?	The implementation plan for each educational program in the agency includes an overview, objectives, learner characteristics, content outline, teaching and learning methods, setting, and resources

It is essential that the educational program's mission or vision, philosophy, and overall goals are congruent with those of the sponsoring agency. The overall goal(s) can be viewed as macro objectives and reflect the overall intent of the program. They are the expected outcomes of the staff education program. They should flow logically from the agency's mission, vision, and philosophy. Based on the overall purpose or goal of the staff development program, objectives are developed to provide the implementation plan for the program. The overall goal and its objectives are usually stated in behavioral terms with measurable outcomes to facilitate the development of the instructional plan and the measurement of the success of the program. The use of behaviorally stated goals and objectives is especially relevant to nurse educators' practice where productivity, quality improvement, evidence-based practice, and cost-effectiveness can determine the continued existence of an educational program or initiation of a new program. Each goal or objective should explain what is to be learned, how the student will learn the material including an action verb that can be measured, when the objective is to be reached, what level of competency is expected, and is learner-centered. The reader is directed to Chapter 5 for a detailed discussion of educational taxonomies and the format for writing goals and objectives.

Individual class objectives flow from the program objectives and provide guidelines for the development of the instructional design for the class. The instructional design should include a brief description of the purpose of the class, characteristics and educational needs of the learner, teaching strategies, a content outline, the learning environment, teaching aids, necessary supplies and equipment, and an evaluation plan for measuring the success of the program.

CURRICULUM DEVELOPMENT APPLIED TO STAFF EDUCATION

Most health care agencies have education departments for the purposes of staff orientation, employee training programs, new graduate programs, continuing education (in-service), and competency assessment and to prepare staff for specialty roles such as the operating room, emergency department, intensive care units, and so forth. The following are overviews of the essential curriculum components for each type of program while recognizing that smaller agencies may not have the resources to support all of the programs mentioned.

ORIENTATION, EMPLOYEE TRAINING PROGRAMS, AND NEW GRADUATE PROGRAMS

Orientation, employee training, and new graduate programs have much in common with the development and evaluation of academic nursing education programs. The major differences are the characteristics of the target learning audiences and the length of the programs according to the learning needs of the participants. Orientation programs are geared to new employees who have the educational and experiential qualifications to assume a specified position in the health care agency. These programs are often scheduled for an initial in-depth, intensive period of time where critical pieces of information are presented such as the agency's mission, purpose, policies, procedures, and specific job functions and expectations. New employee education programs often include content related to specific knowledge, skills, behaviors (professionalism), and attitudes (such as the importance of customer service). The initial training programs vary in length, the length depending upon the nature of the position and the material to be learned.

The complexity of the programs will depend on the positions' job descriptions and performance expectations. It is important for the nurse educator to be aware of state regulations or accreditation standards that require approval of these types of programs or that provide standardized curriculum plans that can be tailored to the health care agency's education needs. Preceptorships with an experienced staff member provide the structure and support to learn the specific job functions and provide a resource to answer any questions that arise as the new staff members adjust to the health care agency. The sessions and preceptorships also provide an opportunity for the agency to evaluate the new employee's performance within the introductory period.

New graduate nursing orientation programs are usually at least 6 weeks long and may be as long as 6 months for specialty areas with periodic follow-up sessions to reinforce learning and introduce new knowledge. Initial centralized content includes an in-depth orientation to the agency's mission, the nursing department's vision, mission and professional practice model, policies, procedures, documentation system, and the physical facility, including the assigned unit(s) or work area. In hospitals, specialty curricula are developed to provide the knowledge, skills, and critical thinking for areas such as critical care, pediatrics, medical/surgical, women's health, operating rooms, and emergency department. These courses provide novice nurses with the opportunity to apply and expand knowledge from their basic curriculum in a safe environment and to increase critical thinking skills. A core part of the orientation process is assigning new graduates to experienced preceptors who guide them throughout their transition into clinical practice, mentor them throughout their orientation period, and continue to provide support as needed after the "official" orientation period has ended. Preceptorship is a vital component of the transition experience of newly graduated nurses into clinical practice. As stated by Nicol and Young (2007), "an empathetic preceptor who is aware of the graduate's needs can make the difference between the graduate nurse enjoying their professional role, surviving the first year, and leaving the profession" (p. 298). Research from the perspective of newly graduated nurses illuminated the importance of the role of the nurse preceptor in orientation programs (Oermann & Moffitt-Wolf, 1997; Orsini, 2005; Schumacher, 2007). In addition to their teaching, supervising, and evaluating responsibilities, preceptors help newly graduated nurses socialize into their professional roles (Baltimore, 2004; Casey, Fink, Krugman, & Propst, 2004). Because of the significance of the role of the preceptor, it is to the advantage of the educational program and the new employees to include classes and ongoing development for preceptors on their role and functions in guiding new employees.

Each of these programs is developed according to its overall goal or purpose, and application of learning and teaching theories that are appropriate to the target audience, specific behavioral learning objectives, the content and type of material to be taught, the strategies for teaching and learning, the specific length of the program and its sessions, the learning environment, necessary equipment and other resources, and an evaluation plan to measure the learning outcomes, learner and instructor satisfaction, cost analysis, and the program's contribution to the agency's mission.

COMPETENCY ASSESSMENT

Competency assessment programs are essential to the delivery of quality care and risk management in health care agencies. As stated by the ANA, the public has the right to expect competency from their health care providers The ANA believes that nursing competence can be defined, measured, and evaluated but no single tool or method can guarantee competence. Competency is defined by the ANA as an expected level of performance that integrates knowledge, skills, abilities, and judgment (ANA, 2010, p. 12).

The first step, therefore, in a competency assessment program is to identify the expected competencies for a specific job description. The ANA provides standards of practice for assessment, diagnosis, outcomes identification, planning, implementation, and evaluation with related competencies for the registered nurse (ANA, 2010, pp. 32–45). The Standards of Professional Nursing Practice are authoritative statements and all registered nurses are expected to perform them competently regardless of the practice setting, role, population, or specialty. Many institutions utilize these standards to form the basis of the registered nurse job description, which is utilized to evaluate initial and ongoing competency. Regulatory and accrediting agencies also require specific competencies for health care staff, for example, care of patients in restraints.

After the expected competencies for each job description are determined, each health care agency develops a system and tools for evaluating initial and ongoing competent practice. Competencies are an integral part of new staff training programs as well as other educational programs that prepare staff members for specialized tasks and the maintenance of skills in their health care provider roles. According to O'Hearne-Rebholz (2006), competency is validation that skills, processes, and concepts are completed or understood correctly as determined by an expert. O'Hearne-Rebholz describes various methods which can be used to validate staff competency including paper and pen competencies, observation competencies, skills laboratory competencies, and scenario competencies. The ANA (2010) expands this list to include direct observation, patient records, demonstrations, skills lab, simulation exercises, computer simulated and virtual reality testing, performance review, peer review, certification, credentialing, targeted continuing education with outcomes measurement, employer skills validation, and practice evaluations.

Although no one method can guarantee competence, each health care agency needs to thoughtfully develop a system that utilizes multiple methods that can be implemented initially for orientation and on an ongoing basis. The paper-and-pen competency described by O'Hearne-Rebholz (2006) utilizes traditional testing techniques. While it may not be the best overall method for assessing competency, it can be useful in situations that require a measurement of staff knowledge such as understanding of a policy, interpreting electrocardiograms, or proper medication calculations. The observation competency allows the expert to actually watch the staff member performing in real time. Though difficult to carry out especially with large groups of staff, observation is an effective method to evaluate processes such as staff–patient interactions and pain assessment and reassessment. Preceptors are critical to the observation and assessment of the competencies of new staff in the patient care arena. The skills laboratory competency takes a significant amount of time, planning, and resources but it is a valuable method to validate proper use of equipment and to test skills such as cardiopulmonary resuscitation and IV insertion. Scenario competencies utilize a case study or storytelling approach to recreate a patient situation. Scenario competencies are useful in evaluating critical thinking and clinical judgment skills (O'Hearne-Rebholz, 2006). Scenario simulation, especially high-fidelity simulation, provides a safe learning environment to assess and develop psychomotor, critical thinking, and clinical judgment skills. With an increased interest in improving patient safety over the past decade, simulation can be effectively utilized to enhance teamwork and communication among clinicians. Simulation incorporates adult learning principles (Nagle, McHale, Alexander, & French, 2009). Active participation by the learner promotes problemsolving and immediate application of new theory and skills to existing practice. Postscenario debriefing provides the adult learner the opportunity to self-reflect, incorporate feedback, and provide feedback to others in a safe environment. This helps the adult learner acquire knowledge, integrate skills into new situations, evaluate ways to improve teamwork, and recognize the consequences of clinical decisions (Nagle et al., 2009).

A competent level of performance is expected for patient, health care provider, and agency safety. Continuing competence mandates a commitment to lifelong learning activities for all professional nurses, and the ANA purports that the individual nurse is responsible and accountable for maintaining his or her own professional competence (ANA, 2010, p.76). However, the employer must provide an environment that is conducive to professional practice. As skills become more complex, experience and additional education are necessary to reach the higher levels of performance. Health care agencies need to provide education programs to promote competence. These programs should include an overall goal, specific behaviorally stated learning objectives, the competencies to be assessed, remediation plans to bring the learner up to competency, periodic recertification plans, and an evaluation plan to measure learning outcomes, satisfaction, and the success of the program in terms of its quality, cost-effectiveness, and contribution to the agency's mission.

BUDGET PLANNING FOR STAFF DEVELOPMENT

Staff development educators have a responsibility for planning, managing, and reporting budgets to the administration of the sponsoring health agency. It is an essential task to justify the existence of the educational program and its relevance to the mission of the agency and its service. It demonstrates cost-effectiveness as well as cost recovery over the long term. For example, well-oriented new staff members and well-prepared new graduates are more apt to become long-term employees rather than entering and exiting through a revolving door. Prior to developing a new business plan or revising an existing one, it is important to develop a business case. A *business case* is a document intended to generate support for the budget from the agency leadership and other key stakeholders. It identifies the need, purpose, and relationship of the program to the overall mission of the organization.

It provides the context and content around the need and lists the desired objectives, outcomes, and its advantages to the health care organization.

When preparing a business case and its related plan, the first item to assess is the source of revenues including the income generated by the health agency through general funds (if government sponsored), patient fees, insurance programs, and Medicare and Medicaid. While historically these sources have been somewhat stable, recent changes in the national and international economy make this income much less dependable while organizations continue to deal with changing patient care demands and ever-changing reimbursement and prospective pay systems. Thus, it is important for staff development educators to investigate other possible sources of income for the program such as grants from other health-related organizations, federal, state, or regional grants, benefactor gifts, and fees for educational programs. The type of revenue will determine how it will be spent. For example, established, long-term income and resources might be used to maintain ongoing programs while new program development, or one-time only programs, may be funded through short-term grants and other gift monies.

On the debit or cost side of the budget, the two largest items are capital expenditures and personnel. Capital expenditures include office, classroom, and laboratory facilities that are usually shared spaces and can be calculated according to the percentage of use by the educational program. Other capital expenditures include "big ticket items" such as instructional support systems (videoconferencing, telecommunications, and web-based technology including learning management systems), computers, audio–visual hardware, mannequins, high fidelity simulators, large software teaching packages, and online nursing reference resources for skills and professional development. While they are usually considered on the debit side, their value can also be considered as assets with only their depreciation added to the costs each year. If the educational program expects to undergo accreditation or certification, the one-time expenses for preparing a readiness evaluation and site visits are included for that year.

Personnel expenses include the salaries and benefits of the educators, administrative support staff, administrators, and in some instances, the costs for released time of staff to attend educational programs. The use of scenario-based simulation is instructor intensive, as low participant-to-instructor ratios are needed for effective learning. Additional or reallocation of resources may need to be considered when implementing innovative educational experiences. Each year, the budget must build in salary increases and concomitant benefit increases for the staff. The time of the staff members who precept new employees is an additional personnel cost to be calculated. Other expenses for the program include online nursing reference resources, learning management systems, office supplies, books, journal subscriptions, teaching supplies, travel expenses for staff, continuing education and professional meetings for the staff development educators, and meals or refreshments for class participants.

The budget is prepared several months in advance of its submission for approval by the administration. Health agency budgets run either on a fiscal year basis (July to June) with quarterly reporting or on a calendar year (January to December) basis with quarterly reporting. It is wise to build in a contingency fund to cover any unexpected costs that the program encounters during the year. When submitting the budget, it is advisable to include an attachment with sufficient justifications for each item.

In the ideal staff development setting, the manager or director of the education department manages the budget and has administrative assistance for tracking expenditures, preparing purchase orders, receiving, cataloging, and keeping inventory of equipment and supplies, and managing the payroll. Careful records are kept so that quarterly and end-of-year reports are easily assembled and provide the agency with the program's accountability as well as trends in income generation and expenditures for future planning. This discussion reviews the major items in budget preparation, management, and reporting. Although each agency has its own budget format, the items in the discussion can be adapted to the agency's specific format. Table 15.4 summarizes the discussion.

TABLE 15.4 EDUCATIONAL PROGRAM BUDGETING

MAJOR BUDGET ITEM	INCOME OR (DEBIT)	ITEMS INCLUDED
Program Maintenance	Income	Agency funds from fees, insurance, reimbursements, general revenues
Program Development or Enhancement	Income	Grants, contributions, gifts, endowments
Personnel	(Debit)	Salaries, benefits, released and/or nonproductive time
Capital Expenditures	Assets and (Debit: Depreciation)	Offices, labs, classrooms, conference rooms, furniture, equipment, simulators, utilities, contracts for maintenance of equipment, major software packages
Supplies and Services	(Debit)	Online nursing references, learning management system, office and teaching supplies, simulation lab supplies, texts, journal subscriptions, travel, food and refreshments

JUSTIFICATION AND FUNDING FOR EDUCATIONAL PROGRAMS IN HEALTH CARE AGENCIES

It is not unusual for health agencies experiencing budget crises to think of cutting personnel and programs associated with "nonessential" services. Educational programs are frequently the targets of such cuts in spite of the impact they have on cost savings and the delivery of quality care to the agency's staff and its clients. In the previous discussion on the budget for education programs, there was mention of the need to demonstrate cost-effectiveness and related cost savings from the educational program to the administration of the health care agency as well as to the public or consumers of the program. For example, the nurse educator can compare the major costs of bringing in traveling RNs to staff the agency to the lesser cost of providing incentives for staff retention derived from the support of new graduates through preceptor and mentorship programs, continuing education programs, and in-service opportunities for core staff. As to the value of the program, the health care agency that has a satisfied staff soon sees gains in the quality of the care delivered which, in turn, translates into patient or customer satisfaction. Magnet hospitals are excellent examples of quality care and part of their successes is staff development and educational program achievements, which contribute to the overall retention of highly engaged employees. Information on Magnet hospitals can be found at http://www.nursecredentialing.org.

EVALUATION OF STAFF EDUCATION PROGRAMS

The principles of total quality management in staff development programs are the same as those applied to evaluation strategies in schools of nursing. The reader is directed to Section V and Chapter 16 of this text for an overview of definitions, concepts, theories, and models that are relevant to educational programs in health agencies. There are two major components of evaluation in staff development. On the micro level are the individual teaching and learning sessions provided to the target audience, and on the macro level is program evaluation to assess the effectiveness and worth of the total education program and its services for the health agency. A brief discussion follows that relates to each of these components of evaluation.

EVALUATION OF INDIVIDUAL TEACHING AND LEARNING SESSIONS

Developing and implementing individual teaching and learning sessions are ongoing processes and it is advised that plans for evaluation of the sessions occur during the initial development. Carefully stated learning objectives serve as one method for measuring the success of the session. If the objectives are learner-centered, include a time frame, how, an action on the part of the learner can be measured, and the level of competency expected, the evaluation becomes quite simple. As discussed previously, this validation can be accomplished through traditional testing methods such as paper and pencil, scenario techniques, and/or through instructor observation in the reality setting or in skills or simulation lab settings.

In addition to learner achievement, there are other aspects of the educational session that the evaluator assesses. These include the effectiveness of the instructor and teaching strategies, the learning environment and materials, and learner and instructor satisfaction with the session. These latter assessments can be measured through surveys of the learners and instructors with rating scale responses to questions or open-ended questions that are subject to content analysis.

EVALUATION OF EDUCATIONAL PROGRAMS

The evaluation of education programs in health agencies is an important activity on the part of nurse educators for several reasons. Positive evaluations provide justification for the education program's place and value of service in the agency. Evaluation activities such as continuous quality assessment lead to improvement of the program and the achievement of excellence. Additionally, evaluation activities and reports contribute to the accreditation, licensure, or certification of the program and the health agency. The elements of program evaluation in staff education are similar to those found in schools of nursing. The first item to assess is the congruence of the health agency's mission and the mission of the education program. They should be in alignment and if not, a rationale for why there is a difference should be prominent in the description of the program, or the mission and purpose of the education program should be adjusted to the parent agency's mission and purpose.

The philosophy statements and conceptual frameworks of the agency and the education program should be compatible and the goals for each should flow from the philosophy, organizational framework (if present), and the mission. Once the goal is assessed for its reflection of the intent of the program, the implementation of the program is assessed and evaluated for its consistency with the mission, purpose, philosophy, and framework. The next step is to determine to what extent the outcomes of the educational program are measured by its goals and objectives, its overall impact on the clients' community served by the parent organization, its cost-effectiveness, its measure of quality compared to other staff development programs, its achievement of benchmarks that the agency and program set for it, and its accreditation, licensure, or certification status.

Table 15.5 summarizes these elements according to evaluation elements and the desired outcomes. As with nursing education programs, a master plan of

TABLE 15.5   THE ELEMENTS OF AN EVALUATION PLAN FOR STAFF DEVELOPMENT

EVALUATION ELEMENT	QUESTIONS FOR DATA COLLECTION	DESIRED OUTCOME
Mission, Overall Purpose, and Philosophy	To what extent are the mission, overall purpose, and philosophy of the agency and its educational program congruent?	The mission, overall purpose, and philosophy of the educational program are congruent with that of the agency
Goals (Long term)	Is it evident that the overall or long-term goal(s) flow from the mission, purpose and philosophy?	The overall or long-term goal(s) flow from the mission, purpose and philosophy
Objectives (Short term) and Implementation Plan	Is it evident that the objectives for the program and each learning session flow from the overall goal(s) and are congruent with the mission and philosophy?	The objectives for the program and each learning session flow from the overall goal(s) and are congruent with the mission and philosophy
	To what extent do the objectives include specification of the learner, the learning content, behavior of the learner, expected outcome, and time frame?	The objectives are stated in such a way that they can be measured for their outcomes
	Is there evidence that the implementation plan flows from the mission, goal(s), and objectives?	The implementation plan flows from the mission, goal(s), and objectives

(continued)

TABLE 15.5 THE ELEMENTS OF AN EVALUATION PLAN FOR STAFF DEVELOPMENT (*continued*)

EVALUATION ELEMENT	QUESTIONS FOR DATA COLLECTION	DESIRED OUTCOME
Cost-effectiveness	What are the major sources of financial support for the program? To what extent is the education program self-sufficient? Have other possible funding resources been identified and are they part of a plan to secure funds? To what extent does the education program contribute to the financial stability of the agency? Is there a plan for either maintaining or reaching financial stability?	The program is supported through multiple means such as organizational budget, fees for services, grants, and so on; the education program is self-sufficient The education program contributes to the quality and financial stability of the agency
Outcomes (Participants and Community)	To what extent do data from the assessment of the outcomes from the education program indicate achievement of its goal and objectives? To what extent do participants report a high level of satisfaction from the program? Is there a plan in place to either maintain or improve outcomes? To what extent is the community aware of the agency's education program? Is there a plan in place for raising the public's awareness of the education program and its contributions to the community?	Outcomes from the education program indicate achievement of its goal and objectives Participants (both learners and instructors) report a high level of satisfaction from the program The community is aware of the agency's education program and holds it in high regard
Comparison to Similar Programs and Benchmarks	To what extent is the education program superior to or on a par with similar education programs? Do the program costs meet budget limits? To what extent does the program meets its goals and objectives each year? Are there plans in place to improve the program or set higher benchmarks?	The education program is superior to or on a par with similar education programs The program costs meet budget limits The program meets its goals and objectives each year and/ or the program is re-evaluated and new benchmarks are set
Accreditation, Licensure, and Certification	Has the program received accreditation, licensure, or certification? If the program is an integral part of the health agency, to what extent does it contribute to accreditation, licensure, or certification? Is there a plan in place to continually assess the program for maintenance of accreditation, licensure, or certification? To what extent is there a record keeping system in place for accreditation, licensure, or certification?	Depending upon the nature of the program, the education program has accreditation, licensure, or certification

evaluation is recommended so that evaluation becomes an ongoing process and guides the activities of the program for total quality management.

An excellent classic model for a comprehensive tool for the evaluation of education programs in health care agencies is the pyramid model of evaluation for continuing education programs described by Hawkins and Sherwood (1999). The model is based upon Donabedian's (1966) structure, process, and outcome model of evaluation and the social science evaluation model developed by Rossi and Freeman (1993). It incorporates all of the elements of program and curriculum development discussed thus far in this chapter including a look at the internal and external frame factors that impact educational programs. In addition to assessing the program design, implementation, outcomes, and impact, it addresses cost-effectiveness issues. It is a highly recommended reading for nurse educators considering the use of a master plan of evaluation for staff education.

ISSUES AND TRENDS IN STAFF DEVELOPMENT

Issues of concern to staff development educators are in part related to the financial challenges faced by health care organizations today. Changes in the economy have resulted in decreased reimbursement to health care organizations; at the same time, increased levels of service are often needed. Organizations are faced with difficult decisions in terms of eliminating programs in order to remain financially solvent; often, funding for staff development programs is reduced or eliminated entirely. Equally concerning is the nursing shortage, which is expected to worsen over the next several years. Certain areas of the country are impacted more drastically by this shortage in which newly graduated nurses have assumed an important role in the recruitment and staffing strategies of hospitals. The transition experience of newly graduated nurses into the workforce is often fraught with stress and disillusionment resulting in a particularly alarming trend of new nurses leaving their first jobs within 2 years and many leaving the nursing profession altogether. The stress associated with this transition is compounded by the fact that it is no longer feasible to assign lower acuity patients to new graduates while they learn their roles in today's health care environment. These lower acuity patients simply do not receive care within the acute care setting. Furthermore, because of the dire need to fill vacant positions, employers are expecting newly graduated nurses to quickly function as competent professionals. A nurse who leaves an organization with less than one year of employment represents a loss ranging from $34,000 to $145,000 in hiring and orientation costs, further contributing to the financial constraints associated with staff development programs (Bowles & Candela, 2005; Casey et al., 2004; Duclos-Miller, 2011; Grochow, 2008; Halfer & Graf, 2006). Another factor to consider is the effect of the aging of the nursing profession and the resulting loss of many of the most experienced nurses in the field due to decreased work hours or retirement. Although this issue has been identified among nursing faculty, health care organizations face a similar issue, both in the clinical practice arena among staff as well as among APNs.

MAINTAINING QUALITY PROGRAMS AND PLANNING FOR THE FUTURE

Heller, Oros, and Durney-Crowley (2000) discuss several trends in health care and nursing that have an impact on nursing education, including staff development. Although the article was published in 2000, it continues to be relevant to the current and future health care system and provides 10 major trends to watch as they influence education. The trends they identify are: changing demographics, technology, globalization, educated consumers, population-based care, health care costs/managed care, health policy and regulation, need for interdisciplinary education and collaboration, nursing shortage, and advances in nursing science and research. Their reflections on these trends are helpful in planning for the future and provide guidelines for factors to assess within each trend.

Consistent with the trends discussed by Heller et al. (2000), the task force to lead the revision of the Scope and Standards of Practice for NPD identified the following education-specific issues that will need to be acknowledged and addressed while moving forward: increased use of technology, global target audience, teaching/learning modalities, evidence-based practice, increased accountability, increased interdisciplinary involvement, fiscal management, need for complex implementation expertise, professional development metrics, decreasing time to achieve competency, generational differences, escalating competing priorities, knowledge management and succession planning, increased need for clinical affiliations and academic partnerships, move toward learning as an investment in human capital, cost avoidance versus expenditure, and focus on transition into practice (presented by Bradley et al. at the 2009 NNSDO Convention, General Session as cited in Health Leaders Media, 2009). Careful attention to these issues and trends will serve staff development educators well as we move into a future filled with economic uncertainty and potentially one of the worst nursing shortage our country has ever faced (American Association of Colleges of Nursing [AACN], 2014).

SUMMARY

Though the discussion in this chapter focused on the role of the staff development educator working in a health care agency, nurse educators are found in a multitude of settings such as academia, public and private school systems, home care agencies, public health agencies, and industry. Regardless of the setting, the global health care needs of society reflect a health care environment where client needs are increasingly complex and patients in clinical settings are of higher acuity. As our country continues to face significant economic challenges and we confront what will potentially be the worst nursing shortage our country has ever experienced, it is imperative that nurse educators in all of these settings join forces to promote their important role in shaping the future of nursing education and public policy to improve health care with the collective goal of reaching optimal health for our society.

DISCUSSION QUESTIONS

1. To what extent do you believe an assessment of the external and internal frame factors influences the development and evaluation of an educational program?

2. Give a rationale for applying the components of curriculum development and evaluation to staff education. Compare the components in the practice setting to those in the academic setting. What are the differences and similarities?
3. Identify an educational program and determine what learning theories, educational taxonomies, and teaching strategies apply to it. Give a rationale for your choices.
4. Why is it important for a staff development educator to be able to prepare, manage, and evaluate the budget of an education program? Explain your answer.
5. Discuss looming issues in the health care system that impact staff development. What strategies would you as a nurse educator take to help bring about solutions to these issues?

LEARNING ACTIVITIES

Select an education program in a health care agency and assess it for its recognition of the impact of the external and internal frame factors on the program. Evaluate the program according to the classic components of curriculum development and evaluation. Include an analysis of the evaluation plan in place for individual sessions and the program as a whole. Is there evidence that the data collected for evaluation are used to revise the program and improve quality? Analyze the budget of the program for its relationship to the mission and goals of the agency and the education program.

REFERENCES

Abruzzese, R. S. (1996). *Nursing staff development: Strategies for success* (2nd ed.). St. Louis, MO: Mosby.

American Association of Colleges of Nursing. (2014). *Nursing shortage.* Retrieved from http://www.aacn.nche.edu/media-relations/fact-sheets/nursing-shortage

American Nurses Association. (2010). *Scope and standards of practice for nursing professional development* (2nd ed.). Silver Springs, MD: Nursebooks.org.

American Nurses Credentialing Center. (2012). *Role delineation study.* Retrieved from http://www.nursecredentialing.org/Certification/NurseSpecialties/NursingProfessional Development/NPD-RelatedLinks/2012-RDS-Survey.pdf

American Nurses Credentialing Center. (2014). *Specialty certifications.* Retrieved from http://www.nursecredentialing.org

Baltimore, J. (2004). The hospital clinical preceptor: Essential preparation for success. *The Journal of Continuing Education in Nursing, 35,* 133–140.

Benner, P., Kyriakidis, P., & Stannard, D. (2011). *Clinical wisdom and interventions in acute and critical care: A thinking-in-action approach* (2nd ed.). New York, NY: Springer Publishing.

Bowles, C., & Candela, L. (2005). First job experiences of recent graduates. *Journal of Nursing Administration, 35,* 130–137.

Burk, G. (2008). Forecasting instead of reacting to educational needs. *Journal for Nurses in Staff Development, 24*(5), 226–231.

Casey, K., Fink, R., Krugman, M., & Propst, J. (2004). The graduate nurse experience. *Journal of Nursing Administration, 34,* 303–310.

Donabedian, A. (1966). Evaluating the quality of medical care. *Milbank Memorial Fund Quarterly, 44*(Part 2), 166–206.

Duclos-Miller, A. (2011). Successful graduate nurse transition: Meeting the challenge. *Nurse Leader, 9*(4), 32–35, 49.

Durham, C., & Sherwood, G. (2008). Education to bridge the quality gap: A case study approach. *Urologic Nursing, 28*(6), 431–453.

Gallagher, R. (2005). National quality efforts: What continuing and staff development educators need to know. *Journal of Continuing Education in Nursing, 36*(1), 39–45.

Grochow, D. (2008). From novice to expert: Transitioning graduate nurses. *Nursing Management, 39*, 10–12.

Halfer D., & Graf, E. (2006). Graduate nurse perceptions of the work experience. *Nursing Economics, 24*(3), 150–155.

Hawkins, V., & Sherwood, G. (1999). The Pyramid model: An integrated approach for evaluation continuing education programs and outcomes. *The Journal of Continuing Education in Nursing, 30*(5), 203–212.

Health Leaders Media. (2009). *What the ANA's new professional development scope and standards mean for nursing staff.* Retrieved from http://www.healthleadersmedia.com/page-2/NRS-243558/What-the-ANAs-New-Professional-Development-Scope-and-Standards-Mean-for-Nursing-Staff

Healthy People 2020. (2010). U.S. *Department of Health and Human Services.* Retrieved from http://www.healthypeople.gov

Heller, B., Oros, M., & Durney-Crowley, J. (2000). The future of nursing education: Ten trends to watch. *Nursing and Health Care Perspectives, 21*(1), 9–13.

Johnson, M. (1977). *Intentionality in education.* (Distributed by the Center for Curriculum Research and Services, Albany, N.Y.). Troy, NY: Walter Snyder, Printer.

Knowles, M. S., Holton, E. F., & Swanson, R. A. (1998). *The adult learner: The definitive classic in adult education and human resource development* (5th ed.). Houston, TX: Gulf Publishing.

Krugman, M. (2003). Evidence-based practice: The role of staff development. *Journal for Nurses in Staff Development, 19*(6), 279–285.

Nagle, B. M., McHale, J. M., Alexander, G. A., & French, B. M. (2009). Incorporating scenario-based simulation into a hospital nursing education program. *The Journal of Continuing Education in Nursing, 40*(1), 18–25.

Nicol, P., & Young, M. (2007). Sail training: An innovative approach to graduate nurse preceptor development. *Journal for Nurses in Staff Development, 23*, 298–302.

Oermann, M., & Moffitt-Wolf, A. (1997). New graduates' perceptions of clinical practice. *The Journal of Continuing Education in Nursing, 28*, 20–25.

O'Hearne-Rebholz, M. (2006). A review of methods to assess competency. *Journal for Nurses in Staff Development, 22*(5), 241–245.

Orsini, C. (2005). A nurse transition program for orthopaedics: Creating a new culture for nurturing graduate nurses. *Orthopaedic Nursing, 24*, 240–246.

Rossi, P., & Freeman, H. E. (1993). *Evaluation: A systematic approach.* Thousand Oaks, CA: Sage.

Schumacher, A. (2007). Caring behaviors of preceptors as perceived by new nursing graduate orientees. *Journal for Nurses in Staff Development, 23*, 186–192.

Smith, M. (2002). *Malcolm Knowles, informal adult education, self-direction and andragogy, the encyclopedia of informal education.* Retrieved from www.infed.org/thinkers/et-knowl.htm

Strickland, R., & O'Leary-Kelley, C. (2009). Clinical nurse educators' perceptions of research utilization: Barriers and facilitators to change. *Journal for Nurses in Staff Development, 25*(4), 164–171.

Program Evaluation and Accreditation

Sarah B. Keating

CIPP
context input process product

OVERVIEW

Section V analyzes theories, concepts, and models used to evaluate nursing education programs and curricula. Although evaluation appears as the last step in curriculum development and evaluation, it occurs throughout the processes of curriculum development and its implementation. Evaluation activities are part of the accreditation processes that schools or health care agencies experience as part of their credibility for consumers of the programs and for documentation of the institution's ability to meet professional and educational standards and criteria. Information from evaluation activities provides the impetus for major and minor changes that must take place to maintain an up-to-date and high-quality curriculum.

Current economic and educational systems in the United States place an emphasis on outcomes and *total quality management*, that is, continually assessing the program, correcting errors as they occur, and thus, improving the quality of the program. Earlier evaluation models in nursing focused on the process phases for delivering education. They spoke of student-centered teaching and learning processes. Faculty's role was to enable the learner to become actively involved and self-directing to acquire new knowledge, behaviors, attitudes, and skills. Outcomes were linked to and measured by the goals and objectives of the curriculum. These processes continue to be vital to evaluation; however, there is a demand for additional information that measures the outcomes in terms of graduates' performance and the quality of the program as compared to professional standards and its competitors.

While evaluation theories, concepts, models, and processes apply to both the academic and practice settings, the discussion in Section V focuses on program evaluation in academe and regional and professional accrediting bodies for nursing education. However, the information presented can be extrapolated from academe to the practice setting. Entities involved in the evaluation and accreditation of community-based education programs and staff development activities include the Joint Commission for Accreditation of Health Care Agencies' programs and the American Nurses Association (ANA), which provides standards for nurse educators and professional practice.

THE ROLE OF FACULTY, STUDENTS, CONSUMERS, AND ADMINISTRATORS IN EVALUATION

As is true for curriculum development, the faculty is key to the assessment of program outcomes and to the collection and analysis of the data. Students are an important part of the evaluation process as measured by their performance on tests and clinical skills, satisfaction with the program, and their assessment of teaching effectiveness and the quality of the courses in which they participate. Evaluation of the program must also come from the major consumers of the program, which include alumni, employers of the graduates, and the recipients of the graduates' nursing care. The program's success is assessed by the graduates' performance on licensure and certification exams, job skills, professional achievement, and promotion of the program to others. Employers of the graduates and the population receiving their services provide invaluable information and serve as a barometer of the program's match to the health care needs of the population and the system's demand for its graduates.

The role of administrators in education programs is to provide the leadership and financial resources necessary for evaluation processes and if indicated, consultation services (internal or external expertise). Administrators must see to it that there is adequate support staff for the ongoing collection of data and analyses and they have responsibility for ensuring that the findings are disseminated in a timely fashion to stakeholders and for follow-up on the recommendations from the findings.

THE MASTER PLAN OF EVALUATION AND PROGRAM REVIEW

Chapter 16 focuses on major evaluation theories, concepts, and models related to program review and assessment. It describes the system of program approval and periodic review within the parent institution. Peer and administrative review bodies and individuals grant approval to initiate programs in academe. Traditionally, established program reviews occur every 5 years within the institution to ensure quality and, in some instances, justify the continuation of the program when enrollments decline or economic times require downsizing of academic programs.

With an emphasis on outcomes, evaluation is essential for measuring success, establishing benchmarks, and continually improving the quality of the program. Because programs need to meet academic and accreditation standards, professional discipline expectations, and consumer demand, most institutions have a master plan of evaluation. The master plan may be organized around an evaluation model or theory or by criteria set by accrediting bodies, or it may choose to use both. The master plan provides the guidelines for collecting information to prepare required reports such as program approval or review, accreditation, and to demonstrate the worth of the program to the parent institution and the community. Institutions use the results of evaluation to continue and to improve the program, demonstrate excellence, and market their programs to the public.

PROGRAM APPROVAL AND ACCREDITATION

While assessment and evaluation activities for program approval/review and for accreditation often involve the collection and analysis of the same information, their purposes are quite different. Chapter 17 reviews regulatory program approval and accreditation activities for schools of nursing. The state board of nursing in which the school of nursing is located is a regulating agency and must approve the program initially and at periodic intervals. While the board looks at quality, its primary charge is to view the program's performance in light of consumer protection. It also determines the program's eligibility for graduates to sit for RN licensure and, in many states, approves nursing programs for advanced practice.

Accreditation is voluntary but at the same time, it gives credibility to the program on the regional, national, and professional levels. Its purpose is to ensure quality as measured by higher education and nursing education accrediting agencies' criteria set by professional peers. An accredited program provides advantages including its reputation for quality, eligibility for grants and other external funding, and for its graduates' eligibility for licensure, certification, admission into higher degree programs, and scholarships. Chapter 17 goes into detailed descriptions of the types of accreditation for higher education and nursing including regional, national, and specialty accreditation. It discusses the pros and cons of accreditation and provides educators with detailed guidelines for preparing for accreditation.

The two major accreditation agencies for nursing education are, one, the Accreditation Commission for Education in Nursing (ACEN) (formerly NLN-AC, a subsidiary of the National League for Nursing (NLN). It accredits practical, associate, diploma, baccalaureate, master's, and clinical doctorate programs. The other major accrediting agency for higher education in nursing is the Commission on Collegiate Nursing Education (CCNE). It accredits baccalaureate, graduate, and residency programs. Both agencies are recognized by the U.S. Department of Education (DOE). The NLN established the Commission for Nursing Education Accreditation (C-NEA) in 2013. C-NEA is undergoing a reorganization by the DOE, which takes a minimum of 2 years.

Program Evaluation

Sarah B. Keating

OBJECTIVES

Upon completion of Chapter 16, the reader will be able to:

1. Analyze common definitions, concepts, and theories of quality assurance and program evaluation
2. Analyze several models of evaluation for their utility in nursing education
3. Compare research to program evaluation processes
4. Justify the rationale for strategic planning and developing a master plan of evaluation for educational programs
5. Compare the roles of administrators and faculty in program evaluation
6. Apply the guidelines and major components of a master plan of evaluation to a nursing education program

OVERVIEW

Chapter 16 reviews definitions, concepts, and theories related to evaluation and quality assurance as they apply to nursing education. Conceptual models of evaluation; utilization of standards, criteria, and benchmarks; comparison of evaluation research and program evaluation; and types of program evaluation and their purposes are included. The chapter continues with a discussion of strategic planning, the roles of administrators and faculty in evaluation, and the development of master plans of evaluation. As discussed in the section overview, educational evaluation occurs while assessing the program for its quality, currency, relevance, projections into the future, and the need for possible revisions in light of these factors. While the administration usually assumes the leadership for strategic planning, faculty becomes part of the process, especially as it relates to responding to the information provided by the evaluation of the curriculum and the future plans for the institution. A master plan of evaluation provides the information necessary for curriculum evaluation and revision if indicated, and for program or institutional strategic planning.

COMMON DEFINITIONS, CONCEPTS, AND THEORIES RELATED TO EVALUATION AND QUALITY ASSURANCE

While many of the terms, concepts, and theories of educational evaluation originated from business models, they have been adapted to education, especially in light of the emphasis on outcomes. The following definitions are commonly used terms in evaluation as they apply to nursing education. To initiate the discussion, the first term to consider is evaluation as compared to assessment. *Evaluation* is a process by which information about an entity is gathered to determine its worth. It differs from assessment in that the end product of evaluation is a judgment of its worth, while *assessment* is a process that gathers information that results in a conclusion such as a nursing diagnosis or problem identification. It does not end with a judgment but rather a conclusion. Weiner (2009) provides an overview of assessment processes and purposes in academe with descriptions of the roles of faculty and administrators in the establishment of a "culture of assessment." He lists some of the curricular and co-curricular activities that need to be part of assessment and that they must be included in the budgeting process. Student learning outcomes in courses and at the end of the program are essential elements in assessment and he provides samples of measurable student outcomes.

Quality is a term that takes on many meanings depending upon the context in which it is used. For the purposes of this chapter and in the interest of simplicity, the Merriam-Webster's Online Dictionary (2014) third definition of quality is used: "a high level of value or excellence." Examples of the measures of quality include the standards, by which an entity is measured, comparison to other like entities, and consumer expectations. *Quality control* is "an aggregate of activities designed to insure adequate quality in … products." *Quality assurance* is "the systematic monitoring and evaluation of the various aspects of a project, service, or facility to ensure that standards of quality are being met" (Merriam-Webster). For the purposes of the evaluation of nursing education and this textbook, *total quality management* is defined as an educational program's commitment to and strategies for collecting comprehensive information on the program's effectiveness in meeting its goals and the management of its findings to ensure the continued quality of the program.

Formative and summative evaluation terms are used frequently when evaluating educational programs. The classic and still used definitions for the terms were developed by Scriven (1996). He describes *formative evaluation* as "intended–by the evaluator– as a basis for improvement" (p. 4). For example, in nursing, the faculty compares students' grades in prerequisites to their grades in nursing courses to determine if certain levels of achievement in prerequisites influence grades in nursing. Scriven describes *summative evaluation* as a holistic approach to the assessment of a program and it uses results from the formative evaluation. Continuing with the examples from nursing, faculty can evaluate the development of critical thinking skills in its graduates as a product of the educational program. In this instance, these skills would need to be measured both before and after the program to determine an increase in the skills. Both formative and summative types of evaluation "involve efforts to determine merit or worth, etc." (Scriven, 1996, p. 6). Scriven points out that summative evaluation can serve as formative evaluation. For example, if a nursing program finds that graduates' clinical decision-making skills are weak (summative evaluation), it can use that information to analyze the program (formative evaluation) for the strategies utilized to promote these skills throughout the program and make improvements as necessary.

Additional definitions commonly used in evaluation are *goal-based evaluation* and *goal-free evaluation*. Scriven (1974) described goal-based program evaluation as that which focuses only on the examination of program goals and intended outcomes while an alternative method could be used to examine the actual effects of the program. These effects (goal-free evaluation) include not only the intended effects, but also unintended effects, side effects, or secondary effects. An unintended effect in nursing might be an increase in the applicant pool owing to the community's interactions with students in a program-sponsored, nurse-managed clinic. While this was not a stated goal of the program, it was a positive, unintended outcome.

CONCEPTUAL MODELS OF EVALUATION

Conceptual Models

For years, nursing education programs used many of the models of evaluation developed in health care and education. Examples were Donabedian's (1996) Structure, Process, and Outcome model for health care evaluation and Stuffle-beam's (1971) Context, Input, Process, and Product (CIPP) educational model. Some of these models continue to serve nursing well but as nursing develops the uniqueness of the discipline, it is using its own models for evaluation. Most of the models are based on accreditation or professional organizations' standards, essentials, or criteria to evaluate outcomes. For example, Kalb (2009) describes using the Three C's Model, that is, context, content, and conduct for a comprehensive evaluation of the curriculum and program. The Kalb's school of nursing used the model to integrate its three nursing programs (associate degree in nursing [ADN], bachelor of science in nursing [BSN], and master of science in nursing [MSN]) according to the National League for Nursing Accrediting Commission's (NLN-AC's) (2008) accreditation standards and there were plans to use it for developing the doctor of nursing practice (DNP) as well. The evaluation processes in addition to the accreditation standards included the organizational structure, the curriculum, courses, faculty, staff, students, and ANAs (2004) professional standards.

DeSilets (2010) describes the use of a hierarchal model, the Roberta Straessle Abruzzese model (RSA), which moves evaluation from the simple to the complex and assesses the processes, content, outcomes, impact, and finally, total program evaluation. The model is comprehensive and the author describes ways in which data are collected, analyzed, and used for programmatic decisions.

Horne and Sandmann (2012) conducted an integrative review of the literature to ascertain if graduate nursing programs evaluate their effectiveness including reaching outcomes, cost effectiveness, student and faculty satisfaction, making decisions based on evaluation outcomes, and measuring the quality of the program. Prior to their report on the findings, they define evaluation and its various processes as well as describing some of the models of evaluation reported in their review of the articles. They found a paucity of articles related to program evaluation but found a few helpful ideas for programs to measure program quality and effectiveness in nursing.

Pross (2010) describes the Promoting Excellence in Nursing Education (PENE) model for program evaluation that centers on the achievement of excellence through three major factors. They are (a) visionary, caring leadership, (b) an expert faculty, and (c) a dynamic curriculum. She goes on to explain the factors in detail with the dynamic curriculum one that not only meets, but exceeds standards, criteria, and regulations. She emphasizes the need for measurable program outcomes. For the dynamic curriculum to succeed, it must have visionary leadership to reach its goals and the expert faculty to continually improve performance, participate in creative and innovative scholarship, and provide exemplary service.

Benchmarking

Programs can set benchmarks to measure their own success and standards of excellence, or compare themselves to similar institutions. Benchmarks can be used in competition with other programs for recruiting students or seeking financial support or they can be used to motivate the members of the institution to strive toward excellence. Yet another function of benchmarking is the ability to collaborate with other institutions to share strengths with each other and to continually improve programs. Benchmarks include the financial health of the institution; applicant pool; admission, retention and graduation rates; commitment to diversity; student, faculty, staff, and administrators' satisfaction rates; NCLEX and certification pass rates; and so forth.

An example of a benchmarking project when developing or revising DNP programs is presented by Udlis and Manusco (2012) from their website survey of DNP programs across the United States. The authors present a summary of the history of the development of the degree and then present their findings from the 2011 website survey of 137 programs. Findings are organized according to type of program, program length and number of credits, location by region of the United States, cost, platform for offering the program, electives availability, number of credits, and the practice course name. Their study provides benchmarks and trends in DNP education programs as programs continue to evolve and increase across the United States.

Evaluation Processes Models

In addition to using conceptual models for program and curriculum evaluation, some institutions choose to use process models for evaluation activities. Holden and Zimmerman (2009) describe the Evaluation Planning Incorporating Context (EPIC) model for the evaluation process. Included in their text are examples of the use of the model for assessing an educational program and a community-based service agency. These can apply to nursing as well. The EPIC model "assesses the context of the program, gathers reconnaissance, engages stakeholders, describes the program, and focuses the evaluation" (p. 2). The model is especially helpful by its provision of guidelines for conducting an evaluation.

The Centers for Disease Control and Prevention (CDC) (2014) developed a framework for program evaluation that is useful for educators. While it focuses on the processes of evaluation, it includes a framework for assigning value or worth to the findings from the process. The major steps of the process are (a) engage the stakeholders, (b) describe the program, (c) focus the evaluation plan, (d) gather credible evidence, (e) justify conclusions and recommendations, (f) ensure use and share lessons learned and, finally, the cycle begins again with engage the stakeholders. The steps of the model incorporate standards against which the program is evaluated. For nursing programs, there are many; they include accreditation standards or criteria and professional/educational essentials or standards.

Formative Evaluation for Nursing Education

Formative and/or process evaluation strategies include course evaluations; student achievement measures; teaching effectiveness surveys; staff, student, administration, and faculty satisfaction measures; impressions of student and faculty performance by clinical agencies' personnel; assessment of student services and other support systems; students' critical thinking development and other standardized tests such as gains in knowledge and skills; NCLEX readiness; satisfaction surveys of families of students; retention/attrition rates; and cost effectiveness of the program. Antecedent or input evaluation items include entering grade point averages (GPAs), American College Testing (ACT) (2014), Scholastic Achievement Test (SAT) (The College Board, 2014), and Graduate Record Examination (GRE) (2014) scores for applicants and accepted students; retention and/or attrition rates; scholarship, fellowship, and loan availability; and endowments and grants for program development and support.

Praslova (2010) responds to a lack of specific criteria to measure student learning outcomes and, therefore, program effectiveness. Measuring student learning outcomes is part of formative evaluation activities that lead to summative evaluation and program outcomes. Praslova takes Kirkpatrick's model for training and adapts it to higher education to measure program effectiveness. She reviews the definition and purpose of assessment and describes the important role of the stakeholders in conducting assessments. The model consists of four criteria, that is, reaction, learning, behavior, and results. The four criteria are then explained and examples of how they are adapted to higher education with suggested assessment tools are offered. The model could be used to assess specific outcomes related to student learning. Another model for formative evaluation is presented by McNeil (2011), who adapts Bloom's taxonomy as a measurement of student learning outcomes. The author presents a 12-step evaluation model with the taxonomy as a guideline for both program and course evaluations. Although the model limits itself to learning outcomes and not necessarily the other factors that influence the quality of the total program including faculty, staff, student characteristics, and the infrastructure that supports the educational program, it is a very useful model for measuring student learning outcomes.

SUMMATIVE EVALUATION USING STANDARDS, ESSENTIALS, AND CRITERIA

Summative evaluation differs from formative evaluation with its purpose to assess and judge the final outcomes of the educational program, while formative evaluation assesses the processes used to achieve the final outcome. The "product" of the educational program can be measured according to the overall goal and objectives of the program/curriculum, standards and criteria of regulating bodies such as boards of nursing, professional standards such as nursing organizations' code of ethics and practice standards, essentials or competencies defined by professional and educational organizations, and last but not least, accreditation standards and criteria.

Measures to determine final outcomes of the program include follow-up surveys of the success rates of the graduates including their pass rates on licensure and certification exams, employers' and graduates' satisfaction with the program, graduates' performance, and alumni's accomplishments in leadership roles, as change agents, professional commitment, and continuing education rates. Additional outcome measures include graduation rates, accreditation and program approval status, ratings of the program by external evaluators or agencies, faculty and student research productivity, community service, and public opinion surveys. Many of these outcome measures can be used to serve as benchmarks for setting achievement levels, for example, 99% pass rates on NCLEX or for comparing the institution to other admired or similar institutions as a measure of quality.

Newhouse (2011) discusses summative evaluation as it applies to assessing computer and technology students' achievement of knowledge and competency in a technology educational program. He questions the use of written exams to measure students' abilities in understanding and working with technology and challenges the validity of such measures. A research team worked on the development of digital measures of achievement for these students including an electronic portfolio developed by the student and a computer-based examination. Newhouse and team found statistically significant results for the two methods including improved reliability and validity of the method and student and instructors' ease of access, marking, and satisfaction.

Stavropoulou and Kelesi (2012) summarize methods of program evaluation with a definition of evaluation that applies to nursing education. They discuss methodologies with a review of quantitative and qualitative evaluation methods, the debate of their use between the two, and the advantages and disadvantages for both. The authors conclude with the idea that both quantitative and qualitative methods should be used and they bring in the notion of triangulation as a method for program evaluation. Schug (2012) describes the process faculty undergoes when developing or revising a curriculum using the NLN's *Accreditation Manual* (2012). She presents a table listing the criteria with questions for the faculty to use as guides to evaluate the curriculum. She also mentions the Three C's Model for assessing and evaluating curricula, that is, context, content, and conduct. There is a plethora of instruments in nursing education programs that are available for measuring graduates' performance and satisfaction as an indication of the program's success. Nurse educators are urged to review the latest literature in a search for the best tools for collecting and analyzing data to measure the outcomes and the processes used to evaluate the achievement of the outcomes of educational programs. At the same time, while student learning outcomes are the core of program success, other summative factors must be considered such as the program's quality of faculty, research and scholarly output, staff, support systems, and infrastructure.

TYPES OF PROGRAM EVALUATION

Basically there are two types of program approval evaluation in academe that differ from regulatory and accreditation processes. They are *program approval* and *program review.*

Program Approval

Before a new program is initiated, its parent institution must approve it. As reiterated throughout this text, it is the faculty who develop the curriculum for a new program and it should be based on a needs assessment that provides the rationale for why it is needed, how it meets the mission of the institution, and who the key stakeholders are. In addition to the curriculum plan, a budget should accompany it and it is expected that it projects the costs and income for at least the next 5 years to justify its start-up and maintenance.

In academe the usual rounds of approval are as follows. The first round is for the faculty within the originating department/school to approve the proposal; its next round depends upon the hierarchal structure of the institution. The following levels of approval are based on a moderate to large-scale institution and it is understood that smaller institutions may not have as many approval rungs. After faculty approval within the originating program, the proposal may go to a curriculum or program approval committee within its college or division. Preliminary approval may have to be granted by administrators before it enters other formal approval levels in order to determine its economic feasibility and its fit to the mission and/or strategic plan.

After approval at the program's local level by committees and faculty as a whole, it proceeds to the next level, which is usually a program or curriculum committee at the division or college level. With its approval, it goes to the overall university or college graduate or undergraduate committee for their review and approval. Next, it goes to a subcommittee of the senate that reviews program proposals. On their approval, the senate reviews it for its input and approval and then sends it to the chief executive for academic affairs such as a vice president or provost. On that person's approval, the president of the institution approves the program. The governing board such as a board of trustees or regents is the final rung of approval and it may have a subcommittee that reviews it with recommendations prior to its going to the full board. These levels of approval are for academic approval only. For professional programs such as nursing, accreditation processes and state board of nursing approvals should be initiated along the way to reassure the academic entities that the program is qualified for professional approval and accreditation.

Program Review

Program review in academe occurs on average every 5 years within the parent institution. The purpose for program review is to ensure the quality and sustainability of the program. Faculty prepares an overview of the program especially related to enrollments, the quality of the faculty, student learning outcomes, and enrollment and graduation projections (Weiner, 2009). When economic times are tough, these reviews help to demonstrate the relationship of the program to the mission of the institution, its contributions to the community, and the quality of the program. Nursing often finds itself having to justify its program owing to the relatively small faculty to student ratios required when clinical supervision is factored in. Nursing programs need data as evidence to support the program, its cost-effectiveness, its place in meeting the mission of the institution (serving the public), and its contributions of student enrollments to the core general education and prerequisite requirements.

The requirements and processes for program approval and review use the same data sets as many of the other assessment and evaluation activities related to professional accreditation and standards of excellence. Thus, it is not unusual for a parent institution to request copies of the most recent self-studies and accreditation reports that either substitute for program review criteria or supplement the requirements. Program approval and review should be integrated into the school's master plan of evaluation so that the data sets can serve all of the required purposes for assessment.

Bers (2011) reviews the purposes of program review for community colleges that applies to other institutions of higher education as well. The major purposes are to assess the program's effectiveness both internally and externally, to meet both internal and external regulation or requirements, to exhibit accountability, and to utilize its public relations. She discusses both formative and summative evaluation as it applies to measuring program outcomes and offers models of evaluation that institutions can use for program review. Bers points out that many of these models are combinations of several models. The models for evaluation that she lists include the Strengths, Weaknesses, Opportunities, and Threats (SWOT) technique; free-form (goal-free) evaluation; outside expert review; self-study; and so on. Her article is very useful with many practical guidelines for programs undergoing program review.

Research and Program Evaluation

Sometimes there is confusion between evaluation research and the process of evaluation. The evaluation process starts with an identification of the program or entity that is to be evaluated, the purpose of the evaluation, and who the stakeholders are within the program. It requires many of the same steps of research including a review of the literature, identification of a theory or model of evaluation to guide the process, collection and analysis of credible data related to the program, synthesizing the analysis to come to a conclusion, and a judgment with recommendations for further assessment and strategies for improvement.

Research in evaluation, on the other hand, differs from the evaluation process. It begins with a description of a problem and a research question, its purpose for investigation, and follows with the usual steps of the research process, that is, literature review, theoretical/conceptual framework, methodology, data collection and analysis, findings, and recommendations.

Research in evaluation is usually viewed as applied research and differs from basic research as it is searching for practical solutions to problems. Donaldson, Christie, and Mark (2009) describe applied research and evaluation processes and the continuing debates among the experts on the validity of quantitative and qualitative methodologies and their application to evaluation. They discuss current emphases in the disciplines on evidence-based practice, what constitutes credible evidence, evaluation theories, and their influences on applied research in evaluation. In the end, their text presents the latest in evaluation theories and their relevance to the search for evidence-based practice in education.

Spillane et al. (2010) provide an example of a combined program evaluation and research project in their study of the use of mixed methodologies for evaluation. The project was an evaluation of a professional development education program for principals of schools. It was a randomized controlled trial (RCT) with two groups of principals, one group randomly assigned to a treatment group and the other group experiencing the training program a year later. The latter group served as the control group. The study was theory driven using a logic model that took into account not only the program but the principals' previous experience, faculty and student characteristics, and the leader's background. The researchers collected both qualitative and quantitative data. Analyses consisted of studying both types of data separately, then combining data to quantify qualitative data and to place the quantitative data into a qualitative context. This resulted in validation and contextualization of both types of data and their mix. Triangulation of the results pointed out the value of mixed methods. It provides an example of the differences between research and program evaluation and how research applies to practice.

Strategic Planning

Strategic planning for an institution provides the guidelines for carrying out the mission of the institution and at the same time can be used to evaluate how well the institution is meeting its mission and goals. Strategic planning usually begins with the top executive and management team providing the leadership for its development. In academe, the parent institution's top administrators (president, vice presidents, provosts, deans, etc.) initiate the plan, which is, in turn, implemented throughout the institution by the various academic divisions. Each division may choose to develop its own strategic plan; however, it should be congruent with that of its parent but unique to the program's mission and goals. The first step in strategic planning is to develop a vision statement. The vision statement presents a description of where the institution will be in the future, usually 3 to 5 years hence, and incorporates the core values of the institution. The leadership team may wish to engage other stakeholders in the process and in the planning to meet the vision.

Varkey and Bennett (2010) discuss the strategic planning process applied to health care agencies but the same processes can be adapted to educational milieus. They advise that the leadership team create a sense of urgency for developing the plan with the first session centered on developing a vision that is of the highest order and reflects the team's belief of where the organization needs to be in the future. Once the vision is developed through brainstorming and coming to consensus, the planning process commences.

A positive, comprehensive, and inclusionary approach to strategic planning is described by Harmon, Fontaine, Plews-Ogan, and Williams (2012) in a summary of the University of Virginia's School of Nursing strategic planning process. They adapted the Appreciative Inquiry (AI) model used in business for planning and promoting a positive milieu (Ludema, Whitney, Mohr, & Griffin, 2003). The authors describe the process they underwent for planning, holding, and summarizing the outcomes from a summit that developed strategic plans for the School of Nursing's future. It is a very useful model for other institutions undergoing the strategic planning process.

Stuart, Erkel, and Schull (2010) tie the analysis of costs of programs and their financial viability to the process of strategic planning. They describe how their College of Nursing at the Medical University of South Carolina examined existing programs, their need, and cost-effectiveness in planning for the future and for providing a rationale for establishing a doctor of nursing practice (DNP) program. This type of analysis contributes to strategic planning for the future that maintains and develops educational programs in response to current and future needs, yet operates within a realistic budget that utilizes existing resources.

Research and scholarly production by faculty and students as part of strategic planning are described by Kulage et al. (2013). The Columbia University School of Nursing dean and faculty undertook a project to update research and scholarly priorities based on new programs in the school, changes in faculty, trends in health care, and calls for interdisciplinary and inter-institutional collaboration. The process they undertook, the workgroups that were organized to carry out the tasks, and the methods for measuring outcomes are described as part of their strategic planning process.

Although nursing programs may not have a strategic plan per se, it is wise to have goals set for the future with action plans to carry them out. These goals and action plans are reviewed at least annually to assess the progress toward the goals and to adjust or develop new goals as the program and its needs and constituencies change. To avoid the pitfall of exquisite planning processes that fail to implement the plan, the use of a master plan of evaluation provides the structure, details, and timelines for assessing and evaluating the progress that the program is making toward reaching its vision and short-term and long-term goals.

MASTER PLAN OF EVALUATION

Rationale for a Master Plan of Evaluation

When developing a master plan of evaluation, one of the major tasks to integrate into the plan is to meet accreditation or program approval standards. These standards or criteria are the baseline requirements of the profession to ensure that programs are of sufficient quality to meet the expectations of the discipline. They also demonstrate to the public that a program is recognized by external reviewing bodies and thus the quality of its graduates meets educational and professional standards. Graduation from an accredited program is usually one of the admission standards for continued degree or education work. Many funding agencies for programs require accreditation as it indicates that the program is of high enough quality to assume the responsibility for the administration of grants and completion of projects. Most accrediting agencies require that a program have a master plan of evaluation and even if it is not required, a master plan helps to identify the components that need to be evaluated, who will do the data collection and when, what methods of analysis of the data will be employed, and the plans for responding to the findings for quality improvement (Accreditation Commission for Education in Nursing [ACEN], 2014 and Commission on Collegiate Nursing Education [CCNE], 2014). Having a master plan of evaluation in place greatly facilitates these processes when submitting accreditation self-study reports, program approval reports, or proposals for funding.

With today's emphasis on outcomes, the evaluation process is essential to measuring success, establishing benchmarks, and continually improving the quality of the program. A master plan of evaluation is used to provide data for faculty's decision making as part of an internal review and for meeting external review standards. It is important to have a master plan that continually monitors the program so that adjustments can be made as the program is implemented and it is part of the total quality management process. It is equally important to measure outcomes in terms of meeting the vision, strategic plans, goals, and objectives of the program, and certain benchmarks that help to pinpoint the quality of the program.

Components of a Master Plan of Evaluation

The master plan must specify what is being evaluated and an organizing framework is useful so that as nearly as possible, no crucial variable is omitted for review. Additionally, it is important to identify the persons who will:

1. Collect the data
2. Analyze the findings
3. Prepare reports
4. Disseminate the reports to key people
5. Set the timelines for collection, analysis, and reporting of the data

Finally, there must be a feedback loop in place for recommendations and decision making. Reports from the evaluation should include:

1. Identification of existing and potential problems
2. Previously unidentified or new needs
3. Successes and why
4. Recommendations for improvement, discontinuance of a program, or proposals for new programs
5. Action plans for changes that include the people responsible and timelines
6. A summary of the evaluation and judgment on the program's success or progress toward meeting its goals

Table 16.1 provides guidelines for developing a master plan of evaluation and the major components to be assessed for evaluation. In addition to including the curriculum and its components, it incorporates external and internal frame factors (Johnson, 1977), the infrastructure, the core curriculum, students, alumni, and human resources. As indicated in the table, these are only the major components. It is possible that as educational evaluation evolves, other components will emerge. The elements within each component are not listed. Each institution must determine which elements fall under the major components.

ROLES OF ADMINISTRATORS AND FACULTY IN PROGRAM EVALUATION

Administrators in academe provide the vision and leadership for the educational program. However, it is imperative for the administration and the major stakeholders of the institution to be in agreement about its mission, vision, purpose, and goals. Stakeholders include the governing board, the chief executive officer, the administrators of the infrastructure and the academic programs, the faculty, students, and consumers served by the institution. These stakeholders make up the "personality" and body of the institution that marks it as unique in its contributions to society and they must be in agreement with the vision and purpose of the institution to maintain a strong educational program. Administration periodically reviews the mission and vision of the institution to match them to current needs and provides the leadership for revising them according to need. Additionally, administration monitors assessment and evaluation activities to ensure program quality and provides adequate resources in a timely manner for accreditation and program evaluation activities.

All faculty members participate in the evaluation of the curriculum and the program through their input into specific areas and needs for assessment, the collection of data, data analyses, and the formulation of recommendations for decision making regarding the program. In many schools of nursing there are evaluation committees who lead the process or, in other cases, curriculum committees may be charged with the evaluation of the curriculum and program. As part of the parent institution, nursing representatives provide input into university/college-wide evaluation activities. As a professional program, nursing faculty has valuable input

TABLE 16.1 MAJOR COMPONENTS AND GUIDELINES FOR DEVELOPING A MASTER PLAN OF EVALUATION

COMPONENT	ACTION PLANS						FOLLOW-UP PLANS	
	RESPONSIBLE PARTY	WHEN & HOW OFTEN	INSTRUMENTS & TOOLS FOR DATA COLLECTION	DATA FINDINGS & ANALYSIS	CRITERIA, OUTCOMES OR BENCHMARKS	REPORTS & RECOMMENDATIONS	MAINTAIN & MONITOR OR IMPROVE	BY WHOM, HOW, & WHEN
External Frame Factors								
Internal Frame Factors								
Infrastructure Systems: Buildings								
Facilities								
Support Systems								
Student Services								
Financial								
Administration								
Technology								
Library								
Baccalaureate Curriculum: Prerequisites								
General Education								
Electives								
Nursing Major								

(continued)

TABLE 16.1 MAJOR COMPONENTS AND GUIDELINES FOR DEVELOPING A MASTER PLAN OF EVALUATION (*continued*)

COMPONENT	ACTION PLANS						FOLLOW-UP PLANS	
	RESPONSIBLE PARTY	WHEN & HOW OFTEN	INSTRUMENTS & TOOLS FOR DATA COLLECTION	DATA FINDINGS & ANALYSIS	CRITERIA, OUTCOMES OR BENCHMARKS	REPORTS & RECOMMENDATIONS	MAINTAIN & MONITOR OR IMPROVE	BY WHOM, HOW, & WHEN
Graduate Curriculum: Prerequisites								
Cognates								
Core Nursing Courses								
Specialty/ Functional Courses								
Curriculum Components: Mission/Vision								
Organizational Framework								
Philosophy								
Overall Purpose/Goal								
End-of-Program (Student Learning Outcomes) and Level Objectives								

Implementation Plan	
Course Objectives & Content	
Learning Activities	
Teaching Effectiveness	
Graduate Curriculum: Prerequisites	
Cognates	
Core Nursing Courses	
Specialty/ Functional Courses	
Curriculum Components: Mission/vision	
Organizational Framework	
Philosophy	

(continued)

TABLE 16.1 MAJOR COMPONENTS AND GUIDELINES FOR DEVELOPING A MASTER PLAN OF EVALUATION (*continued*)

COMPONENT	ACTION PLANS						FOLLOW-UP PLANS	
	RESPONSIBLE PARTY	WHEN & HOW OFTEN	INSTRUMENTS & TOOLS FOR DATA COLLECTION	DATA FINDINGS & ANALYSIS	CRITERIA, OUTCOMES OR BENCHMARKS	REPORTS & RECOMMENDATIONS	MAINTAIN & MONITOR OR IMPROVE	BY WHOM, HOW, & WHEN
Overall Purpose/Goal								
End of Program (Student Learning Outcomes) and Level Objectives								
Implementation Plan								
Course Objectives & Content								
Learning Activities								
Teaching Effectiveness								

into evaluation processes owing to the necessity for meeting professional accreditation and organizations' standards and criteria.

SUMMARY

Chapter 16 reviewed classic definitions, concepts, and models of evaluation with definitions of commonly used terms. The rationale for strategic planning and a master plan of evaluation was presented. Types of tools and instruments for data collection for evaluation of educational programs and the roles of administrators and faculty were reviewed.

DISCUSSION QUESTIONS

1. Explain the differences between conceptual models of evaluation and the use of benchmarks. Give examples of their application to the evaluation of an educational program.
2. To what extent do you believe faculty should be involved in a strategic planning process? Explain why.
3. Describe how a master plan of evaluation contributes to the external review of a nursing program.

LEARNING ACTIVITIES

STUDENT LEARNING ACTIVITY

Utilizing Table 16.1, develop a master plan of evaluation for the case study of a fictional school of nursing outreach program found in Chapters 6, 7, and 9.

NURSE EDUCATOR/FACULTY DEVELOPMENT ACTIVITY

Utilizing Table 16.1, find your school of nursing's evaluation plan and assess it for any missing components or action plans.

REFERENCES

Accreditation Commission for Education in Nursing. (2014). *Accreditation manual.* Retrieved from http://www.acenursing.org/accreditation-manual

American College Testing. (2014). *Homepage. ACT Assessment.* Retrieved from http://www.act.org/products/k-12-act-test

American Nurses Association. (2004). *Nursing: Scope and standards of practice.* Washington, DC: Author.

Bers, T. (2011). Program review and institutional effectiveness. *New Directions for Community Colleges, 152,* 63–73.

Centers for Disease Control and Prevention. (2014). *A framework for program evaluation.* Retrieved from http://www.cdc.gov/EVAL/framework/index.htm

The College Board. (2014). *SAT program. Higher education.* Retrieved from The College Board http://professionals.collegeboard.com/higher-ed

Commission on Collegiate Nursing Education. (2014). *About CCNE.* Retrieved from http://www.aacn.nche.edu/accreditation/AboutCCNE.htm

DeSilets, L. (2010). Another look at evaluation models. *Journal of Continuing Education in Nursing, 41*(1), 12–13.

Donabedian, A. (1996). Quality management in nursing and health care. In J. A. Schemele (Ed.), *Models of Quality Assurance* (pp. 88–103). Albany, NY: Delmar Publishers.

Donaldson, S. I., Christie, C. A., & Mark, M. M. (2009). *What counts as credible evidence in applied research and evaluation practice?* Los Angeles, CA: Sage.

Graduate Record Examination. (2014). GRE *website.* Retrieved from http://www.ets.org/gre

Harmon, R. B., Fontaine, D., Plews-Ogan, M., & Williams, A. (2012). Achieving transformational change: Using appreciative inquiry for strategic planning in a school of nursing. *Professional Nursing, 28,* 119–124.

Holden, D. J., & Zimmerman, M. A. (2009). *A practice guide to program evaluation planning.* Los Angeles, CA: Sage.

Horne, E. M., & Sandmann, L. R. (2012). Current trends in systematic program evaluation of online graduate nursing education: An integrative literature review. *Journal of Nursing Education, 51*(10), 570–576.

Johnson, M. (1977). *Intentionality in education.* (Distributed by the Center for Curriculum Research and Services, Albany, NY.). Troy, NY: Walter Snyder, Printer, Inc.

Kalb, K. (2009). The three Cs model: The context, content, and conduct of nursing education. *Nursing Education Perspectives, 30*(3), 176–180.

Kulage, K. M., Ardizzone, L., Enlow, W., Hickey, K., Jeon, C., Kearney, J., … Larson, E. L. (2013). Refocusing research priorities in schools of nursing. *Professional Nursing, 29,* 191–196.

Ludema, J. D., Whitney, D., Mohr, B. J., & Griffin, T. J. (2003). *The appreciative inquiry summit.* San Francisco, CA: Berrett-Koehler Publishers, Inc.

McNeil, R. C. (2011). A program evaluation model: Using Bloom's taxonomy to identify outcome indicators in outcomes-based program evaluations. *Journal of Adult Education, 40*(2), 24–29.

Merriam-Webster's Online Dictionary. (2014). Retrieved from http://www.m-w.com

National League for Nursing Accrediting Commission. (2012). *NLNAC accreditation manual.* Retrieved from www.nlnac.org/manuals/NLNACManual2008.pdf

Newhouse, C. P. (2011). Using IT to assess IT: Towards greater authenticity in summative performance assessment. *Computers & Education, 56,* 388–402.

Praslova, L. (2010). Adaptation of Kirkpatrick's four level models of training criteria to assessment of learning outcomes and program evaluation in higher education. Educational *Assessment and Evaluation, 22,* 215–225.

Pross, E. A. (2010). Promoting excellence in nursing education (PENE): Pross evaluation model. *Nurse Education Today, 30*(6), 567–581.

Schug, V. (2012). Curriculum evaluation. Using national league for nursing accreditation commission standards and criteria. *Nursing Education Perspectives, 33*(5), 302–305.

Scriven, M. (1974). Evaluation perspectives and procedures. In W. J. Popham (Ed.), *Evaluation in education. Current applications.* Berkeley, CA: McCutchan Publishing Corporation.

Scriven, M. (1996). Types of evaluation and types of evaluator. *Evaluation Practice, 17*(2), 151–161.

Spillane, J. P., Pareja, S., Dorner, L., Barnes, C., May, H., Huff, J., & Camburn, E. (2010). Mixing methods in randomized controlled trials (RCTs): Validation, conceptualization, triangulation, and control. *Education, Assessment, Evaluation, Accountability, 22*, 5–28.

Stavropoulou, A., & Kelesi, M. (2012). Concepts and methods of evaluation in nursing education–A methodological challenge. *Health Science Journal, 6*(1), 11–23.

Stuart, G. W., Erkel, E. A., & Shull, L. H. (2010). Allocating resources in a data-driven college of nursing. *Nursing Outlook, 50*(4), 200–206.

Stufflebeam, D. L., Foley, W., Gephart, W., Guba, E., Hammond, R., Merriman, H., & Provus, M. (1971). *Educational evaluation and decision making.* Itasca, IL: Peacock.

Udlis, K. A., & Manusco, J. M. (2012). Doctor of nursing practice programs across the United States: A benchmark of information. Part I: Program characteristics. *Journal of Professional Nursing, 28*(5), 265–273.

Varkey, P., & Bennet, K. (2010). Practical techniques for strategic planning in health care organizations. *Physician Executive, 36*(2), 46–48.

Weiner, W. (2009). Establishing a culture of assessment. *Academe, 95*(4), 28–32.

Planning for Accreditation: Evaluating the Curriculum

Abby Heydman

Arlene Sargent

OBJECTIVES

Upon completion of Chapter 17, readers will be able to:

1. Analyze the various forms of accreditation and typical accreditation processes that are used to indicate a program meets specific standards and criteria
2. Outline a plan for accreditation, developing a timeline, and providing for involvement of faculty, students, and other stakeholders in the self-study and site visit
3. Apply principles of continuous quality improvement in accreditation activities
4. Evaluate current issues in accreditation within higher education, particularly those related to the increasing role of federal agencies in establishing accreditation standards and policies, the impact of technology, and the development of a global market place in higher education

OVERVIEW

Accreditation is a process that educational programs and curricula undergo to receive recognition for meeting standards or criteria set by national, regional, or state organizations. Programs undergo accreditation to demonstrate their quality to consumers (students, alumni, and employers) of their products. Because programs such as nursing prepare students for the practice of a profession involving activities that have a direct impact on public health and safety, there are rigorous standards and more numerous types of accreditation reviews that are common for other academic programs. For this reason, it is important for faculty and program directors to have a broad understanding of accreditation and the significant role they play in evaluating the program and curriculum to meet accreditation standards.

Chapter 16 explored the broader areas of educational program evaluation and presents examples of models used in nursing education. Selecting a model for evaluation can assist faculty members in focusing and organizing their work and in expressing their particular philosophy of education. Use of a particular model also provides a comprehensive framework to guide the work of faculty and staff in the evaluation process. In Chapter 16, readers were introduced to the benefits of developing a master plan for program and curriculum evaluation. The development of a master plan for evaluation indicates that faculty thoughtfully considered key learning outcomes and the importance of determining the extent to which these outcomes were attained. Optimally, the master plan provides data that can be used for both formative and summative evaluation, with evidence being used for continuous improvement of the program.

Chapter 17 explores the world of accreditation and the external requirements that must be satisfied in order for a nursing program to operate successfully in the context of the state or province in which it exists, within its region, within the larger boundaries of the country, and within the special world of a profession. Trends toward globalization of accreditation are explored.

DEFINITION OF TERMS

1. *Institutional accreditation*—provides a comprehensive review of the functioning and effectiveness of the entire college, university, or technical institute. The state mandate or institutional mission provides the lens used to guide the review.
2. *Programmatic accreditation*—focuses on the functioning and effectiveness of a particular program within the larger institution (e.g., nursing, medicine).
3. *Specialized accreditation agencies*—focus on the functioning or effectiveness of a particular kind of program (e.g., nursing, nurse anesthesia) or review a specialized, single-purpose college or postsecondary school.
4. *Regulatory*—a form of approval, recognition, or accreditation required by a federal, state, or provincial government agency.
5. *Voluntary*—a form of accreditation not required by law or regulation. Voluntary accreditation processes are managed by private, voluntary organizations composed of peer member institutions or programs.
6. *National accreditation agency*—any accreditation agency that accredits colleges, universities, or technical institutes within an entire country. These include agencies that accredit faith-related or career-related institutions.
7. *Regional accreditation agency*—One of seven private, voluntary accreditation agencies within six defined regions of the United States, formed for the purpose of peer evaluation and setting of standards for higher education.
8. *State-regulatory agencies*—Agencies with a mandate to recognize or approve colleges, universities, or programs for operation within a state as governed by state statutes.
9. *CQI (Continuous quality improvement)*—The implementation of a system designed to provide for ongoing evaluation, analysis of findings, and implementation of plans for improvement within an organization.

NATIONAL ACCREDITING BODIES

The United States is distinctive in that historically its accreditation efforts have been managed by private, voluntary organizations formed by peer institutions for the purpose of judging quality and setting standards to guide educational practice. Although the federal and state governments play a role, particularly as it relates to eligibility for licensure and state or federal financial aid, the independent accrediting agencies are key figures in quality assurance through accreditation of colleges, universities, and technical schools. In Canada, as is generally true in the international community, institutions are granted the right to operate within their respective province according to statutes established by provincial legislatures and the Ministry of Education (Ontario Ministry of Education, 2010). Since 1987, collegiate nursing programs in Canada that offer the baccalaureate in nursing may also apply for specialized accreditation from the Canadian Association of Schools of Nursing (CASN, 2014a).

Though the structure of accreditation may differ from country to country, universities and nursing education programs are generally required to be accredited or approved by regulatory bodies within the country, state or province in which they operate. Other forms of accreditation, even regional accreditation in the United States, are voluntary, that is, the institution or nursing program may choose to seek accreditation in order to demonstrate that it has a particular commitment to meeting high standards. Some would argue that it is a euphemism to say that regional accreditation and specialized accreditation are voluntary today, since eligibility for student financial aid in the United States is tied to these approvals, but technically, most forms of accreditation, except those that authorize a college or university to operate within a state, remain voluntary in the United States.

Depending on their purposes, accreditation agencies evaluate institutions or specialized units within an institution. Thus colleges or universities have institutional accreditation, and programs, departments, or schools within larger institutions have specialized or programmatic accreditation. Specialized accreditation is common among professional health science programs, as well as among other professions, and there are numerous specialized accrediting agencies. A few specialized accreditation agencies also accredit single-purpose institutions of higher education, such as colleges of chiropractic medicine, acupuncture and oriental medicine, and colleges of nursing, some of which are hospital-based.

Over the years, as the number of students enrolled in postsecondary institutions increased dramatically, and as higher education received increased funding both for direct operations and for student financial aid, accreditation requirements and expectations for accountability increased (Eaton, 2010). As a result, accreditation processes and standards continue to become more demanding and costly to address (Eaton, 2008b).

ROLE OF THE U.S. DEPARTMENT OF EDUCATION

Unlike many other countries, the United States does not have a central ministry of education that controls postsecondary institutions of higher education. States assume a role in the approval and control of colleges and universities within their boundaries and approval processes and regulations vary widely among them. Thus American colleges and universities have operated with a great deal of autonomy and independence as reflected in their diverse missions and organizational structures.

A distinctive feature of American higher education, and one that may be considered both a strength and a weakness, is the diversity in type and kind of institution operating with considerable variation in quality and reputation.

Although the states have primary jurisdiction over U.S. colleges and universities, the federal government, through the U.S. Department of Education (USDE), has begun to play a larger role in higher education in the past decade. One of the USDE's primary roles is to ensure that federal student aid funds, administered under the provisions of Title IV of the Higher Education Act of 1965 as amended, are used to provide access for students enrolling in academic programs and courses of high quality (Eaton, 2012b; USDE, 2009). It does this by reviewing and approving both regional and specialized accrediting agencies. USDE's recognition process for accrediting agencies uses standards that address recruitment and admission practices, fiscal and administrative capacity, facilities, curricula, faculty, student support programs, records of student complaints, and success in student achievement. Only those colleges and universities accredited by a USDE-recognized accrediting agency are eligible to receive federal financial aid for students (Eaton, 2012b). The USDE maintains a list of approved accreditation agencies and maintains a comprehensive website with detailed information on accreditation, as well as a listing of all accredited postsecondary education programs in the United States (USDE, 2014).

Regional and specialized accrediting agencies are periodically reviewed by the USDE and/or a private organization, the Council for Higher Education Accreditation (CHEA). The recognition process for institutional and specialized accrediting agencies is a part of the federal regulatory mandate in the United States (Eaton, 2008a).

Accreditation agencies are not only approved by the USDE and CHEA but their scope of authority is also determined. For example, an accreditation agency may be approved to accredit programs only at the certificate or baccalaureate level, but not at the master's or doctoral level. Approval may also be extended to include accreditation of programs offered through distance learning modalities. Abuses in federal financial aid have led to increasingly stringent oversight of all forms of accreditation that provide access to federal financial aid.

In the United States, there are six regions within defined geographical areas, which are served by seven regional accreditation agencies (New England Association of Schools and Colleges Commission on Institutions of Higher Education, 2014). A region may have separate and autonomous commissions, which accredit institutions offering degree programs at different levels or for technical institutes. For example, the Senior Commission of the Western Association of Schools and Colleges (WASC) accredits colleges and universities offering baccalaureate and higher degrees within California, Hawaii, Guam, and the Pacific Islands, while the WASC Commission for Community and Junior Colleges accredits institutions offering associate degrees in the same region. Refer to Table 17.1, Regional Accrediting Agencies in the United States, for a complete listing of the regional accrediting agencies and a description of the geographic areas they cover.

In recent years, more colleges established campuses across state lines from the original campus and more programs are offered using technology that makes time and location unimportant. For this reason, among others, the regional accreditation agencies have formed the Council of Regional Accrediting Commissions (C-RAC).

C-RAC develops policies on accrediting institutions that cross regional accrediting boundaries, and builds consensus on accreditation policies and best practices on issues such as distance learning (New England Association of Schools and Colleges Commission on Institutions of Higher Education, 2014). In recent years, the USDE has become increasingly active in establishing rules and regulations to be followed by accreditation agencies. At regular intervals, the USDE appoints representatives from the various accrediting bodies to a negotiated rule-making team. Negotiated rule-making is the process for developing recommendations for proposed regulations governing accrediting agencies. The proposed regulations, which reflect a consensus of the team members, are then considered by USDE. Topics considered in negotiated rulemaking include the definitions of the credit hour, a high school diploma, satisfactory academic progress, "gainful employment" and matters such as state authorization for online programs, and issues surrounding institutions' management of federal student aid funds (CHEA, 2013a; Eaton, 2012a; USDE, 2009). USDE regulations resulted in less flexibility for accrediting agencies, including definitive timelines by which institutions must come into compliance with accreditation standards. Colleges and universities are monitored in regard to their financial performance each year and eligibility for financial aid is dependent on evidence of fiscal health. Fears of increasing oversight by the USDE have led to growing concern about the fate of the historical autonomy of higher education in the United States (Eaton, 2012a, 2013).

THE COUNCIL FOR HIGHER EDUCATION ACCREDITATION

The CHEA was formed in 1996 as a private, nonprofit, national organization designed to coordinate accreditation activities in the United States. CHEA accomplishes its purposes by providing formal recognition of regional, national, and specialized higher accreditation bodies. The Council's focus is on academic quality, whereas the USDE'S concern is on quality and accountability as it relates to student financial aid. Accreditation agencies may be recognized (approved) by both the USDE and CHEA or by only one of these organizations depending on the accreditation agency's role and focus (Eaton, 2008a). In all, there are 80 recognized institutional and specialized accrediting organizations operating in the United States (Eaton, 2012b). Sixty accrediting agencies are recognized by CHEA (CHEA, 2013b).

PURPOSES OF ACCREDITATION

The primary purpose of accreditation is to ensure that at least minimum standards of quality are met. Most voluntary accreditation agencies state that they aim to achieve higher than minimum standards as determined by peers in the field. Accreditation provides recognition that the program was evaluated by peers who found it to meet the standards established by the profession. A second purpose of accreditation is to provide recognition for funding and student financial aid, which can significantly aid in student recruitment and retention. A third rationale for accreditation is to ensure consistency in quality across academic programs, thus facilitating transfer of academic credit from one institution to another and the acknowledgment of the comparability of one degree to another in the same field across institutions. Accreditation can also assist employers who seek graduates who are competent nurses as well as fulfilling the eligibility requirements for applicants seeking advanced certification. Accreditation reflects commitment to standards and continuous improvement through reflection and analysis. Accreditation as well as licensure and certification are the means used to regulate the professions. The goal of nursing licensure and accreditation is to assure the public that nurses are providing safe and competent care (Rounds, 2010).

In the United States, where voluntary accreditation is the norm, accreditation is distinguished by emphasis on both self-regulation and peer evaluation. In this environment, accreditation processes tend to be both formative and summative, seeking continuous improvement rather than being oriented only to compliance. Accreditation standards typically require institutions or programs to develop evaluation plans and to write comprehensive self-studies to ensure that a system is in place to ensure CQI. These activities facilitate assessment and reflection on findings. Peer evaluation is a core value in voluntary accreditation where peers work on setting standards, participate in site visits, and serve on review panels, appeal panels, and commissions.

In recent years, there has been some dissatisfaction with traditional accreditation processes and practices. Concern has been raised about whether quality is really assured by the current process of voluntary accreditation in the United States. In 2013, the U.S. House of Representatives Subcommittee on Higher Education and the Workforce proposed exploring reform of traditional accreditation and encouraging innovation in higher education. One factor that precipitated this proposal is the rapid growth of massive open online courses (MOOCs) and other online offerings from noneducational providers. It seems clear that there is significant support for some kind of alternative accreditation process especially for extra-institutional providers of educational offerings (CHEA, 2013a). MOOCs are largely offered by top universities and companies but, in most cases, without credit. Yet the quality of instruction and the rigor of examination rival that of traditional online classes used in many for-credit degree programs (Thrun, 2013). "These classes might easily be leveraged into degree programs if the providers were accredited" (Thrun, 2013, p. 1). The large impact of technology in higher education, specifically online learning, paved the way for significant educational and accreditation reform. Technology greatly impacted accreditation by challenging the brick and mortar approaches that have been utilized for many decades. Accreditation increasingly is being conducted in a disaggregated world and enhanced dialogue is occurring on how best to assess new delivery models and determine success while achieving programmatic and student outcomes (LeBlanc, 2013).

For-profit postsecondary institutions of higher education and institutions offering degrees through distance learning modalities have proliferated and their students have participated heavily in federal financial aid. Of particular concern to government officials and legislators is the high dropout rate and high student loan default rate among students enrolled in these programs or institutions (Marklein, Upton, & Kambhampati, 2013). In response to these concerns, in 2011, the USDE passed a regulation that requires any educational program receiving federal financial aid to seek authorization from the state or states in which it operates. This rule, it was argued, could make it easier for states to identify and regulate colleges operating within their jurisdictions. The rule was contested by colleges and was struck down but it is being appealed by the USDE. The significant amount of attention given to institutions who receive federal financial aid is a result of the billions of dollars the government currently expends on student financial aid and its desire to implement increased quality control.

Increasingly, institutions of higher education are asked to demonstrate to the USDE (through regulations imposed on regional and professional accreditation agencies) that they are tracking trends in key performance indicators such as student graduation rates, graduates' loan default rates, and postgraduation employment (Morgan, 2012). In addition, accreditation agencies are beginning to require that these data be readily accessible to potential students so that they can make informed choices about the institutions to which they apply. As a result of additional requirements from the USDE, accreditation agencies are posting accreditation decisions and sometimes the summative site team report and commission action letters on their websites. Eaton urges colleges to embrace this "public accountability imperative" to increase the transparency and credibility of accreditation outcomes (Eaton, 2012c).

Data on these trends are requested by regulatory agencies such as boards of nursing as well as by accrediting agencies. In 2010, the National Council of State Boards of Nursing's (NCSBN) Board of Directors convened a committee to assess this redundancy and to make recommendations to the NCSBN's board. This resulted in a commitment to a more collaborative engagement with national accreditors recognizing that accreditation, education, and regulation all have the same goal of providing safe and competent nurses to meet the needs of society (Spector & Woods, 2013).

PROS AND CONS OF ACCREDITATION

Faculty will undoubtedly engage in discussions about the pros and cons of accreditation, such discussions being particularly common when in the midst of a self-study or a site visit. In addition to providing eligibility for student financial aid, there are multiple other benefits that accreditation offers to an institution or a program. Accreditation demonstrates to the public the program's quality and effectiveness. It can assist potential students to identify appropriate programs for their goals, assuring students that they have selected a college, university, or program that meets high standards in its operations. In addition, accreditation typically assures students that their coursework will be acceptable for transfer credit to another institution of higher education. This is important for students who find they want to change colleges or universities (for whatever reason) or who want to go on to graduate school.

The biggest benefit to accreditation is the strong emphasis it places on self-evaluation, re-evaluation, and continuous improvement. As noted by Spector and Woods in a recent article, "national nursing accreditation ensures the quality and integrity of nursing education programs and serves the public interest by assessing and identifying programs that engage in effective educational practices" (Spector & Woods, 2013).

Achieving and maintaining accreditation provides recognition that a program's graduates are sufficiently prepared and qualified to compete in an ever-challenging environment.

Critics of accreditation express concern about increasing demands on faculty time required by accreditation activities and the resulting impact on faculty and staff workload as compared to some decades ago when accreditation was in its infancy. It should be remembered, however, that accreditation came about not just because of the public demand for accountability and quality, but because peers felt a responsibility to work collaboratively to establish standards that would guide their practice. Although time intensive, involvement in accreditation provides the opportunity for faculty to become increasingly familiar with the accreditation standards and to review a program in light of these standards.

Perhaps the biggest complaint about accreditation is its cost. Staff and faculty time involved in planning for either institutional or specialized accreditation is significant and costly. Often institutions or programs must postpone major initiatives while they are working on a major accreditation review. This highlights the "opportunity cost" that may be attendant to accreditation. In a time where resources are perceived to be scarce, institutions and programs sometimes feel these resources should be used for more important activities or initiatives. Duplication of effort with overlapping requirements in regional and specialized accreditation is yet another frequent complaint of current accreditation systems (Spector & Woods, 2013). Preparation of faculty for assessment of student learning, educating them about accreditation standards and policies, and involving them in the self-study and site visit present yet more challenges. Some see these as distractions from their primary role in teaching and research. Accreditation is also charged with being inflexible, parochial, failing to take institutional diversity into account, stifling innovation, and being too focused on inputs. Some critics have expressed the viewpoint that accreditation does not ensure quality (Morgan, 2012).

The use of technology in higher education and the overt development of higher education as a market commodity created new issues and criticism surrounding accreditation. As noted earlier in this chapter, technology permits institutions to offer programs outside of their traditional state, provincial, or regional boundaries. More institutions are offering programs through distance learning strategies that provide global access to degree programs. Thus questions arise about which agency has jurisdiction in accreditation of these out-of-region programs. The entry of for-profit colleges and universities into the realm of higher education also brought attention to the vast financial and economic enterprise of higher education. Consider the case of the University of Phoenix (UOP), the largest independent college in the United States. In 2010, UOP enrolled more than 450,000 students, operating campuses in 40 states plus Puerto Rico and Canada (Alberta and British Columbia). A large portion of its students are enrolled in programs that are offered totally online (UOP, 2010). This is just one of the for-profit institutions that has generated concern due to low graduation and high student loan default rates (Marklein et al., 2013).

CONTINUOUS QUALITY IMPROVEMENT

In recent years, concerns about the deficiencies in accreditation and the very episodic nature of accreditation led to consideration of alternative evaluation methods for educational programs. Higher education has begun to adopt concepts and processes of CQI from the corporate world in its evaluation systems. Building a culture in which CQI is a core value enables a college or department to create a system of evaluation, which is inclusive, systematic, and reliable (Suhayda, 2006). CQI calls on institutions or programs to identify customers clearly. Customers include students, alumni, clinical agencies, the profession, and consumers. Establishing key requirements for the satisfaction of these stakeholders is an important step in the CQI process. Typically, evaluation strategies in CQI include evaluating satisfaction of students and other customers, as well as establishing whether key requirements have been met (i.e., benchmarks for graduates' performance and learning outcomes). Cross-functional teams (staff and faculty) work to assess whether systems are optimal to produce best practices and results. A major advantage in the CQI process is that it provides a systematic process for continuous activity in which organizational data are evaluated regularly in order to target results needing improvement. Key performance indicators are established to provide a set of metrics that a program can monitor on a regular basis.

THE GLOBAL ENVIRONMENT

Developments in recent years highlighted the growing competition for the international market of higher education as evidenced by universities offering high demand programs around the world. Increasingly higher education is becoming a "commodity" with value added because of the opportunities presented to those who receive credentials through higher education. Recognizing these developments, a number of regional and specialized accreditation agencies began to accredit institutions or programs offered in various parts of the world. Accreditation often enhances the economic value of the credential received, thus increasing the marketability of an institution's programs.

POLITICAL REALITIES

A key question being asked today is whether all the money being spent on higher education is really worth the investment. Would this funding be better spent on health care, housing, or other pressing social needs? The accountability question is driving the federal appetite to become more directly involved in accreditation in the United States, particularly as it relates to an institution's eligibility to handle student financial aid awards. This debate is likely to become even more intense in the United States given reauthorization of the Higher Education Act of 1965 with the passing of the Higher Education Opportunity Act in 2008 (Eaton, 2008b). This legislation included many new provisions regarding student financial aid, along with new regulations for colleges and universities. As a result of the growing importance of student financial aid, regional and specialized accreditation agencies feel a sense of urgency about demonstrating that voluntary accreditation processes are effective. Growing governmental intrusion is also viewed with some alarm (Eaton, 2008b, 2013). Regional accreditation agencies have been responding to this threat with a number of new initiatives that focus on evidence of quality (Higher Learning Commission, 2010).

ORGANIZATIONAL OVERVIEW OF THE STRUCTURE OF ACCREDITATION

As noted earlier in this chapter, legitimate accrediting agencies in the United States must be recognized by the USDE or CHEA. There are two major types of accreditation bodies, institutional and specialized or programmatic. Institutional accreditation agencies include seven regional associations covering six regions (see Table 17.1). A regional accreditation agency in the United States is a voluntary organization composed of member schools from a defined geographic region of the country. These include the following regional accreditation agencies and the commissions that accredit postsecondary schools and colleges:

- Middle States Association of Colleges and Schools Commission on Higher Education
- New England Association of Schools and Colleges Commission on Institutions of Higher Education Commission on Technical and Career Institutions
- North Central Association of Colleges and Schools Commission on Institutions of Higher Education
- Northwest Association of Schools and Colleges Commission on Colleges
- Southwest Association of Colleges and Schools Commission on Colleges
- Western Association of Schools and Colleges Senior Commission of Colleges and Universities
- Western Association of Schools and Colleges Accrediting Commission for Community and Junior Colleges

TABLE 17.1 SIX REGIONS AND SEVEN REGIONAL ACCREDITING AGENCIES IN THE UNITED STATES

REGIONAL ACCREDITING AGENCY	SCOPE OF RECOGNITION
WASC Senior Commission for Colleges and Universities	Accreditation and pre-accreditation ("Candidate for Accreditation") of senior colleges and universities in California, Hawaii, the U.S. territories of Guam and American Samoa, the Republic of Palau, the Federated States of Micronesia, the Commonwealth of the Northern Mariana Islands and the Republic of the Marshall Islands, including distance education programs
WASC Accrediting Commission for Community and Junior Colleges (ACCJC)	Accreditation and pre-accreditation ("Candidate for Accreditation") of 2-year, associate degree-granting institutions located in California, Hawaii, the U.S. territories of Guam and American Samoa, the Republic of Palau, the Federated States of Micronesia, the Commonwealth of the Northern Mariana Islands, and the Republic of the Marshall Islands, including the accreditation of such programs offered via distance education at these colleges

(*continued*)

TABLE 17.1   SIX REGIONS AND SEVEN REGIONAL ACCREDITING AGENCIES IN THE
UNITED STATES (*continued*)

REGIONAL ACCREDITING AGENCY	SCOPE OF RECOGNITION
Southern Association of Colleges and Schools, Commission on Colleges	Accreditation and pre-accreditation ("Candidate for Accreditation") of degree-granting institutions of higher education in Alabama, Florida, Georgia, Kentucky, Louisiana, Mississippi, North Carolina, South Carolina, Tennessee, Texas, and Virginia, including distance education programs offered at those institutions
Middle States Association of Colleges and Schools	Accreditation and pre-accreditation ("Candidacy status") of institutions of higher education in Delaware, the District of Columbia, Maryland, New Jersey, New York, Pennsylvania, Puerto Rico, and the U.S. Virgin Islands, including distance education programs offered at those institutions
North Central Association of Colleges and Schools, the Higher Learning Commission	Accreditation and pre-accreditation ("Candidate for Accreditation") of degree-granting institutions of higher education in Arizona, Arkansas, Colorado, Illinois, Indiana, Iowa, Kansas, Michigan, Minnesota, Missouri, Nebraska, New Mexico, North Dakota, Ohio, Oklahoma, South Dakota, West Virginia, Wisconsin, and Wyoming, including tribal institutions, and the accreditation of programs offered via distance education within these institutions
Northwest Commission on Colleges and Universities	Accreditation and pre-accreditation ("Candidacy status") of postsecondary degree-granting educational institutions in Alaska, Idaho, Montana, Nevada, Oregon, Utah, and Washington, including the accreditation of programs offered via distance education within these institutions
New England Association of Schools and Colleges	**Commission on Institutions of Higher Education** Accreditation and pre-accreditation ("Candidacy status") of institutions of higher education in Connecticut, Maine, Massachusetts, New Hampshire, Rhode Island, and Vermont that award associate's, bachelor's, master's, and/or doctoral degrees, including the accreditation of programs offered via distance education **Commission on Technical and Career Institutions** Accreditation and pre-accreditation ("Candidate status") of secondary institutions with vocational-technical programs at the 13th and 14th grade level, postsecondary institutions, and institutions of higher education that provide primarily vocational/technical education at the certificate, associate, and baccalaureate degree levels in Connecticut, Maine, Massachusetts, New Hampshire, Rhode Island, and Vermont. Recognition extends to the Board of Trustees of the Association jointly with the Commission for decisions involving pre-accreditation, initial accreditation, and adverse actions

Source: U.S. Department of Education website: Regional and National Institutional Accrediting Agencies.

Regional accreditation agencies offer institutional accreditation following a comprehensive review of the mission and goals, infrastructure, resources, and evidence of educational effectiveness of the institution seeking accreditation. Degree-granting institutions of postsecondary education are usually accredited by a regional accreditation body in the United States. However, some single-purpose professional schools and proprietary and/or technical schools are accredited by various national or specialized agencies that provide institutional accreditation. Nonetheless, regional accreditation is generally held to be the optimal standard required to ensure transferability of academic credit from one postsecondary institution of higher education to another in the United States.

INTERNATIONAL ACCREDITATION

In many countries, a centralized Ministry of Education governs post-secondary education, including quality standards and quality assurance. In Canada, the Constitution Act provides authority to each province to make laws and statutes governing education, including higher education. Each of the provinces typically has its own Minister of Education or a comparable official who is charged with the oversight of universities and degree programs within the province. Institutions may not operate without the approval of the provincial ministry or some other authority such as an agency authorized to accredit independent colleges or universities. An example of this type of agency in Canada is the Campus Alberta Quality Council (CAQC), to which the provincial government delegated accreditation authority. The CAQC reviews all proposals for new degree programs from both public and private institutions to ensure they are of high quality before they are approved. The Council also conducts periodic evaluations of approved degree programs to ensure that quality standards continue to be met (Government of Alberta, 2014).

Accrediting agencies in the United States are also involved in international accreditation. In many cases, this involves U.S. programs that are being offered overseas but in some cases, agencies actually accredit programs from other countries upon request (Eaton, 2008a). Cooperation between and among accreditation agencies is occurring globally as is evident in the Mutual Agreement on Accreditation between the CASN and the Commission on Collegiate Nursing Education (CCNE) in the United States (CCNE, 2009a).

SPECIALIZED ACCREDITING AGENCIES

Accreditation of nursing education programs in the United States began in 1893 with the founding of the American Society of Superintendents of Training Schools of Nurses, whose purpose was to establish universal standards for training nurses (Kalisch & Kalisch, 1995). In 1912, this organization became the National League for Nursing Education and in 1917, it published *Standard of Curricula for Schools of Nursing*. In 1952 the National League for Nursing (NLN) was established and assumed responsibility for accrediting nursing education programs (National

League for Nursing Accrediting Commission [NLN-AC], 2008). From 1952 to 1998, the NLN was the only professional accrediting agency for nursing.

The NLN operated its accreditation functions through four councils that established criteria for programs at various levels (practical, diploma, associate, and baccalaureate and higher degree). Subsequently, the NLN reorganized its accreditation structures, founding the independent NLN-AC (Bellack, O'Neil, & Thomsen, 1999). In 1996, the American Association of Colleges of Nursing announced its intention to establish an accreditation body, the CCNE, which would accredit only baccalaureate and higher degree programs. In 2013, the NLNAC announced that the organization had changed its name to the Accreditation Commission for Education in Nursing (ACEN). Both the ACEN and CCNE are approved by the DOE and CHEA. It is important to note that only those programs whose institutions are not part of a regionally accredited college or university may use ACEN accreditation to establish eligibility for federal student financial aid assistance. ACEN is the only USDE and CHEA recognized accrediting agency to offer accreditation for all six types of nursing programs.

Both ACNE and CCNE have established accreditation criteria that programs must meet in order to become accredited. These criteria are reviewed and revised on a regular basis by the respective constituencies. Both accrediting bodies operate through a peer review system whereby accreditation site visitors from comparable educational institutions serve as the on-site evaluators. In addition to peer educators, CCNE also includes a practicing nurse whose experience is congruent with the program as part of the evaluation team. The site visitors provide a written report, upon completion of the site visit, to the Board of Review of the respective accrediting agency. In recent years, both nursing accrediting agencies developed criteria for the clinical doctorate, as well as for programs at other levels. However, only the ACNE accredits practical, diploma, and associate degree nursing programs. Table 17.2 lists the accreditation agencies for nursing in the United States and Canada.

There are a few additional specialized nursing accreditation agencies for advanced practice nursing programs in the United States. These include the Council on Accreditation of Nurse Anesthesia Educational Programs and the Accreditation Commission for Midwifery Education. Additional information on these agencies is provided in Table 17.3. Information on eligibility, standards, and policies for accreditation for these agencies are available on the web. New programs in Nurse Midwifery and Nurse Anesthesia require a pre-approval process prior to enrolling students.

In 2006, the Alliance of Advanced Practice Registered Nurse (APRN) Credentialing was established because of concerns that the accreditation of multiple specialties was costly and duplicative for programs. The Alliance, composed of numerous advanced nursing specialties, works toward common processes, common data sets, and commonly accepted standards and norms in order to reduce duplication of efforts. Because of the rapid expansion of some advanced practice nursing programs, there has been growing concern about the quality of advanced nursing education. Culminating in 2009, a new consensus model for the regulation,

TABLE 17.2	NATIONAL NURSING ACCREDITATION AGENCIES IN THE UNITED STATES AND CANADA

AGENCY NAME	SCOPE OF ACCREDITATION	YEAR ACCREDITATION OF SCHOOLS INITIATED	RECOGNIZED BY DEPARTMENT OF EDUCATION AND/OR CHEA
Accrediting Commission for Education in Nursing (ACEN) Sharon J. Tanner Executive Director 3343 Peachtree Road NE Suite 850 Atlanta, Georgia 30326 Tel. (404) 975-5000 Fax (404) 975-5020 E-mail address: sjtanner@acenursing.org Web address: www .acennursing.org	Accreditation of nursing education programs and schools, both postsecondary and higher degree, which offer a certificate, diploma, or a recognized professional degree including clinical doctorate, masters, baccalaureate, associate, diploma, and practical nursing programs in the United States and its territories, including those offered via distance education. **Title IV Note:** Practical, diploma, associate, baccalaureate, and higher degree nursing education programs that are not located in a regionally accredited institutions may use accreditation by this agency to establish eligibility to participate in Title IV programs.	1998*	Recognized by DOE & CHEA
CCNE Jennifer L. Butlin Director One Dupont Circle NW Suite 530 Washington, DC 20036-1120 Tel. (202) 887-6791 Fax (202) 887-8476 E-mail address: jbutlin@ aacn.nche.edu Web address: www .aacn.nche.edu/ accreditation/index. htm	Accreditation of nursing education programs in the United States, at the baccalaureate and graduate degree levels, including programs offering distance education. **Title IV Note:** Accreditation by this agency does not enable the entities it accredits to establish eligibility to participate in Title IV programs	2000	Recognized by DOE & CHEA

(continued)

TABLE 17.2	NATIONAL NURSING ACCREDITATION AGENCIES IN THE UNITED STATES AND CANADA (*continued*)

AGENCY NAME	SCOPE OF ACCREDITATION	YEAR ACCREDITATION OF SCHOOLS INITIATED	RECOGNIZED BY DEPARTMENT OF EDUCATION AND/OR CHEA
Canadian Association of Schools of Nursing (CASN) Lise Talbot Director of Accreditation 99 Fifth Avenue Suite 15 Ottawa, ON K1S 5K4 Tel: (613) 235-3150 Fax: (613) 235-4476 Tel:(613) 235-3150 Ext. 24 E-mail address: ltalbot@casn.ca	Accreditation of undergraduate nursing programs. CASN accreditation is a combination of institutional and specialized accreditation in which educational units and nursing education programs are assessed against predetermined standards.	1987	Not applicable

* The NLN originally engaged in accreditation in 1952. The independent NLNAC was established in 1998, and in 2012 retitled Accrediting Commission for Nursing Education.

TABLE 17.3	SPECIALIZED NURSING ACCREDITATION AGENCIES IN THE UNITED STATES

AGENCY NAME	SCOPE OF RECOGNITION	YEAR ESTABLISHED/ RECOGNITION STATUS
Council on Accreditation of Nurse Anesthesia Educational Programs (AANA) Francis Gerbasi Director of Accreditation and Education 222 South Prospect, Suite 304 Park Ridge, Illinois 60068-4010 Tel. (847) 692-7050, Fax (847) 692-7137 E-mail address: fgerbasi@aana.com Web address: www.aana.com	The accreditation of institutions and programs of nurse anesthesia within the United States at the post master's certificate, master's, or doctoral degree levels, including programs offering distance education.**Title IV Note:** Only hospital-based nurse anesthesia programs and freestanding nurse anesthesia institutions may use accreditation by this agency to establish eligibility to participate in Title IV programs.	1952 Recognized by DOE & CHEA
Accreditation Commission for Midwifery Education (ACNM) Heather L. Maurer Executive Director 8403 Colesville Road, Suite 1550 Silver Spring, Maryland 20910 Tel. (240) 485-1803 Fax (240) 485-1818 E-mail address: hmaurer@acnm.org Web address: www.acnm.org	The accreditation and pre-accreditation of basic certificate, basic graduate nurse-midwifery, direct entry midwifery, and pre-certification nurse-midwifery education programs, including those programs that offer distance education. **Title IV Note:** Only freestanding institutions of midwifery education may use accreditation by this agency to establish eligibility to participate in Title IV programs.	1982 Recognized by DOE

licensure, accreditation, certification, and education of advanced practice registered nurses was published. The consensus model was completed through the work of the Advanced Practice Registered Nurse Consensus Work Group and the National Council of State Boards of Nursing APRN Advisory Committee. The consensus model for APRN regulation requires APRNs to be educated, certified, and licensed to practice in one of four APRN roles (Kleinpell & Hudspeth, 2013).

ACCREDITATION OF SCHOOLS OF NURSING IN CANADA

Specialized accreditation for nursing in Canada is under the auspices of the CASN. The CASN Board on Accreditation is authorized to review and approve policies. It makes decisions on candidacy and accreditation reviews within established policies and procedures. CASN accreditation is conducted according to the guiding principles of the Association of Accrediting Agencies of Canada (AAAC) of which it is a founding member. CASN accreditation policies were last revised and approved by the Board of Directors in 2007 and were reviewed with minor editing in 2010. The policies are available online (CASN, 2014b).

THE ACCREDITATION PROCESS

The accreditation process typically involves five major elements. These include an institutional self-study, peer review, site visit, action by the accrediting association, and periodic monitoring and oversight (Eaton, 2012b). The self-study is a self-analysis of performance completed by the school based on the standards of the accrediting association. Peer review occurs because of the broad involvement of the various stakeholders in the educational environment: faculty, administrators, key partners, and the public. Site visits are typically conducted to verify the information provided in the self-study and to provide additional clarification to the accrediting agency. The action of the accrediting agency occurs after the submission of the self-study and the site visit with consideration of the entire body of evidence by the review panel for the accrediting agency. Programs or schools are normally reviewed in a cycle of 5 to 10 years, with monitoring and oversight occurring through the submission of annual reports by the schools and substantive change reports to the agency when major change occurs.

CURRICULUM PLANNING AND ACCREDITATION

Curriculum planning should take accreditation requirements and statements of essential competencies into account from the onset (American Association of Colleges of Nursing [AACN], 2008; AACN, 2011; ACEN, 2014; CCNE, 2009b; CCNE, 2012). A basic understanding of accreditation requirements enables faculty to develop a program that is in compliance with key requirements established by accreditation agencies. Although such agencies generally attempt to avoid being overly prescriptive, there may be specific criteria or standards that must be met by a program to be approved. Accreditation standards for professional programs, for example, will often outline a minimum set of academic and clinical requirements that must be included in the program. Thus, the minimum number of credits for the entire professional component of the program may be prescribed, and even the minimum number of credits or hours of clinical practice within a specialized clinical area may be indicated. These requirements were established by the accreditation agency or regulatory board based on broad input from the profession as well as other constituents including public consumers. Among the many considerations in developing a new or revised curriculum are the standards and criteria established by those agencies that accredit the college or university as well as those required by nursing accrediting bodies (CCNE, 2009b; ACEN, 2013).

The development of the organizing curriculum framework warrants consideration of accreditation standards. Daggett, Butts, and Smith (2002) describe the development of an updated organizing framework by one faculty in its long-term preparation for accreditation. Seager and Anema (2003) and Heinrich, Karner, Gaglione, and Lambert (2002) describe the benefits of using a matrix or audit process to ensure curriculum integrity in preparation for accreditation and as a part of continuous improvement efforts.

PLANNING FOR ACCREDITATION

Developing an Evaluation Plan

The previous chapters provided guidance on the development of a school or program evaluation plan. It is a good idea to formulate this plan early on in order to begin collecting baseline data when students first begin a nursing program. Thompson and Bartels (1999) review the literature on assessment and describe one school's response to the development of a systematic plan for outcomes assessment. Similarly, Davenport and co-authors offer a step-by-step process for curriculum review to aid in preparation for accreditation (Davenport, Spath, & Bauvelt, 2009). It is also important that this plan focus on learning outcomes and not just program outputs. Ewell (2001) describes this shift in emphasis to learning outcomes in a CHEA publication on accreditation and student learning outcomes. Ingersoll and Sauter (1998) describe how accreditation criteria can be integrated effectively into the evaluation plan. Accreditation standards, criteria, procedures, and policies are readily available from the accrediting associations and their websites.

Theoretical Framework for Evaluation

Several evaluation theories are available to provide a framework for the evaluation plan. The use of a theoretical approach helps provide an organizing lens for identification and analysis of data. Refer to theories described in the previous chapter for guidance in this area.

Developing a Timeline

Accreditation is like any major project. The scope and size of the work can be overwhelming. A way to deal with this effectively is to break this task up into manageable bits that can be delegated and timed over a lengthy preparation period.

Often the accrediting agency will provide some useful direction about possible key dates in a planning timeline. These are just general guides however and must be modified based on the particular situation for each program or school. Preparation time may need to be extended if it must include faculty development for the director and/or faculty who do not have prior experience with the accreditation process.

ROLE OF ADMINISTRATORS, FACULTY, STUDENTS, AND CONSUMERS

Everyone has a role in the accreditation process. Administrators provide leadership and direction, supporting the efforts of the taskforce or faculty committee assigned to conduct the self-study. Faculty aid the work of the team by becoming familiar with the accreditation standards, providing timely information needed for the self-study, providing critical feedback on the draft of the report, and preparing to participate in the site visit. Students participate by learning about accreditation, cooperating with the site visitors during visits to classes and clinical sites, and by participating in school committees engaged in CQI. Other stakeholders include clinical partners and consumers who participate by responding to evaluation surveys and serving on advisory committees. One of the major recommendations of a national taskforce on accreditation of health professions (and a key principle in CQI) is that programs should be required to establish effective linkages with their stakeholders, including the public, students, and professional organizations reference. When developing the evaluation plan, faculty should give thoughtful consideration to how these linkages can be effectively established. As the focus of accreditation shifted to the evaluation of evidence of achievement of program outcomes rather than inputs, linkages with alumni and employers became increasingly important, as these groups are often a key source for evaluation evidence.

PREPARING THE ACCREDITATION REPORT

Assignments should be given to teams or individuals to prepare drafts of the various sections of the self-study report. It is expected that faculty be deeply engaged in preparation of the self-study, thus it is not advisable to hire a consultant to take on this work (Tanner, 2011). Funds spent on a consultant would be better used to hire additional part-time faculty to provide release time for regular faculty to engage in developing the self-study report if needed. The drafts should be widely circulated for discussion among faculty. An open forum for faculty, students, and other stakeholders may be offered to provide maximum opportunity for constructive criticism and shaping of final recommendations. This process provides the opportunity for faculty members to refocus on the accreditation criteria and analyze how their respective courses reflect the accreditation criteria and fit into the overall curriculum plan. One person should do the final writing of the report in order to provide a coherent and consistent voice to the document. It is also recommended that someone be asked to do a final editing of the report before printing. The report should be candid and accurate. You do not want the site visitors to find that the report glossed over major issues or controversies. The self-study document is the primary document used by the site visit team, the review panels, and the Board of Commissioners and must accurately present evidence that clearly indicates how the standards are met.

PREPARING FOR THE SITE VISIT

The purpose of the site visit is to provide an opportunity for external reviewers (site visitors) to verify the information provided in the self-study and to provide supplemental information to aid the review panel in making the accreditation decision. Thus, planning for the site visit is a key part of the accreditation process. Faculty, students, and staff will need to be oriented to the site visit process and procedures. Faculty and academic administrators are the primary sources of judgment about what constitutes quality education and how their programs meet accreditation standards, and they are critical participants in the planning process (Eaton, 2012b).

Approximately 2 to 3 months before the site visit, planning begins to shift to the site visit phase of accreditation. The designated chair of the institution's accreditation process should follow the guidelines of the accreditation agency in making hotel accommodations for site visitors. This information may be available on the agency's website.

Faculty and support staff members who have not been involved in the self-study process should be oriented to the accreditation process and procedures prior to the site visit. This process provides an opportunity to review the organizing framework of the curriculum and key policies (e.g., grievance procedures) with both students and faculty. It is also advisable to make an appointment with administrators such as the president, academic vice president, and dean of the division, if nursing is a part of a larger academic unit, to familiarize them with the date and purpose of the visit, providing a context for their involvement and likely interviews by the site visitors. It is very important to provide significant advanced notice of the site visit to these individuals to ensure that they will be available at some point during the visit if requested by the site visitors.

Some programs find that arranging a mock site visit a month or so before the actual site visit is a valuable exercise if the majority of faculty have never experienced an accreditation visit previously. A mock site visit can be arranged by having one or two peers who have experience in accreditation visit the institution to conduct interviews and to make class and clinical visits just like the official site visitors will do. A mock visit is like a dress rehearsal and can be a learning experience for less seasoned faculty as well as for students. Often this experience motivates faculty to read the self-study with more care than they might otherwise exercise.

It is highly recommended that accommodations be provided that are not too distant from the campus in order to save travel time. Depending on the size of the team, it is often feasible that the chair of the team be provided with a larger hotel room or suite to accommodate team conferences and writing of the summative report. A meeting space at the hotel is important as the team will often spend long evening hours discussing the materials and interviews scheduled for each day and for writing the report.

An exhibit room on campus should provide displays of evidence and supplemental materials that the site visitors can use to verify information presented in the Self-Study report. It is helpful to provide a matrix of the display materials according to the standards and criteria so that the visitors can quickly find materials. Typically, the materials in the exhibit room are those materials that are too large or too numerous to be included in the self-study report and may not be available on the college or university website. These may include the faculty handbook, samples of examinations or of student work with the student's identity removed for confidentiality purposes, institutional data such as fact books, institutional and departmental strategic plans, recruitment materials, departmental newsletters, university publications, and so on. Careful attention to the selection and organization of materials can be important in showcasing program strengths and creating a favorable impression (McDaniel, 2010). The exhibit room should provide a computer and printer for the site visitors' use on campus since much of the supporting information can be obtained online through the college or university website. The availability of a conference table in the exhibit room for meetings of the team is also recommended.

Site visitors themselves usually make travel arrangements. Institutions and programs are discouraged from entertaining or providing gifts to site visitors other than some small token such as items with the institution's logo (e.g., a mug or portfolio). Sometimes even this type of courtesy is prohibited and site visitors may even be required by the agency to pay for their own meals in order to ensure that there is no perception of conflict of interest. It is important to remember that site visitors do not make the accreditation decision themselves. It is the site visitors' responsibility to prepare a report that presents an objective assessment of the accuracy of the self-study information as well as any additional information obtained during the visit that may be beneficial to the review panel and Board of Commissioners in making a decision regarding accreditation. Programs are usually provided an opportunity to respond to the site visitors report and to provide any additional documentation demonstrating additional progress made toward ongoing quality improvement. Typically, the site visitors describe findings and may note strengths or weaknesses in the program, but the review panel of the accrediting body will be the actual decision maker. For this reason, site visitors may recommend that supplemental materials be sent to the review panel if they find information that has not been included in the self-study but that may be important to demonstrating that an institution or program is meeting accreditation standards.

Typically, the board or designated review panel of the accrediting agency or regulatory body meets at regular intervals to review the entire body of evidence provided by the institution and the site visitors. A few members of the review panel may be assigned as primary readers and reviewers of the materials. Following a summation of evidence, the review panel will make its decision. Review panels usually only meet a few times a year so programs may not learn about the final outcomes of their accreditation report and site visit until several months after the team left campus. Normally, programs will be given some indication by the site visitors on whether there are any major deficiencies or recommendations to address. It is often advantageous to begin work on these items shortly after the visit because these items are very salient to faculty who are motivated to respond to the recommendations. It should be remembered, however, that the review panel makes the final recommendations and they may not come to the exact same conclusions as the site visitors.

Once the accreditation commission reviews the program, a formal decision will be received from the accrediting agency. This may, in some cases, include a set of recommendations. A copy of this report is usually sent to the president or chancellor of the institution as well as to the dean or director of the school. Follow-up activities may include a progress report after a defined period of time if deficiencies have been noted or if institutional capacity to sustain its present positive state is not clearly demonstrated.

Once initial accreditation is achieved, faculty and administration benefit from viewing accreditation as an ongoing process. Faculty has the responsibility to evaluate the curriculum in light of the accreditation standards on a regular basis. Administration and faculty share the responsibility of evaluating data related to student outcomes as well as other survey data that reflect the achievement of program goals and adherence to accreditation standards. Documentation of evaluation activities, including decisions made to improve program quality, is essential. Minutes of committee and departmental meetings should reflect the fact that data on program outcomes have been analyzed regularly and that an action plan for improvement has been implemented.

SUMMARY

Preparation for accreditation is a core activity for the current generation of nursing faculty. An effective way to build the collective expertise of faculty in accreditation is to plan for orientation and faculty development on this topic on a regular basis. Engagement in regular activities that demonstrates the principles of CQI are recommended to ensure faculty and student appreciation and cooperation in accreditation activities. Development of an evaluation plan, which uses selected tools such as a curriculum matrix or audit, is identified as a best practice in preparation for accreditation. Student, alumni, and employer surveys to assess stakeholder key requirements and satisfaction are other elements that should be used regularly rather than episodically to enhance program improvement. Data on program outcomes such as comprehensive exams, licensure results, analyses of capstone projects, and employer evaluations are a few examples of evidence of educational effectiveness that should be gathered and analyzed over time. Development of an accreditation timeline with definitive deadlines is strongly recommended as a tool to manage the accreditation process.

DISCUSSION QUESTIONS

1. What are ways in which students and faculty can be motivated to participate actively in preparation for accreditation?
2. What strategies can be used to begin to imbed a culture of CQI within a school of nursing?
3. What data would provide credible evidence that a nursing program is being successful in achieving its mission and stated learning outcomes?

LEARNING ACTIVITIES

STUDENT LEARNING ACTIVITIES

1. In a small group, explore the implications of accreditation for you as a student. What difference would it make if your nursing school does not have accreditation?
2. Go to a website for specialized nursing accreditation and review the standards for accreditation. Describe how these standards focus on achievement of learning outcomes and educational effectiveness.
3. Pick one standard and write a draft report on how your program meets that standard. Indicate what information you would have to collect to provide evidence that your program meets that standard.

NURSE EDUCATOR/FACULTY DEVELOPMENT ACTIVITIES

1. Take the evaluation plan for your nursing program or school and develop a timeline for the next accreditation visit.
2. Develop an orientation program for new faculty to accreditation and the accreditation process.
3. Describe the two issues and challenges facing accreditation in the rapidly changing environment of higher education today.
4. Describe three strategies faculty can engage in each semester/term to verify continued compliance with accreditation criteria.

REFERENCES

Accrediting Commission for Nursing Education. (2014). *ACEN accreditation manual.* Retrieved from http://acenursing.org/accreditation-manual/

Advanced Practice Registered Nurse Joint Dialogue Group. (2008). *Consensus model for APRN regulation: Licensure, accreditation, certification & education.* Retrieved from http://www.aacn.nche.edu/Education/pdf/APRNReport.pdf

American Association of Colleges of Nursing. (2008). *The essentials of baccalaureate education for professional nursing practice.* Washington, DC: Author.

American Association of Colleges of Nursing. (2011). *The essentials of master's education in nursing.* Washington, DC: Author.

Bellack, J., O'Neil, E., & Thomsen, C. (1999). Responses of baccalaureate and graduate programs to the emergence of choice in nursing accreditation. *Journal of Nursing Education, 38*(2), 53–61.

Canadian Association of Schools of Nursing. (2014a). *Accredited nursing education programs.* Retrieved from https://www.casn.ca/vm/newvisual/attachments/856/Media/AccreditedCanadianNursingEducationPrograms.pdf

Canadian Association of Schools of Nursing. (2014b). *CASN Mission. Accreditation: Recognition of Excellence.* Retrieved from http://www.casn.ca/CASN/ACEST Mission: Canadian Association of Schools of Nursing.

Commission on Collegiate Nursing Education. (2009a). Mutual recognition agreement on accreditation between the Canadian Association of Schools of Nursing (CASN/ACESI) and the Commission on Collegiate Nursing Education 2009–2012. Washington, DC. Retrieved from https://www.aacn.nche.edu/ccne.../MutualRecognition.pdf

Commission on Collegiate Nursing Education. (2009b). *Standards for accreditation of baccalaureate and graduate nursing education programs.* Washington, DC. Retrieved from http://aacn/nche.edu/accreditation

Commission on Collegiate Nursing Education. (2012). *Procedures for accreditation of baccalaureate and graduate degree nursing programs* (amended April 28, 2012). Washington, DCRetrieved from http://www.aacn.nche.edu/ccne-accreditation/Procedures.pdf

Council for Higher Education Accreditation. (2013a). *Federal update. U.S. House of representatives holds hearing on Accreditation 35: June 13, 2013.* Retrieved from http://www.chea.org/Government/FedUpdate/CHEA_FU35.html

Council for Higher Education Accreditation. (2013b). *Recognized accrediting organizations* (September 2013). Retrieved from http://www.chea.org/pdf/CHEA_USDE_AllAccred.pdf

Daggett, L. M., Butts, J. B., & Smith K. K. (2002). The development of an organizing framework to implement AACN guidelines for nursing education. *Journal of Nursing Education, 41*(1), 34–37.

Davenport, N. C., Spath, M. L., & Bauvelt, M. J. (2009). A step by step approach to curriculum review. *Nursing Education, 34*(4), 181–185.

Eaton, J. S. (2008a). *Accreditation and recognition in the U.S. council for higher education accreditation.* Retrieved from http://www.chea.orga

Eaton, J. S. (2008b). The higher education opportunity act of 2008: What does it mean and what does it do? *Inside Higher Education CHEA 4, 1.* Washington, DC: Council for Higher Education Accreditation.

Eaton, J. S. (2010). *Accreditation 2.0 Inside Higher Education.* Washington, DC: Council on Higher Education Accreditation.

Eaton, J. S. (2012a). *Accreditation and recognition in the United States.* Washington, DC: Council on Higher Education Accreditation. Retrieved from. http://www/chea/org/pdf/AccredRecogUS_2012.pdf

Eaton, J. S. (2012b). *An overview of U.S. accreditation.* Washington, DC: Council for Higher Education Accreditation. Retrieved from http:/www.chea.org/OverviewofUSAccreditation2012 pdf

Eaton, J. S. (2012c). *The future of accreditation: Planning for higher education* (pp. 8–15). Ann Arbor, MI: Society for College and University Planning.

Eaton, J. S. (2013). The changing role of accreditation: Should it matter to governing boards? *Trusteeship. 6* (21). Retrieved from http://www.chea

Ewell, P. T. (2001). *Accreditation and student learning outcomes: A proposed point of departure.* Washington, DC: Council for Higher Education Accreditation Occasional Paper.

Government of Alberta, Alberta Learning Information Service. (2009). *Education in Alberta, types of institutions.* Retrieved from http://alis.alberta.ca/et/studyinalberta/institutions.html

Government of Alberta. (2014). *Innovation and Advanced Education, Campus Alberta.* Retrieved at http://eae.alberta.ca/post-secondary/campusalberta.aspx

Heinrich, C. R., Karner, K. J., Gaglione, B. H., & Lambert, L. J. (2002). Order out of chaos: The use of a matrix to validate curriculum integrity. *Nurse Educator, 27*(3), 136–140.

Higher Learning Commission. (2010). *HLC pathways construction project: A proposed new model for continued accreditation.* (Draft Version 6, January 31, 2010) Retrieved from http://www.ncahlc.org

Ingersoll, G. L., & Sauter, M. (1998). Integrating accreditation criteria into educational program evaluation. *Nursing and Health Care Perspectives, 19*(5), 224–229.

Kalisch, P. A., & Kalisch, B. J. (1995). *The advance of American nursing.* Philadelphia, PA: J.B. Lippincott.

Kleinpell, R. & Hudspeth, R. S. (2013) Advanced practice nursing scope of practice for hospitals, acute care/critical care, and ambulatory care settings: A primer for clinicians, executives and preceptors *AACN Advanced Critical Care, 24*(1), 23–29.

LeBlanc, P. (2013). *Thinking about Accreditation in a Rapidly Changing World.* WASC Concept Papers: The Changing Ecology of Higher Education and Its Impact on Accreditation. Alameda, CA: Western Association of Schools and Colleges.

Marklein, M., Upton, J., & Kambhampati, S. (2013, July 2). College default rates higher than grad rates. USA Today,

McDaniel, T. R. (2010, March 22). Five tips for surviving accreditation: A tongue-in cheek reflection. Faculty focus. Retrieved from http//:facultyfocus.com/?p=11956

Morgan, J. M. (2012). Regulating for-profit nursing education programs. *Journal of Nursing Regulation, 3*(2), 24–30.

National League for Nursing Accrediting Commission. (2008). *National League for Nursing Accrediting Commission Accreditation Manual.* Atlanta, GA: Author. Retrieved March 6, 2010, from http://www.nlnac.org

National League for Nursing Accreditation Commission. (2009). *Executive director appointed to a second U.S. DOE negotiated rulemaking team.* Retrieved from http://nlnac.org/home.htm

New England Association of Schools and Colleges Commission on Institutions of Higher Education. (2014). *U.S. Regional accreditation: An overview.* Retrieved from http://cihe.neasc.org/about-accreditation/us-regional-accreditation-overview

Ontario Ministry of Education. (2010). *Degree authority in Ontario. Ontario ministry of training, colleges, and universities.* Retrieved from http://www.edu.gov.on.ca/eng/general/postsedc/degreegauth.html

Rounds, L. (2010). Integrating regulation into nursing curricula. *Journal of Nursing Regulation, 1*(3), 4–8.

Seager, S. R., & Anema, M. G. (2003). A process for conducting a curriculum audit. *Nurse Educator 28*(1), 5–6.

Spector, N., & Woods, S. (2013). A collaborative model for approval of prelicensure nursing programs. *Journal of Nursing Regulation, 3*(4), 47–52.

Suhayda, R., & Miller, J. M. (2006). Optimizing evaluation of nursing education programs. *Nurse Educator, 31*(5), 200–206.

Tanner, S. J. (2011). About accreditation. *Nursing Educational Perspectives, 32*(1), 63.

Thompson, C., & Bartels, J. E. (1999). Outcomes assessment: implications for nursing education. *Journal of Professional Nursing, 15*(3), 170–178.

Thrun, S. (2013). *Changing ecology: Towards accreditation for institutions offering courses, not degrees.* WASC Concept Papers, 2nd series, The changing ecology of higher education and its impact on accreditation. Alameda, CA: Western Association of Schools and Colleges.

University of Phoenix. (2010). *Just the facts.* Retrieved from http:/.edu/about_us/media_relations/just-the-facts.html

U.S. Department of Education. (2009). *An overview of the U.S. department of education.* Retrieved from http://www2.ed.gov/print/about/overview/ficys/what.html

U.S. Department of Education. (2014). *An overview of the U.S. department of education.* Retrieved from http://www2.ed.gov/print/about/overview/ficys/what.html

Van Damme, D. (2002). Quality assurance in an international environment: National and international interests and tensions. *International Quality Review: Values, Opportunities, and Issues.* Washington, DC: Council for Higher Education Accreditation. CHEA Occasional Paper, August, 2002. Retrieved from http://ccne.org

Western Association of Schools and Colleges Senior Commission. (2009). *Guidelines for the evaluation of distance education [on-line learning]- C-RAC).* Retrieved from http://www:wascsenior.org

Issues and Trends in Curriculum Development and Evaluation

Sarah B. Keating

OVERVIEW

Section VI reviews current issues and trends in nursing education for their effect on curricula and the priorities derived from them that influence curriculum development and evaluation activities now and in the future. This section of the text addresses specific trends in nursing education related to the growth of technology-driven distance education programs, informatics, and the utilization of clinical simulations and other high technology devices for the acquisition of nursing knowledge and skills. These phenomena had a dramatic effect on the delivery of nursing education and raise issues related to quality, cost-effectiveness, and competitiveness of programs in the marketplace.

Chapter 18 examines informatics and technology and their influence on nursing education. It traces the history of distance education from the early home study programs to today's high technology–based programs delivered from home campuses to distant satellite campuses as well as virtual campuses in cyberspace. The chapter goes on to examine realistic clinical simulation programs that allow students to acquire basic, advanced, and critical thinking nursing skills in a safe environment prior to actual clinical practice. Other high-tech devices and systems such as electronic record systems, smart phones, electronic tablets, and advanced communication systems add to the rapid changes in the delivery of health care and education and the need for students and faculty to keep abreast of the newer innovations.

Chapter 19 reviews the current state of research in nursing education, specifically as it applies to curriculum development and evaluation. The need for research that provides the basis for evidence-based educational practice is reviewed. Possible research questions are posed based on a summary of the scholarly/research-based articles found in the nursing and education literature and presented throughout this text. While qualitative research generates useful information, the numerous qualitative studies relating to nursing education should serve as a foundation for further quantitative, qualitative, and mixed methodology studies that are geographically diverse and reflect various types of programs. Such studies can lead to evidence-based educational practice for the development of relevant nursing programs that center on the learner and program outcomes and meet the needs of the profession and health care system.

Chapter 20 reexamines some of the issues raised in the text and offers possible solutions that could affect the future of nursing education. A look at nursing education in hindsight leads to a forecast of the future including several scenarios for education and their impact on the profession. Members of the nursing profession are asked to discard old prohibitive ways of thinking about nursing education and its mandate to provide knowledgeable, competent, and caring professionals and move into the future with additional innovative and creative nursing programs that continue to educate nurses ready for the challenges of the health care system. A unified nursing curriculum is proposed with ways to embrace the traditional career ladder features of nursing and at the same time, facilitate a nonstop quality education ending in a doctorate that produces nurse researchers, theorists, educators, advanced practice nurses and clinicians, advocates for health care policy change, and leaders. The proposed curriculum is not meant as a template, but rather as a stimulant for discussion among nurse educators and those in practice to bring about needed changes now and in the future. Nursing must continue to move its trajectory for higher education or find itself out of sync with other professionals and the health care system. Section VI begins the discussion for nursing educators and their role in conducting meaningful research, scholarship, translational science, and evidence-based practice in nursing education to meet the challenges and plan for the future.

CHAPTER 18

Effects of Informatics and Technology on Curriculum Development and Evaluation

Sarah B. Keating

OBJECTIVES

Upon completion of Chapter 18, the reader will be able to:

1. Analyze the various types of distance education programs that are utilized in the delivery of nursing education programs
2. Analyze the application of technology and informatics and their effectiveness on the implementation of the nursing curriculum
3. Review the literature related to the efficacy of distance education programs
4. Examine the issues facing nurse educators that relate to the application of informatics and technology in nursing education

OVERVIEW

Chapter 18 discusses the effects of informatics and technology on curriculum development and evaluation. Distance education formats are reviewed including land-based satellite campuses of home institutions, broadcasting by teleconferences and videoconferences, and web-based platforms. Other technological advances such as smart classrooms, patient simulations, electronic medical record systems, and information systems applied to education and health care, are analyzed. A brief review of the research findings on the efficacy of these programs and student satisfaction is presented and issues related to distance education and technology are introduced.

DISTANCE EDUCATION PROGRAMS

Distance education is defined as any learning experience that takes place a distance away from the parent educational institution's home campus. It can be as close as a few blocks away in an urban center to as far away as another nation(s). It implements the curriculum through a planned strategy for the delivery of courses or classes that can include off-site satellite classes managed by the home faculty or credentialed off-site faculty, broadcast of classes through videoconferencing and teleconferencing to off-campus sites, web-based instruction, and faculty-supervised clinical experiences including preceptorships and internships. Distance education offers continuing education programs, degree programs, single academic courses, or a mixture of on-campus and off-campus course offerings.

The following discussion reviews satellite campus programs with land-based facilities and programs that use video- and teleconferencing to broadcast the programs. Distance education formats through cyberspace follow the discussion on video- and teleconferencing.

Needs Assessment and Compatibility With the Components of the Curriculum

When planning for a distance education program, nurse educators must have supporting data from an assessment of the external and internal frame factors that document the need for a program. It should include the projected success of the program based on a business case, cost analysis, assured applicant pool, and a business plan. Once the needs assessment is completed and a time frame is in place, planners review all of the components of the curriculum to ensure congruence with the originating educational program. For details on conducting a needs assessment, budgeting, and the components of the curriculum see Sections III and IV. In addition, an evaluation plan should be developed to ensure the quality of the program and to meet accreditation standards.

External Frame Factors

Utilizing the components of assessment from the internal and external frame factors, a needs assessment reveals the feasibility for mounting a distance education program. If the program plans an off-campus but on-land satellite, the external frame factors include an assessment of the community where the program is to take place with such factors as community location and receptivity to distance education, the population's characteristics and its sophistication in technology, the delivery of education far from the home campus, and the ability to create an academic setting away from the home campus. Additional external frame factors consideration include the political climate and body politic, that is, the openness to off-site educational programs and possible competitive issues from vendors of distance education programs and other nursing education programs that serve the region. The health care system and health needs of the populace have an influence on the program as to how graduates of the program can serve them. It is necessary to learn if there are potential collaborative opportunities to supply the program with students who are staff in the off-site health care agencies and who are interested in furthering their education for career opportunities.

A demonstrated need for a distance education program includes an adequate student body that will continue for at least 5 to 10 years; support from members of the nursing profession in the region that is to be served; national, regional, and state regulations; and accreditation agencies' approvals. Usually, the sponsoring program must notify all accrediting and approval agencies of its plans to offer the distance education program with each of these agencies requiring specific descriptions of the program including the potential student body, faculty, curriculum plan, academic and capital infrastructure support systems, timelines, plans for evaluation, and most importantly, financial feasibility with a business plan.

Internal Frame Factors

Much like the external frame factors, a review of the internal frame factors provides additional information in the planning for a distance education program. Of prime concern is the support of the parent academic institution and its experience with distance education programs. If it has a history of managing these types of programs, it is more likely to be supportive of the nursing program. Even more advantageous is an established distance education program from the parent institution that exists in the proposed delivery site. A check with the mission and purpose, philosophy, and goals of the parent institution and the nursing program is in order to ensure the distance education's program's congruence with those of the parent. The internal economic situation and its influence on distance education programs are critical to the financial feasibility of the program.

Cost Issues

If the recommendations from the needs assessment demonstrate that the distance education program is viable, the school of nursing administration prepares a business case to present to the parent institution. The purpose for a business case is to persuade key administrators and stakeholders that establishing a distance education program meets the mission of the institution, has a substantial potential student body, and adapts the existing accredited program to a satellite format without compromising its quality. The business case describes the program in detail and demonstrates that it is economically feasible. If prior distance education programs demonstrated success in bringing revenues to the program or are, at the least, self-sufficient, it is more likely that new programs will be supported. After presentation to and approval by the administration, the business case is developed into a detailed business plan.

The first and foremost cost issue to address in the business plan is the economic feasibility of the distance education program based upon an analysis of expected start-up costs, administrative costs, required number of faculty and staff, capital expenses (on-site facilities and technology support systems), and academic support (recruitment, admission, records, library access, and student support systems). Many times the needs assessment becomes a write-off at the expense of the nursing program and is financed through contingency funds or program development funds generated from grant overhead costs. The plan should include possible initial grant support for start-up funds and plans for eventual self-sufficiency. The resources that are required from the parent institution are listed and include off-site offices, laboratories, and classrooms; clinical-experience facilities;

technological support systems for videoconferencing, teleconferencing, and/or web-based instruction; administrative, faculty and staff expenses; and academic support systems such as library, academic, and student services. Included in the assessment is a list of potential administrators, staff, faculty, and the proposed program's student body characteristics.

The administration's role and costs include supervisory or management functions to implement the program such as budget and personnel management, liaison activities with regional stakeholders, public relations, coordination, marketing plans, and preparation of reports to seek approval and accreditation of the distance education program from relevant agencies. Some of the staff and/or faculty cost considerations are the required full-time and part-time equivalents, benefits, travel and other expenses, supplies, and equipment.

These expenses vary according to the selected method of delivery of the educational program. For example, off-site offices, classrooms, and lab facilities are necessary for courses or classes conducted by on-site faculty or traveling faculty from the home campus. Expenses for this type of program are rent, telephones, computer support for faculty, staff, and students, and the usual office and classroom teaching supplies, hardware, and software such as computers, printers, audio–visual hardware and software, laboratory supplies, paper, correspondence materials, desks, chairs, laboratory clinical equipment and supplies, and so on.

Curriculum and Evaluation Plans

In addition to the economic feasibility for the program, an analysis of the curriculum is in order to ensure that the proposed distant program is congruent with the mission, goals, organizational framework, and student learning outcomes of the parent program. Although, the format and delivery of the curriculum may differ from the original, it must meet the same goals and objectives of the program. Administrators and faculty must make decisions regarding the format and have a rationale for why certain formats are chosen, for example, on-land satellites, video and/or teleconferencing, and/or web-based platforms.

The new program should be integrated into the master plan of evaluation of the parent program to ensure its quality. Additionally, it should have its own evaluation plan for monitoring the program as it is implemented for corrections along the way (formative evaluation) and to have summative evaluation plans in place that measure the success of the program in terms of student learning outcomes and success, satisfaction of the stakeholders, and its continued congruence with the components of the parent program's curriculum. See Table 18.1 for guidelines for the development of distance education programs.

TYPES OF DISTANCE EDUCATION PROGRAMS

The following is a description of the major types of distance education program. Some of the pros and cons for them are listed.

Satellite Campuses

For the purposes of this discussion, *satellite campuses* are defined as those programs that offer the curriculum in whole or in part on off-campus sites from the parent institution. While they can incorporate technology methods such as videoconferencing and web-based instruction, the majority of the teaching and learning takes place in classrooms and involves in-person interactions between the faculty and students. For nursing, clinical experiences may occur in health care facilities in the community in which the satellite campus is located. Faculty members who teach in the parent institution serve as on-site faculty or act as consultants to off-site faculty who teach the same curriculum. For those faculty members on the home campus who actually teach on the satellite campus, travel costs and the related time it takes for travel are included in the costs for implementing the program. These costs are weighed against the cost of the salary and benefits for hiring on-site faculty.

There are added challenges for finding off-site faculty who are qualified to teach the subject content as they must be oriented to the curriculum to ensure its integrity. Thus, it is not unusual for the parent institution to have an academic manager for the satellite campus program(s) who can serve as the curriculum and academic services coordinator. In the instances of off-site satellite campuses, the course content and materials for both theory and clinical are identical to that of the home campus. Special events to link the off-site and home campuses are often planned to foster the socialization process for students and faculty so that there is a milieu of all people belonging to the same institution.

Additional resources are needed to implement the distant satellite campus such as students' access to texts either through the home bookstore or other resources such as online book companies; library access; online access if it is part of the curriculum; and student services including academic, financial aid, and personal counseling usually through the on-site coordinator and support staff. Recruitment, admission, and enrollment services are additional resources that can be served by on-site personnel if the program is large or by home-campus staff who travel periodically to the satellite campus.

Some of the arguments against these types of program are the loss of students on the home campus, possible incongruence between the implementation of the courses in the curriculum owing to a loss of interactions among students and faculty with the home campus, a danger that the majority of the faculty and staff are part time and therefore some of the commitment to the institution is lost, and the possibility that the program is too costly and cannot become self-sufficient. Some of the arguments for these types of distance education programs include the interpersonal communications and relationships between faculty and students, a sense of belonging to the parent institution through face-to-face encounters on campus or other on-land locations, increasing student enrollments for the program, and serving a community need. If there is a careful plan for implementing the curriculum, there is an assurance that the curriculum remains intact. Some cost savings for students and the institution can be realized in travel and personnel expenses if some of the faculty and staff are part time.

TABLE 18.1 GUIDELINES FOR THE DEVELOPMENT OF A DISTANCE EDUCATION PROGRAM

GUIDELINE TOPIC	QUESTIONS FOR DATA COLLECTION AND ANALYSIS	DESIRED OUTCOME
Needs Assessment: External Frame Factors	To what extent are the distant sites supportive of the program and sophisticated in the use of technology? To what extent has the health care system demonstrated support for the program and the nursing profession? To what extent is the health care system open to student clinical experiences and what resources do they have available for the experiences? To what extent is the program competitive with other educational program at the site(s)? To what extent is there a potential student body at the site(s) and is there an indication that it will continue for at least 5 to 10 years?	The community is receptive to distance education programs, sophisticated or open to the technology of distance education, and has a health care system supportive of the program, the nursing profession, and student clinical experiences, if indicated The program is competitive with other programs There is a potential student body that will continue for at least 5 to 10 years
External Frame Factors	Have program approval and accreditation bodies been notified of the program and do they approve or is there an indication that they will approve the program in the future?	Relevant program approval and accrediting agencies have been notified and approve the program or there are indications for approval in the future
Needs Assessment: Internal Frame Factors	To what extent does the distance education program's mission, philosophy, organizing framework, goals, and objectives reflect those of the parent institution? To what extent does the parent institution have experience in the selected modality(ies) of distance education and/or have the resources to support it? Are there plans in place that indicate adequate resources for the program including infrastructure, human resources, and academic program support?	The mission, purpose, philosophy, organizing framework, goals, and objectives of the distance education program are congruent with the parent institution The parent institution has experience with and/or the resources to support the program Plans are in place and resources are adequate for academic infrastructure, human resources, and academic program support

(continued)

TABLE 18.1 GUIDELINES FOR THE DEVELOPMENT OF A DISTANCE EDUCATION PROGRAM
(*continued*)

GUIDELINE TOPIC	QUESTIONS FOR DATA COLLECTION AND ANALYSIS	DESIRED OUTCOME
Economic Feasibility	To what extent will the parent institution support a needs assessment for the distance education program? If there are no funds from the institution, are there other possible resources?	There is support from the parent institution or other sources for a needs assessment
	Are there start-up funds available from the institution or are there other sources such as funds from partner health care or educational institutions?	There are start-up funds from the parent institution or other sources
	Does the business case justify the need for the program including its congruence with the mission of the institution, u demonstrated need for the program in the community, an adequate potential student body, and assurance of the maintenance of its quality?	The business case is persuasive and includes justification for the development of the program, that is, meets mission, meets a need, has an adequate potential student body, and maintains quality
	Has the business plan accounted for personnel costs (staff, technicians, and faculty); administrative costs; facilities (if indicated); academic support systems, for example, library, enrollment services, financial aid, and so on; and the required technology system(s)?	The business plan includes funds for the required personnel, administrative costs, facilities (if indicated), academic support systems, and the required technology system
	To what extent are there plans for self-sufficiency? Are there projections for the size of the student body and other resources necessary to maintain the program?	There are financial plans in place for self-sufficiency and maintenance of the program
Congruence With the Components of the Curriculum	To what extent does the curriculum plan for the distance education program reflect that of the parent institution, for example, course descriptions, credits, objectives, and content?	The distance education program's curriculum plan is congruent with that of the parent institution

(*continued*)

TABLE 18.1 GUIDELINES FOR THE DEVELOPMENT OF A DISTANCE EDUCATION PROGRAM (*continued*)

GUIDELINE TOPIC	QUESTIONS FOR DATA COLLECTION AND ANALYSIS	DESIRED OUTCOME
Delivery Model Options	Have all modalities been considered including off-site, on-land satellite campuses, videoconferencing and/or teleconferencing, and online or web-based methods?	All modalities for the delivery method are reviewed to lead to a rationale for the selected model or combination of several
Delivery Model Options: Selection and Its Rationale	To what extent does the selected model fit the learning needs of the students?	The selected model fits the learning needs of the students.
	To what extent are there faculty who can utilize the model(s)? If not, are there faculty development plans and technical support in place?	The selected model is within the scope of the faculty's expertise or there are faculty development plans in place
	To what extent is the selected model "user- friendly" for students and faculty?	The selected model is "user-friendly" for students and faculty
Delivery Model: Implementation Plan	To what extent is the selected model(s) congruent with the curriculum plan?	The selected model is congruent with the curriculum plan
	Does the selected model fit the implementation plan of the curriculum, that is, is it possible to deliver theory, lab, and clinical experiences?	The curriculum plan can be implemented through utilization of the selected model(s)
Delivery Model: Evaluation	Is there an evaluation plan in place and to what extent is it congruent with the master plan of the parent institution?	There is an evaluation plan in place and it is congruent with the master plan of evaluation for the parent institution
	Does the evaluation plan include both formative and summative evaluation measures?	The evaluation plan includes both formative and summative measures
	To what extent does the evaluation plan include strategies and personnel for follow-up and revisions if necessary based upon the data analyses and recommendations from the evaluation plan?	The evaluation plan has mechanisms in place to revise the program according to data analyses and recommendations from evaluation activities
	Is the selected delivery model(s) relevant to current education practices?	The selected delivery model is relevant to current education practices and adaptable to future changes in the education, profession, and health care systems
	To what extent is the selected model adaptable to future changes in the profession and education and health care systems?	

Videoconferencing and Teleconferencing

Some distance education programs are delivered to off-campus sites through video-conferencing and/or telecommunications. Videoconferencing requires dedicated classrooms that can send and receive digital data both on-site at the home campus and off-site at the distant campus(es). The ideal videoconferencing system has classrooms located on all sites with the ability to send and receive, thus facilitating live interactive teaching and learning experiences among students and faculty. However, some off-site campuses might have only reception ability, thus limiting live interactions with other students and faculty except perhaps by telephone to facilitate audio communi-cation or communicating by computer using live chat rooms, e-mail messages, or class roster/contact lists systems.

While the videoconferencing method of distance education is expensive, the rate of success is high for state and regionally supported academic programs with satellite capabilities among the various levels of higher education, for exam-ple, community colleges and state university systems. Additionally, partnerships between educational institutions and health care organizations that use satellite campus videoconferencing for staff development and patient and family educa-tion services are of benefit to both partners. The advantage to academic nursing programs for entering into these types of arrangements with established health care systems is the tremendous cost savings for mounting and maintaining the pro-gram. The disadvantage is that unless nursing was an early pioneer in the delivery system and has a major role in it, it may face implementation problems such as least desirable times for broadcasting and possible displacement of class times owing to the priority rights of the sponsoring agency.

Videoconferencing and teleconferencing require an infrastructure for cable television or closed-circuit television, dedicated classrooms that can both broad-cast and receive communications, and technological support staff who manage the broadcasting and hardware and software for instructional support purposes. Unless the sessions are recorded and can be shown after the session for independ-ent viewing, the scheduling of the classes is time certain and cannot be changed owing to the demand for the services by other entities. A fairly recent form of vide-oconferencing is the use of Internet networking services for audio and video inter-actions. Examples include Skype (2014), instant messaging that provides real-time text messages between participants, and FaceTime, an application for Apple prod-ucts such as iPhones and iPads. These services provide real-time opportunities for faculty and students to interact through existing Internet services and personal cell phones, tablets, and computers and if needed, supplementary teleconferencing. This method is inexpensive as it uses existing Internet services and it is useful for international communications as well as local and regional areas, but reception can be spotty if there are multiple users on the same network.

Revatis and Egger (2013) describe the use of FaceTime in a classroom with nurse researchers in a nearby hospital who interacted on FaceTime hardware (cell phone or tablet) with faculty and undergraduate students. The interactions were projected onto a screen in the classroom. The students were able to dialogue with the researchers about their studies' results and application to practice. According to the authors, students were very positive about the experience and developed an enthusiasm for research.

As with all delivery modes, the courses and/or classes offered through video-conferencing must be congruent with the curriculum and follow its goals and objectives. Videoconferencing includes all of the usual teaching methods and resources such as lectures, the use of overhead projectors, slides, videotapes, movies, and PowerPoint (PPT) presentations. Students and faculty interact in real time through exchanges via camera, telephone, tablet, or web-based live chat rooms. These types of interactions require telecommunication and web-based systems as well as satellite broadcasting systems. Negative aspects to this type of delivery of distance education programs are the expenses related to it such as the hardware and technical staffing, inflexible time frames (although they are no different than traditional scheduled classes on the home campus), and the need for faculty expertise in a variety of teaching media. Positive aspects include real-time, live interactions between faculty and students; the wide array of available resources; the delivery of the same subject matter to more than one audience and therefore more students; and the likelihood that the integrity of the curriculum is maintained.

CLINICAL COURSES AND DISTANCE EDUCATION

It is possible to provide quality clinical experiences for students through distance education modalities. For example, the off-site satellite campus with on-site faculty usually provides clinical experiences in the "traditional" mode. Faculty develops the clinical courses, including skills laboratory courses, according to the implementation plan of the curriculum. Students are assigned to clinical laboratories for the acquisition of assessment and clinical skills as well as to health care agencies for supervised clinical experiences. The latter are under the supervision of faculty who either directly supervise a group of students in the clinical setting or coordinate student preceptorships with students assigned to qualified staff nurse preceptors.

With careful planning, it is possible to provide clinical experiences for students enrolled in courses through videoconferencing or teleconferencing and web-based instruction. Keeping in mind that course objectives must remain the same to ensure the integrity of the curriculum, faculty responsible for clinical courses can design the course so that the didactic and discussion components of the course are delivered through the selected distance education technology. Assignments, logs or journals describing the clinical experiences, examinations, and pre- and postconferences can also take place through technology and can be *asynchronous* (occurring at various times) or *synchronous* (simultaneous). The actual clinical experiences occur through faculty-coordinated preceptorships, local faculty hired by the institution for clinical supervision of students, or by faculty traveling to the clinical site to supervise a group of students.

If faculty serve as coordinators for clinical experiences with off-site preceptors and students, they must secure agreements between the educational program and the health care agency and preceptor; set standards for the qualifications of the preceptors; orient the preceptors to the curriculum, the course, and the role of preceptors; provide guidance throughout the experience to the preceptors and students; develop a communications network for all participants; supervise preceptors and students; assign the grades with input from the preceptors; and evaluate and revise the program based on feedback.

Grady (2011) discusses the use of videoconferencing for providing a virtual but real-life clinical experience for students in a rural setting with limited access to clinical experiences. The project she describes took place through the collaboration of a VA medical center and an associate degree in nursing program. A videoconference was set up for a small group of students in a classroom who interacted with a patient, his family, and the staff nurse providing care. The experience occurred though distance communications with telephone and online support to troubleshoot and provide ancillary services. The program was successful from a student satisfaction standpoint and provided the opportunity for students to interact with an expert nurse and other health care professionals. It is an adjunct to simulated laboratory experiences and real-life, hands-on experiences.

Simulated clinical experiences in a laboratory setting can take place with the use of high- and low-fidelity mannequins accompanied by case scenarios to prepare for hands-on clinical experiences in the reality setting. Gore, Hunt, Parker, and Raines (2011) studied anxiety levels in undergraduate students who were about to enter their first clinical experience. Half of the group participated in a 4-hour simulated clinical experience on campus and the other half (control group) were assigned directly to the clinical experience in the health care agency. Using the Spielberger, Gorsuch, Lushene, Vagg, and Jacobs State-Trait Anxiety Inventory (1983) to measure anxiety levels, they found that students exposed to the simulated experiences had lower scores on the inventory than the control group. This study is an example of how simulated clinical experiences can assist students in preparing for hands-on practice in clinical agencies. As with all distance education, clinical experiences must be congruent with the curriculum plan and follow course objectives and projected student learning outcomes.

THE GROWTH OF INFORMATICS AND TECHNOLOGY

Technology in the Classroom

The utilization of technology in the classroom and through distance education guides the implementation of the curriculum by determining the format for delivery of its courses. Technology applied to the classroom and distance education programs has grown exponentially over the past few decades. It moved from teacher-centered lectures accompanied by movies and slide shows in the classroom to the use of videotapes, online PPT presentations with voice-over features, and portable compact disks and flashdrives containing course materials for faculty and students' personal computers. Additional student-centered devices include electronic clickers for classroom participation and electronic note-taking software that links to course syllabi, materials, and lectures. Online technology is available through eLearning software that provides the educator with the ability to broadcast lectures or brief discussions complemented by movies, slides, website access, and so on. Examples of these software packages are Atriculate, Camtasia, and Lectora. The development of these multimedia teaching/learning aids promotes active student participation in the learning process and facilitates the change from teacher-focused strategies to student-centered learning processes.

Klein and Kientz (2013) describe the use of student response systems (SRS) in the classroom. They suggest an orientation process for faculty's and students' use of the devices and how faculty should plan for their use in enhancing the classroom learning experience. In addition, they reported on the successes from utilization of the system including positive student learning outcomes, increased learner participation, and the faculty's ability to assess learning that is taking place. The authors describe application of behavioral and constructivist learning theories to this method.

Critz and Knight (2013) describe the "flipped classroom technique" as it applied to their graduate level pediatric course. Instead of the traditional lecture, students prepared for class in advance by completing reading assignments and listening to short lectures. To test their level of understanding of the material, students took online quizzes following the assignment activity and prior to attending class. The classroom sessions consisted of group activities, discussions, role-playing, and analysis of case studies. The authors found that students reported high satisfaction with this new approach that supported learner-centered pedagogy.

A description of integrating technology into a nursing program by an interdisciplinary team is offered by Griffin-Sobel et al. (2010). The authors describe their experiences with a project to integrate laboratory simulation technology, electronic reference databases, videoconferencing, computer-aided learning tools, and informatics systems into the curriculum. Essential to the process was the team approach and the involvement of the faculty in the process. The interdisciplinary team consisted of a librarian, the laboratory manager, the director of technology, and the project director. The project was in response to the changes in the health care system to prepare nursing students for practice including the use of electronic records, evidence-based practice, drug reference materials, and personal digital assistants (PDAs) utilization.

Electronic library resources provide faculty, researchers, and students with Internet access to journals, electronic versions of textbooks, and reference databases. The most frequently databases used in nursing are CINAHL, Cochrane Database of Systematic Reviews, Health Sciences, Medline, Nursing and Allied Health, Ovid Nursing Journals Full Text, and PubMed. Social sciences and the sciences databases such as Behavioral Sciences and ScienceDirect are frequently used as well as ERIC for references on education.

So-called "Cloud" Internet databases store files and other data in remote computer servers in order to synchronize and download them onto other electronic devices. They provide a virtual place for faculty, researchers, and students to store and exchange files, databases, and to submit and grade written assignments such as papers, journals, and logs. These services can be free or, if there is a large amount of data to store, a fee may be charged. Examples of some of these virtual files Internet services are Apple's iCloud, DropBox, Google Drive, and SugarSync.

Day-Black and Watties-Daniels (2006) describe the application of technology to contemporary classrooms including smart classrooms (in-class computers, overhead projectors, access to the web, and electronic software programs that allow students to revisit lectures and take electronic notes). The authors liken the early days of technology to Socrates' concerns shared with Plato when the first written words were recorded that took the place of oral communication and the sharing of knowledge. He voiced concern that students would come to rely on the written word rather than using their intellectual skills. This concern echoed through the ages as calculators began to replace handwritten mathematics, computers replaced the typewritten word, and smart phones, laptop computers, and electronic tablets provided access to myriad communications and systems. One can only imagine the future as technology continues to expand.

Online/Web-Based Programs

Online and web-based instruction had its beginnings through faculty and student use of communication tools such as list serves, e-mail, and access to resources and references on the World Wide Web. In the 1990s and early 21st century, the use of web-based instruction through learning management systems became more prevalent. They proved so popular with students that some courses were mounted as a combination of web-based and on-campus instruction classes for home campus students as well as off-campus students. Web-based instruction is usually delivered through the use of learning management systems with which the institution has a contract, although some institutions develop their own. As the popularity of this method of teaching and learning increased, the systems grew in complexity and at the same time became more user-friendly. Delivery of web-based programs and courses grew to the extent that in 2013, over 6.7 million students were enrolled in higher education online courses and online enrollment accounted for 33.5% of total enrollment in 2013 as compared to 9.6% in 2002 (Allen & Seaman, 2013, 2014).

Allen and Seaman (2013) in their report *Changing Course: Ten Years of Tracking Online Education in the United States* offered the following definition of online education:

> Online courses are those in which at least 80 percent of the course content is delivered online. Face-to-face instruction includes courses in which zero to 29 percent of the content is delivered online; this category includes both traditional and web facilitated courses. The remaining alternative, blended (sometimes called hybrid) instruction has between 30% and 80% of the course content delivered online. While the survey asked respondents for information on all types of courses, the current report is devoted to only online learning. (p. 7)

While not a new phenomenon, the growth of massive open online courses (MOOCs) has implications for the future for granting credits toward degrees. MOCCs first appeared in 1988 but are growing in numbers available with free course offerings open to anyone. Several well-known institutions such as Harvard, MIT, Stanford, and the U.K. Open University offer the courses. In 2013, the primary objective for institutions' offering MOOCs was to increase the institution's visibility followed by a drive for student recruitment, innovative pedagogy, and flexible opportunities (Allen & Seaman, 2014).

Courses vary by discipline and topic and they usually offer a certificate of completion if the student opts to finish the course. Some universities grant academic credit for completed courses based on competency-based models. It is likely that MOOCs will have an impact on higher education in the near future including quality, faculty development for new technology, instructional design and strategies, and how students learn (Allen & Seaman, 2013; Mazoue, 2013; Tuomi, 2013).

Development of Online Programs

The American Distance Education Consortium (ADEC) (2014) provides classic teaching and learning principles applied to distance and web-based education. It is an overview of what should be considered and part of distance education and online programs. Web-based teaching and learning require a learning management system, computer access to the web by faculty and students, technological support through the use of instructional support staff, and training sessions for faculty and students who are not familiar with the system. Some institutions of higher learning use experienced instructional technology staff and faculty who mount and manage courses for teachers whose only responsibility is for the actual teaching of the course. This method provides technical support for teaching faculty; however, it may remove some of the academic freedom from the teacher-of-record. For example, the teacher does not have the ability to change course assignments or formats without going through the support staff to make the changes. It can also prove to be expensive since the institution is paying for several staff members when only one may be required.

The initial time spent in converting a traditional course or a new course to a web-based course is great and, as with all courses, requires updating and revisions each subsequent time that it is taught. Multiple learning activities are available through the Internet such as synchronous real-time chat rooms and live classrooms where students and faculty meet at a prearranged time and discuss topics or review questions about course assignments. Asynchronous entries (occurring at various times and also labeled as threaded discussions) about selected topics provide the students and faculty with opportunities to discuss topics and present their ideas and views on them. The assignments related to these usually require reading assignments and/or a review of the literature so that the discussions are scholarly treatises on the subject at hand. Faculty can post a lecture through an essay or PPT presentation that includes notes, illustrations, references to URLs, videotapes, movies, and other audiovisual media and pose thought questions for discussions related to the "lecture." Group work assignments are possible through the use of chat rooms, live classrooms, threaded discussions, and e-mail communications.

Jones and Wolf (2010) provide an overview of the role of faculty in integrating technology and online learning into the curriculum. Many learning management systems have programs that allow faculty to develop surveys and examinations that are secure and provide statistical analyses of the results. A few examples of web-based educational and live-time platforms are Blackboard (2014), eCollege (2014), Moodle (2014), and Wimba (2014).

Learning Theories for Online Formats

Most distance education programs employ *andragogy* (adult learning) strategies for the delivery of courses and classes through off-campus satellite sites, videoconferencing, telecommunications, online, and web-based technology. The majority of teaching and learning strategies offered in these formats is learner centered and facilitates active student participation in the process rather than the traditional pedagogical methods for presenting information to the student. See Chapter 4 for learning theories that apply to online educational formats and for ideas for research on the use of learning theories for online instruction.

Kala, Isaramalai, and Pohthong (2010) offer a conceptual model for developing courses online. They discuss major learning theories that apply to electronic learning including behaviorism, cognitivism, and constructivism. They apply constructivism theory to the development of learning activities in their model. They argue that the constructivism theory applies well to electronic learning since the theory centers on the ability of the learner to build on previous knowledge, assimilate new knowledge, and interpret the knowledge gained to the surrounding environment. It requires active learner participation, reflection, and social interaction with faculty and peers. The authors offer examples of learning activities that can occur synchronously or asynchronously online and with a wide variety of teaching–learning strategies such as problem based learning gaming, and stimulated experiences.

Guimond, Salas, and Sole (2011) discuss the development of computerized patient simulator learning experiences and propose that metacognition (thinking about thinking) is a learning theory appropriate to simulated learning experiences that call for the development of critical thinking, which leads to clinical decision-making. They list the acronym KSA (knowledge, skills, and attitudes) as the desired outcomes to be achieved from simulated learning experiences.

Research Findings on the Efficacy of Online Formats

The U.S. Department of Education (2009) in a meta-analysis of the literature related to online education found that online delivery of content results in better student learning outcomes than traditional classroom instruction. In addition, the blending of the online format with face-to-face meetings was even more effective; although, it was pointed out that in those instances, additional materials may have enriched the learning experience. Allen and Seaman (2013) in their national survey of academic programs with online programs reported that over three quarters of academic leaders believe that online education is "just as good as or better" than face-to-face courses (p. 24).

Horne and Sandmann (2012) conducted a literature review of nursing studies related to program evaluation of graduate nursing education online programs. They identified few articles that systematically evaluated programs including not only student learning outcomes, but also, program support systems and stakeholders' satisfaction with the format. They have an extensive list of research questions related to program evaluation of online educational programs as well as recommendations for comprehensive program evaluation that is necessary to ensure quality programs.

Disadvantages and Advantages of Web-Based Education

Some of the disadvantages of online systems are the need for technological support; initial and on-going costs related to contracts for learning management systems and computers; the lack of face-to-face encounters between faculty and students; the large amount of faculty time consumed in mounting the course; the need for faculty and student development is the use of technology, the possible loss of nursing values such as visible and tactile communications; and a minimal sense of belonging to the home campus. Advantages include flexible times for students and faculty, multiple learning and teaching strategies, active participation on the part of all students, personal/individual communications between students and faculty, moderate maintenance times for managing and updating the course once it is mounted, and relative assurance of curriculum integrity.

APPLICATION OF TECHNOLOGY TO EDUCATION

Simulated Clinical Experiences

The application of technology to the implementation of the curriculum occurs both on-campus and through distance education delivery systems. An example is the use of realistic interactive patient simulations in the laboratory setting for students to practice skills in a safe environment prior to providing nursing care in the clinical setting. Patient simulators come with ready-made case scenarios or faculty can develop their own scenarios that can be programmed into the simulators. Many schools of nursing located on multidisciplinary health sciences campuses pool resources with other disciplines that result in shared state-of-the art facilities to practice skills and foster interprofessional education opportunities.

Other simulated experiences include human patient simulation/standardized patient experiences with real people who have been programmed to present with a health problem(s). Students interview and examine the patients for diagnosing health problems and although real patients cannot simulate actual symptoms, they can provide realistic opportunities for history taking and communication skills. Brewer (2011) reviewed the literature for the use of standardized patients in nursing education and found only a few studies to demonstrate their effectiveness. However, the ones identified reported that they were effective and can be useful for developing clinical skills. Brewer provides some suggestions for developing human patient simulations and makes the point that the method for evaluation of student performance must be included in the simulation. She points out the need for studies to measure the effectiveness of this method of clinical simulation learning. Many of these experiences have become interprofessional with medical and nursing students sharing the same patients and approaching the situation from each discipline's perspective.

Newer models of mannequins available for nursing skills labs consist of low-fidelity or high-fidelity models. Examples of low-fidelity models are partial models such as an arm for practicing insertion of an intravenous line or a pelvis for physical examination. Whole body mannequins can be low fidelity for practicing such skills as bathing, turning, and positioning. High-fidelity mannequins are programmed to exhibit symptoms of bleeding, irregular pulses and respirations, emotions such as cries of pain and tears, and so forth. They are programmed according to preset scenarios and can be controlled by faculty in a booth adjacent to the simulated patient room. Founds, Zewe, and Scheuer (2011) describe how they developed scenarios for high-fidelity clinical experiences for their baccalaureate students. The process they describe includes planning for the scenario and how the outcomes from the experience can be evaluated.

Guimond et al. (2011) describe high-fidelity simulation as a technique for providing students with realistic clinical experiences based on scenarios that create or replicate health care situations in a laboratory setting. Although the high-fidelity mannequins can simulate realistic symptoms of disease or distress that require technical skills, they can also be programmed to induce non-hands-on skills such as communication skills, cultural assessment, psychosocial aspects, and interprofessional collaboration. These situations allow students to make clinical decisions in a situation that does not place the patient at risk. The authors describe the process for developing scenarios for clinical simulations with the first step of identifying a learning theory that supports the situation. They provide a model for the development of simulations with a checklist to help guide faculty as they create the learning experience.

Research Findings on the Efficacy of Case Scenario Simulations

Reese, Jeffries, and Engum (2010) measured multidisciplinary (medical and nursing) students' learning outcomes when interacting with a simulated postsurgical patient that was experiencing cardiac arrhythmias. The simulation case study was based on the Jeffries's (2005) Nursing Education Simulation Framework (NESF). Reese et al. found that students reported increased confidence in the care of patients with these problems when transferred to reality and they had positive experiences in working with another discipline. Furthermore, the simulated experiences assisted their learning in a safe environment.

Onello and Regan (2013) discuss some of the issues related to high-fidelity simulation and measuring student learning outcomes. They point out that many studies report increased confidence levels in students who experience simulated clinical practice situations but the authors raise a concern about the preponderance of simulated scenarios that emphasize emergency situations for student reaction and response. They question if students might expect that all patient situations will call for rapid response compared to the more common patient care situations calling for cognitive skills as well psychomotor skills. The authors suggest that scenarios include situations that reflect common patient care problems as well as emergency conditions. In summary, the authors list important questions and suggestions for research related to high-fidelity simulations. The suggestions include validity and reliability studies of instruments used to measure student confidence and competence and the need for quantitative studies to measure learning outcomes. The authors call for standardized simulation frameworks in order to build evidence-based, best practice models for the delivery of student learning experiences.

Electronic Medical Records and Information Systems

As electronic patient records and information systems become more prevalent in the health care system, it becomes necessary for schools of nursing to provide the theoretical and technical knowledge related to these systems for nursing students. Skiba (2009) provides an overview of the integration of informatics and technology into specific nursing curricula. She provides ideas and resources for faculty development for schools to provide learning experiences for students such as simulated patient information systems, electronic documentation, and patient records. Skiba promotes the need for faculty development workshops for instructors to gain the expertise to integrate these concepts and experiences into the curriculum.

Lucas (2010) describes a collaborative program between a health care facility and an associate degree in nursing program that provided simulated experiences for students to practice patient care and use an electronic medical record system for documenting care. The agency's staff training program was adapted for use by nursing faculty and students and, although it consumed faculty time in helping to develop the scenario, it proved to be cost-effective and provided an opportunity for students to practice with an actual medical record system.

Flood, Gasiewicz, and Delpier (2010) provide an example of a baccalaureate program that integrated informatics throughout the curriculum. After a review of the literature, the authors found scanty information on the integration of informatics into the curriculum in spite of the growing need for it and recommendations from the report of the Technology Informatics Guiding Education Reform (2009). The authors describe the introduction of informatics in the baccalaureate program by assignments that have students interact with electronic reference databases. Later in the curriculum, they have access to complex patient clinical records and if possible, meet with an informatics manager to see the influence of this technology in the health care system.

TRENDS, ISSUES, AND CHALLENGES FOR THE FUTURE

To remain competitive and current in the higher education market, nursing programs need to determine how they will expand their programs to meet the needs of students who may live and work some distance away from the home campus. Although entry-level programs, especially undergraduate programs, will continue to take place on traditional home campuses supplemented by technology, there is a need to offer higher education programs for licensed personnel and other experienced learners far from home campuses. Distance learning through technology offers the best opportunity for working nurses to continue their education and, as described earlier in the chapter, has been successful. Through consortia of varying levels of education, regional collaboratives, and the health care industry, these programs can be cost-effective and reach many more nurses than ever imagined.

The increasing market for learning management systems provides cost-effective, quality educational delivery programs through web-based technology and in many ways is proving to be an effective modality for engaging students in transformative learning experiences. These types of programs are far less expensive than videoconferencing and telecommunications; however, they require the technology, staffing, and faculty development programs to realize their full potential.

No matter the modality, the program must be within the context of the program's mission, philosophy, organizational framework, and goals and objectives. As with all curriculum development projects, faculty must examine the purpose of the distance education program in light of these components. In some cases, the program may not be compatible with the mission and therefore is not an option. For those programs that are compatible, the usual formative evaluation strategies must take place to ensure that the planning and implementation phases of the program are congruent with the overall curriculum plan. An evaluation plan to measure outcomes must be in place to maintain quality, meet program approval and accreditation standards, and ensure a quality program for its stakeholders such as students, consumers, and faculty.

The majority of distance education programs have copyright and intellectual property policies in place that are congruent with the parent institution. For new programs, along with faculty development and implementation support, it is advised that these policies be developed early in the process. The ideal policy is one that gives the individual faculty member the rights to the course syllabus and learning activities; however, the course description and objectives remain the property of the institution.

Privacy issues are addressed through the maintenance of the same policies of the parent institution. For web-based courses, owing to identification theft and computer hackers, many institutions issue identification numbers for students, staff, and faculty rather than social security numbers. Most learning management systems have built-in privacy safety and security mechanisms allowing only students and faculty access to courses through personal identification numbers and passwords, and to protect debit and credit card information when paying tuition and fees.

Often, videoconferencing is delivered through closed-circuit television or public broadcasting system and thus is open to public access. However, only students officially enrolled in the courses can receive academic credit and have access to the supplemental material necessary for the course such as library services, course resources, e-mail, list serves, and chat rooms.

An issue infrequently addressed in the literature is the matter of faculty to student ratios in distance education programs and their effect on quality education, faculty workload, and method of instruction. Videoconferencing leads other technologies in reaching the greatest numbers of students while web-based courses, except for MOOCs, are limited in size per faculty member, usually to a maximum of 20 to 25 students. Web-based instruction requires high intensity interactions among students and faculty for effective learning to take place. Videoconferencing can reach many students in multiple sites, but as with all lecture-type classes, fosters minimal student participation unless active learning assignments are included. All of these factors must be taken into consideration when planning the delivery choice.

As distance education programs increase in the future, new issues and challenges face faculty and institutions of higher learning. Less attention will be needed on the actual technology of the delivery systems and more attention will be necessary on the quality of the programs as they match the mission and purposes of the educational programs. Outcomes from distance education programs will be measured by increased opportunities for nurses to continue their education and the continued partnerships between education and service that result in a nursing workforce ready to meet the challenges of an ever-changing health care system and the health promotion and disease prevention needs of the populace.

SUMMARY

Chapter 18 reviewed the various types of distance education programs and their relationship to curriculum development and evaluation. The influence of informatics and technology on nursing education was discussed. Some of the issues facing these types of programs were reviewed including cost-effectiveness, faculty workload, the application of teaching and learning principles, and student learning outcomes.

DISCUSSION QUESTIONS

1. To what extent do you believe that technology-supported distance education programs changed nursing education for the 21st century?
2. Of the multiple technology-supported distance education programs, which do you believe:
   a. Is most cost-effective?
   b. Meets desired outcomes?
   c. Reaches the highest number of students?
   d. Fosters faculty development?
Explain your rationale
3. Discuss the pros and cons for the delivery of clinical courses through distance education strategies.

LEARNING ACTIVITIES

STUDENT LEARNING ACTIVITIES

Search the current literature (past 5 years) for at least three research articles on distance education programs, web-based education, or the application of informatics and technology on nursing education. Analyze them for a description of the outcomes for specific distance education modalities. Compare the modalities according to the outcomes that relate to teaching and learning effectiveness and student and faculty satisfaction.

NURSE EDUCATOR/FACULTY DEVELOPMENT ACTIVITIES

Select one course that you teach and adapt it to either videoconferencing or web-based technology. Explain your rationale for selecting one or the other as it applies to the course.

If you teach a course(s) online, evaluate it for its student learning outcomes and other measures of its effectiveness. Compare it to the program mission and program goals/objectives. Develop a plan for revising the course based on your evaluation.

REFERENCES

Allen, I. E., & Seaman, J. (2013). *Changing course: Ten years of tracking online education in the United States.* Retrieved from http://www.onlinelearningsurvey.com/reports/changingcourse.pdf

Allen, I. E., & Seaman, J. (2014). *Grade change. Tracking online education in the U.S.* Wellesley, MA: Babson Survey Research Group and Quahog Research Group, LLC.

American Distance Education Consortium. (2014). *ADEC guiding principles for distance teaching and learning.* Retrieved from http://www.adec.edu/admin/papers/distance-teaching_principles.html

Blackboard. (2014). *Blackboard. Higher education.* Retrieved from http://www.blackboard.com/Solutions-by-Market/Higher-Education.aspx

Brewer, E. P. (2011). Successful techniques for using human patient simulation in nursing education. *Journal of Nursing Scholarship, 43*(3), 311–317.

Critz, C., & Knight, D. (2013). Using the flipped classroom in graduate nursing education. *Nurse Educator, 38*(5), 210–213.

Day-Black, C., & Watties-Daniels, A. (2006). Cutting edge technology to enhance nursing classroom instruction at Coppin State University. *ABNF Journal, 17*(3), 103–106.

eCollege. (2014). *Pearson.* Retrieved from http://www.ecollege.com/index.php

Flood, L., Gasiewicz, N., & Delpier, T. (2010). Integrating information literacy across a BSN curriculum. *Journal of Nursing Education, 49*(2), 101–104.

Founds, S. A., Zewe, G., & Scheuer, L. A. (2011). Development of high-fidelity clinical experience for baccalaureate nursing students. *Journal of Professional Nursing, 27*(1), 5–9.

Gore, T., Hunt, C. W., Parker, F., & Raines, K. H. (2011). The effects of simulated clinical experiences on anxiety: nursing students' perspectives. *Clinical Simulation in Nursing, 7*(5), e175–e180.

Grady, J. L. (2011). The virtual clinical practicum: An innovative telehealth model for clinical nursing education. *Nursing Education Perspectives, 32*(2), 189.

Griffin-Sobel, J. P., Acee, A., Sharoff, L., Cobus-Kuo, L., Woodstock-Wallace, A., & Dornbaum, M. (2010). A transdisciplinary approach to faculty development in nursing education technology. *Nursing Education Perspectives, 31*(1), 41–43.

Guimond, M. E., Salas, E., & Sole, M. L. (2011). Getting ready for simulation-based training: A checklist for nurse educators. *Nursing Education Perspectives, 32*(3), 179.

Horne, E. M., & Sandmann, L. R. (2012). Current trends in systematic program evaluation of online graduate nursing education: An integrative literature review. *Journal of Nursing Education, 51*(10), 570–576.

Jeffries, P. R. (2005). A framework for designing, implementing, and evaluating simulations used as teaching strategies in nursing. *Nursing Education Perspectives, 26*(2), 96–103.

Jones, D. P., & Wolf, D. M. (2010). Shaping the future of nursing education today using distant education and technology. *ABNF Journal, 21*(2), 44–47.

Kala, S., Isaramalai, S., & Pohthong, A. (2010). Electronic learning and constructivism: A model for nursing education. *Nurse Education Today, 30*, 61–66.

Klein, K., & Kientz, M. (2013). A model for successful use of student response systems. *Nursing Education Perspectives, 34*(5), 334.

Lucas, L. (2010). Partnering to enhance the nursing curriculum: electronic medical record accessibility. *Clinical Simulation in Nursing, 6*, e97–e102.

Mazoue, J. G. (2013). The MOCC model: Challenging traditional education. *EDUCAUSE Review Online.*

Moodle. (2014). *Moodle home.* Retrieved from http://moodle.org/about

Onello, R., & Regan, M. (2013). Challenges in high fidelity simulation: Risk sensitization and outcome measurement. *Online Journal of Nursing, 18*(3).

Reese, C., Jeffries, P., & Engum, S. (2010). Learning together: Using simulations to develop nursing and medical student collaboration. *Nursing Education Perspectives, 31*(1), 33–37.

Revatis, M., & Egger, S. (2013). FaceTime: A virtual pathway between research and practice. *Nurse Educator, 38*(5), 186–187.

Skiba, D. (2009). Emerging technologies center. Teaching with and about technology: Providing resources for nurse educators worldwide. *Nursing Education Perspectives, 30*(4), 255–256.

Skype. (2014). *About Skype.* Retrieved from http://www.skype.com/en

Spielberger, C. D., Gorsuch, R. L., Lushene, R. E., Vagg, P. R., & Jacobs, G. A. (1983). *State-trait anxiety inventory for adults.* Menlo Park, CA: Mind Garden.

Technology Informatics Guiding Education Reform. (2009). *TIGER Informatics Competencies Collaborative (TICC). Final Report.* Retrieved from http://tigercompetencies. pbworks.com/f/TICC_Final.pdf

Tuomi, I. (2013). Open educational resources and the transformation of education. *European Journal of Education, 48*(1), 58–78.

U.S. Department of Education, Office of Planning, Evaluation, and Policy Development. (2009). *Evaluation of evidence-based practices in online learning:* A Meta-analysis and review of online learning studies. Washington, DC: Author.

Wimba. (2014). *Wimba classroom.* Retrieved from http://www.wimba.com/solutions/ highereducation/wimba_classroom_for_higher_education

CHAPTER 19

Research and Evidence-Based Practice in Nursing Education

Sarah B. Keating

OBJECTIVES

Upon completion of Chapter 19, the reader will be able to:

1. Deliberate on the faculty role in scholarship, translational science, and research in nursing education and its influence on curriculum development and evaluation, evidence-based practice in nursing, health care policy, and delivery of care
2. Analyze current research in nursing education that applies to curriculum development and evaluation
3. Identify topics needing investigation and research in curriculum development and evaluation based on the National League for Nursing's (NLN) recommendations for research in nursing education

OVERVIEW

Nursing faculty have three major roles in academe: teaching, scholarship/research, and service. This chapter examines the roles of scholar and researcher as they apply to nursing faculty. A scholar reviews the current state of knowledge in the discipline and applies that knowledge to practice, while at the same time observing phenomena in practice (nursing and education) that need further investigation, searching for the truths that surround them, and bringing them to the attention of others for further study and research if indicated. Scholars share these observations with others through reflection, discussion, debate, and writing scholarly papers/articles that are based on evidence surrounding the topic. Their scholarly works should lead to research that generates new knowledge and builds the sciences of the profession and education.

Researchers likewise observe the environment, raise questions about phenomena and, by exploring the factors surrounding them, ask questions that merit further investigation. The research questions generate inquiries and/or hypotheses that result in proposals for investigation. They require in-depth literature reviews to identify concepts and theories that relate to the topic and help to shape the nature of the proposed research from a pilot study to in-depth studies that include qualitative, quantitative, and mixed-methodology approaches. Faculty members in research-focused programs are usually expected to engage in research, and although it usually holds higher value than scholarly activities, both are respected. Faculty members in multipurpose institutions are not held to as high expectations for research but scholarly activities and research are still part of their academic responsibilities. Research and scholarship competencies play into the responsibilities associated with faculty positions when tenure and promotion are under consideration. Nursing faculty seeking teaching positions need to investigate the institution's policies on scholarship and research prior to accepting a position in order to be aware of the expectations of the institution.

Bridging scholarship and research is translational science that applies research and leads to evidence-based practice. It crosses all disciplines and hence leads to interdisciplinary collaboration and evidence-based practice based on the newest breakthroughs and research in science and, specifically for nursing, in health care, nursing, and education. It plays an increasingly important role in its contributions to nursing practice and specifically to the professional doctorate role (doctor of nursing practice [DNP]). Chapter 19 examines the role of nursing faculty in nursing education research and scholarly activities, reviews the literature related to nursing education and indications for further study, and lists possible topics for investigation that relate to curriculum development and evaluation.

FACULTY ROLE IN NURSING EDUCATION RESEARCH

Faculty Qualifications

Although the National Council for State Boards of Nursing (NCSBN, 2009) recommends that nursing faculty have at least a master's degree to teach in nursing programs and preparation in pedagogy as well as the science of nursing, the faculty shortage in some states resulted in the necessity to hire clinically experienced baccalaureate-prepared nurses. To ameliorate this situation, administrators, faculty peers, and the individual faculty member have a responsibility to support baccalaureate-prepared faculty (and master's-prepared faculty) to complete advanced degrees including the master's and/or doctorate. At the same time, doctorally prepared faculty members are encouraged to further their postgraduate scholarly work by becoming certified as nurse educators, continuing their clinically focused research, and conducting research related to nursing education, that is, curriculum development, evaluation, and instructional design and strategies.

Importance to Personal Professional Development

Depending on faculty's educational preparation and experience, it is expected that they engage in scholarship that relates to their expert knowledge and serves as content expertise for sharing with students in the teaching/learning process.

In addition to content expertise, educators should have knowledge and skills in the art of teaching and learning, student assessment, and program development and evaluation. Each individual should conduct a personal assessment of these knowledge foundations and skills and identify those that need updating, strengthening, or assimilating.

Notwithstanding personal motivation, need, and responsibility for scholarship and research activities, support for these activities is also a responsibility of the academic administration and the institution. Released time, costs for attendance at professional meetings and conferences, and in some cases, tuition for advanced degree or specialty certifications are included as employment benefits. Many research-focused institutions expect faculty to generate studies that will fund not only research activities, but also the individual faculty position, which is bought out by replacing the faculty member's teaching assignments with adjunct faculty for the duration of the funding. As Roberts and Glod (2013) point out, nursing faculty in research-focused institutions face the dilemma of meeting teaching responsibilities but at the same time, those in tenured or tenure-track positions are expected to produce scholarship and research to either retain or gain tenure. Their research activities take away from assigned clinical and theory teaching responsibilities, leaving those activities to adjunct faculty who have the clinical expertise and knowledge, but not necessarily the time for scholarship. This results in a two-tier faculty system that can affect the curriculum, student learning and program outcomes, and faculty morale.

Faculty in schools of nursing based in non-research-focused institutions has a responsibility for scholarship, evidence-based practice, and research as well. For those without the terminal degree required for the discipline or faculty position qualifications, enrolling in and completing the required degree is an expectation. It is hoped that the employer will support this activity through released or flexible time and, in some cases, tuition support. In addition, to maintain the curriculum's currency and relevance, faculty must engage in scholarly activities that keep them updated and enriched in their content and pedagogical knowledge base and skills. Attending workshops and conferences in education and the clinical specialty should be an expectation, and the school should include support for faculty development to update educational skills. Research activities are not precluded in these institutions and have an important role for educators to advance their knowledge in nursing and education and to contribute to the science of the discipline. Since financial support and released time might not be as available as in research-focused institutions, collaborative research among faculty members, other disciplines, practice colleagues, and other schools of nursing offer scholarly opportunities for faculty.

Martin and Hodge (2011) describe their experience in developing a research model for faculty to meet the scholarship and research expectations in a non-research-focused institution. The authors list the expectations for faculty in their school and describe how a model for mentoring faculty research was implemented. Major components of the model included, among others, administrative support and a culture of support for scholarship and research, assigned time for research, goal setting and clear expectations, the mentorship and collaboration of other faculty, and external resources. Klemm (2012) described a research project that took place in an undergraduate research course. Throughout the semester, a faculty member acted as mentor for the students to study women's adjustment to breast cancer. The qualitative research experience was successful with students learning about the research process as well as participating in a faculty member's research through the collection and analysis of data.

An issue in nursing research when students conduct independent research, usually for thesis or dissertation purposes or when they assist faculty with the faculty's research, is the authorship of scholarly works resulting from the research. Welfare and Sackett (2011) surveyed faculty and students at research-intensive institutions to study their beliefs about authorship of research findings when students assisted faculty or conducted independent research. Welfare and Sackett developed case scenarios that described student research activities from collecting data and analysis to collaborative or independent research. They found differences between students' and faculty's perceptions about authorship and the order of the list of authors. While the instrument they developed was checked for content validity, the authors point out that similar studies using the tool should be conducted for validity and reliability of the tool. However, their findings brought forth many recommendations including an understanding or contract between faculty and student prior to initiating the research. They refer to student and faculty responsibilities and eventual authorship as listed by several professional organizations, which have guidelines and principles of ethical conduct (American Psychological Association [APA], 2014; Association for the Study of Higher Education [ASHE], 2014). With the growth of doctoral programs and research in nursing, this becomes a pressing issue to address for the profession, educators, and students.

The Scholarship of Teaching and Application to Nursing

Conducting research or earning an advanced degree in one's own clinical or functional area of nursing lends credence to the faculty member's knowledge and skills in that specialty and contributes to the curriculum's currency in nursing science and practice. At the same time, adding to the knowledge base of learning theories, pedagogy, student assessment, and program development and evaluation is equally as important. Boyer's theory of scholarship in teaching (1990) comes to mind with its four components that promote faculty's application of teaching activities to research and scholarship. The four components are the scholarship of *discovery, integration, application,* and *teaching* and are succinctly described by Boyer in his *Scholarship Reconsidered* document. The model provides a framework for faculty as they carry out their activities in teaching and search for scholarship and research opportunities. Such activities contribute to the disciplines of nursing and education, and research findings when disseminated and translated can lead to evidence-based practice in the art of curriculum development, evaluation, and teaching and learning.

Briefly, Boyer (1990) describes the scholarship of *discovery* as those activities that result in the generation of new knowledge from experiences and phenomena observed while developing and evaluating programs and during the interactions and delivery of teaching and learning between the educator and the student. The scholar studies the new knowledge discovered and tests it for its usefulness and application to practice. The scholarship of *integration* is the summation of activities and interactions that occur in the educational environment and cause the educator to observe and synthesize the information into new approaches and knowledge. It is closely related to discovery and Boyer makes the case for its application to interdisciplinary studies, an issue that nursing has long been affiliated with but not always successful in carrying out. The scholarship of *application* refers to the application of new knowledge to teaching activities to test it for validity and reliability. It is evidence-based practice and deserves to be tested, studied for its relevance, and perfected as it evolves. Translational science has a close relationship to this concept. *Teaching* as scholarship is a way of viewing the activity as a scholarly pursuit for sharing knowledge with the learner and discovering new knowledge and ways of applying it to the sciences of nursing and education.

Examples of the application of Boyer's model to nursing education can be found in the American Association of Colleges of Nursing's (AACN) *Defining Scholarship for the Discipline of Nursing* paper (AACN, 1999). The definition of nursing scholarship that helps to guide nursing educators' research and scholarship is as follows:

> Scholarship in nursing can be defined as those activities that systematically advance the teaching, research, and practice of nursing through rigorous inquiry that 1) is significant to the profession, 2) is creative, 3) can be documented, 4) can be replicated or elaborated, and 5) can be peer-reviewed through various methods. (AACN, 1999)

Using Boyer's (1990) and the AACN's (1999) models for nursing research, scholarship, and translational science as they apply to curriculum development and evaluation, the following fictional examples are offered to illustrate opportunities for faculty research and scholarship. *Discovery* occurred when members of a curriculum committee analyzed accelerated bachelor of science in nursing (BSN) and basic BSN graduates' and their employers' ratings of clinical performance. The findings indicated that for the most part, employers' and accelerated BSN ratings of performance were similar ($P < .001$), while basic BSN graduates rated their performance as lower than their employers' ratings ($P < .001$). Based on these findings, several members of the committee agreed to investigate the findings by randomly selecting 10 representatives from each class and interviewing the graduates and their employers to identify what factors in their curricula, demographics, and academic records influenced these differences. Depending on the results, revisions of the curriculum or changes in instructional strategies would be recommended.

Integration opportunities occurred during a semester when medical, nurse practitioner, and pharmacy students worked together in a standardized patient-learning lab. The disciplines were brought together to practice in a case scenario of an elderly patient, recently widowed and presenting with multiple chronic disease diagnoses. Instructors from the three disciplines supervised their discipline-specific students. In the process, both students and instructors identified crossovers of knowledge and skills among the three types of professions. This effect brought about some confusion to the standardized patient, students, and faculty. Based on the situation, the faculty team decided to review the literature in the disciplines and in interprofessional science to identify other studies conducted, and to invite other faculty from other disciplines to review the case scenario and observe the interactions that occurred during the student practice sessions. Based on the findings, the faculty developed several models of interdisciplinary education and practice to test in a scenario. As numbers of participants grew as well as enthusiasm, the group decided to apply for a grant to support the project and the research related to it.

The scholarship of *application* took place in a doctor of nursing practice program when faculty and students studied the process of influencing health care policy as it applied to state legislation and regulations related to the definition and regulation of nursing practice. Both advanced practice and nursing administration students raised the issue of independent practice for nurses in their state in an analysis of health care policy course. Through an integrated review of the literature, analysis of other states' legislative history on the issue, and meetings with legislators, other stakeholders, professional organization representatives, and possible adversaries, the students and faculty developed a plan of action to bring about change. The plan was carried out and proved to be successful in bringing about legislative and regulatory changes. Analyses of the literature and detailed records of their processes and actions were documented and resulted in authorship of articles in refereed professional journals as well as presentations for other nursing groups and organizations across the country.

Teaching scholarship was illustrated in an associate degree in nursing program when faculty members were in the process of curriculum revision. The school of nursing recently received a fully furnished simulation lab for clinical skills including several high-fidelity mannequins (an infant, child, and adult) as a gift from an anonymous benefactor. The gift meant that instructional strategies for acquiring clinical skills and their application to practice would change with the implication that the curriculum's courses would need realignment. The curriculum committee members and the faculty teaching clinical skills met to review the needs for integrating the new lab into the plan of study. A task force was assigned to review the literature for curriculum development/revision models and instructional strategies for the use of simulation labs. Several instructional models were identified that would be tested and compared for the best fit to the school's curriculum. A research proposal for comparing the models was developed and approved by the institution's insitutional review board (IRB). The faculty involved in the change and those teaching in the skills lab reported on results from the study to the faculty as a whole. The curriculum plan of study was revised and plans were in place for formative and summative evaluations of the revision. The process for curriculum revision was described and the evaluation findings were summarized in an article published in a refereed professional journal. Although these are fictional scenarios, they provide ideas for research and scholarship activities that nursing faculty can generate and participate in to meet scholarship expectations of the faculty role.

Importance to the Profession

Nursing faculty scholarship, translational science, and research contributions to the profession are innumerable. Clinical specialty and functional areas (administration, quality assurance, risk management, epidemiology, etc.) translational science, and research lead to evidence-based practice in the health care setting. Collaborative research with nursing colleagues and other health disciplines in the health care setting fosters positive patient outcomes, quality/safe health care, and changes in health care policy. An example of interprofessional collaboration and research occurred at Columbia University. The social media interactions of PhD and DNP students and faculty during one semester were studied by Merrill, Yoon, Larson, Honig, and Reame (2013). Merrill et al. described the curriculum enhancements that were added during the study, which included required seminar meetings during the time of the study and the PhD and DNP students took two courses together (Ethics and Quantitative Statistics). The students' and faculty's utilization of social networks among themselves during the semester was collected. It was found that during the first week, most communications occurred among faculty but by the end of the study (10 weeks later), the number of interactions and their distribution among the groups increased. This was one of the first studies to use social networks as a source of information and also to analyze relationships between doctoral students and faculty.

Research in nursing education allows for the sharing of best practices in the delivery of nursing education and types of programs that produce graduates ready for practice in the health care system. Scholarship, translational science, and research findings contribute to the profession's advocacy for higher education for nursing to meet the health care needs of the populace and to assume leadership roles in the health care delivery system. Research helps to identify the types of educational programs best suited to levels of responsibility in the health care system and the role of nursing.

CURRENT RESEARCH IN THE LITERATURE ON CURRICULUM DEVELOPMENT AND EVALUATION

Curriculum Development and Revision

Throughout the update of this textbook the author and contributors reviewed the literature for classic and current research and studies in curriculum development in nursing. Many of these studies focused on one program and can serve as pilots for further research to be generalized across types and levels of program and geographical areas. Table 19.1 lists some of the references reviewed in this text that relate to curriculum development. As one can see, additional research-based studies are needed that can inform faculty as they consider revising existing curricula or developing new programs.

TABLE 19.1 STUDIES THAT APPLY TO CURRICULUM DEVELOPMENT

TOPIC	AUTHOR(S)/DATES	TYPE OF PROGRAM	TYPE OF STUDY	RECOMMENDATIONS
		PRELICENSURE		
National surveys of undergraduate programs to determine what physical examination skills are taught	Giddens, Wright, & Grey, 2012	Prelicensure	National survey of prelicensure programs	Replicate for changes in curricula, program outcomes, effect on patient care. Replicate through concept analyses of other specific concepts, e.g., patient safety, cultural competence, etc.
	UNDERGRADUATE ADN, BSN, SECOND-DEGREE BSN, RN TO BSN			
A curriculum development model using learning as central for all stakeholders; response to the NLN's call for curricular transformation	Davis, 2011	ADN	Description of the curricular change process using ta curriculum development model	Utilize the model and analyze its effectiveness in curricular revision for similar programs. Compare to other models and programs.
Changes in curricula to include evidence-based practice, quality, improvement approaches, safety standards, competency frameworks, informatics, and interdisciplinary education	Andre & Barnes, 2010	BSN	Review of curricular needs	Analyze concepts in the curriculum. Comparisons among programs for content and outcomes. Efficacy of instructional strategies among programs.
Shared decision-making model for curriculum revision	D'Antonio, Brennan, & Curley, 2013	BSN	Description of the curricular change process using the model	Utilize the model and analyze the effectiveness in curricular revision for similar programs. Compare to other models and programs.

(*continued*)

TABLE 19.1	STUDIES THAT APPLY TO CURRICULUM DEVELOPMENT (*continued*)			
TOPIC	AUTHOR(S)/DATES	TYPE OF PROGRAM	TYPE OF STUDY	RECOMMENDATIONS
Process for mapping an undergraduate program to the AACN *Essentials*	Dearman, Larson, & Hall, 2011	BSN	Process and how the model tied into NCLEX success rates	Review the literature for similar models, apply the model to several programs and compare results according to student demographics, type of program, student learning outcomes, curricular differences, etc.
A model for integrating technology into the curriculum based on a review of the literature	Flood, Gasiewicz, & Delpier, 2010	BSN	Review of the literature and model development	Replicate for generalizability
Management of curricular content to avoid content saturation; encourages concept teaching	Giddens & Brady, 2007	BSN	Literature review	Compare geographically representative and varying types of curricula that are concept–based and taught in other types of curricula and teaching strategies
Description of a model residency program and its outcomes that resulted in increased confidence, competence, leadership, etc.	Goode, Lynn, & McElroy, 2013	BSN Residency	Evaluation of student learning outcomes	Replicate for validity, reliability, and generalizability
Cognitive scaffolding model for curricular revision. (task, metacognitive, and sociocommunicative)	Hagler, Morris, & White, 2011	BSN	Description of the curricular change process using the scaffolding model	Utilize the model and analyze the effectiveness in curricular revision in similar programs. Compare to other models and programs.

(*continued*)

TABLE 19.1 STUDIES THAT APPLY TO CURRICULUM DEVELOPMENT (*continued*)

TOPIC	AUTHOR(S)/DATES	TYPE OF PROGRAM	TYPE OF STUDY	RECOMMENDATIONS
Faculty and students who champion curricular change also facilitate implementation of the change	Powell-Cope, Sedlak, & Nelson, 2008	BSN	Survey of faculty perceptions	Compare geographically representative and varying types of curricula
A model for arranging clinical experience agreements between health care agencies and schools of nursing including cost factors	DeGeest et al., 2010	Predominantly BSN	Description of a model when complex factors must be taken into account; includes cost and personnel factors	Utilize the model to demonstrate its validity and reliability and to compare to other models and programs. Study its effectiveness for program planning
Incorporating technology into the curriculum from low- to high-fidelity technology; extent to how it will be used, resources, and faculty development	Skiba, 2012; Thompson, & Skiba, 2008	Predominantly BSN	Recommendation for integrating technology into curriculum when undergoing change	Conduct studies to demonstrate student learning outcomes using various technologies. Surveys of schools for levels of integration of technology in the curricula and effects on student learning outcomes and patient care.
Comparison of second-degree and traditional graduates	Brewer, Kovner, Poornima, Fairchild, Kim, & Djukic, 2009	Second-degree and traditional BSN	Survey of employers of BSN, traditional and second degree	Replicate for validity, reliability, and generalizability and investigate for factors that lead to differences
Managers' perceptions of second-degree graduates' clinical skills; comparison of managers' and graduates' perceptions of performance	Rafferty & Lindell, 2011; Regan & Pietrobon, 2010; Ziehm, Cunningham, Fontaine, & Scherzer, 2011	Second-degree BSN	Survey of nurse managers of graduates	Replicate for reliability and validity and investigate for factors influencing perceptions, and generalizability

(*continued*)

| TABLE 19.1 | STUDIES THAT APPLY TO CURRICULUM DEVELOPMENT (*continued*) |

TOPIC	AUTHOR(S)/DATES	TYPE OF PROGRAM	TYPE OF STUDY	RECOMMENDATIONS
Managers' perceptions of second-degree graduates' performance and retention rates	Weathers & Hunt Raleigh, 2013	Second-degree BSN	Survey of nurse managers of graduates	Replicate for reliability and validity and investigate for factors influencing perceptions, and generalizability
Experiences of second-degree BSNs	Penprase & Koczara, 2009	Second-degree BSN	Survey of students	Replicate for generalizability
A model to examine the Q (quality), P (potential), and C (cost) (QPC) of programs to compare disciplines from a cost-benefit perspective	Booker & Hilgenberg, 2010	RN to BSN	Description of a cost analysis model to compare disciplines	Utilize the model to demonstrate its validity and reliability and to compare to other models and disciplines/ programs; study its effectiveness for program planning
RN to BSN and BSN students' perceptions of the value of liberal arts to nursing	DeBrew, 2010	RN to BSN and BSN	Comparison of survey results	Replicate for reliability and validity and investigate for factors influencing perceptions, and generalizability
INTERDISCIPLINARY				
An interdisciplinary program for health sciences students to share patient-centered care and learn about other disciplines	Dacey, Anderson, & McCloskey, 2010	Undergraduate Interdisciplinary	Description of the program and outcomes	Utilize the curriculum to compare for similarities. Compare to other programs, geographical locations, types of students and programs, and measure student outcomes.
Measure students' interprofessional attitudes across medicine, nursing, and pharmacy	Sheu et al., 2012	Interdisciplinary	Mixed qualitative and qualitative on student interprofessional attitudes	Replicate for reliability and validity and investigate for factors influencing attitudes, and generalizability

(*continued*)

TABLE 19.1   STUDIES THAT APPLY TO CURRICULUM DEVELOPMENT (*continued*)

TOPIC	AUTHOR(S)/DATES	TYPE OF PROGRAM	TYPE OF STUDY	RECOMMENDATIONS
ENTRY-LEVEL MASTER'S				
Special needs and socialization of entry-level master of science in nursing (MSN) students	Klich-Hartt, 2010	Entry-level MSN	Review of the literature	Update review of literature; survey students in the programs for validation with representative sample; investigate support programs and their success; replicate
Entry-level MSN students' lived experiences	McNeisch, 2011	Entry-level MSN	Qualitative survey of students	Investigate factors apply to larger sample size and varying geographical areas
MASTER'S				
A master's program that presents leadership theories to advanced practice nurses as well as those in leadership to apply in the health care system	Aduddell & Dorman, 2010	MSN	Description of the program and outcomes	Utilize the curriculum or compare for similarities; compare to other programs, geographical locations, types of students and programs, and measure student outcomes
A master's level curriculum that prepares nurse leaders to deliver culturally diverse and linguistic services in the health care system	Comer, Whichcello, & Neubrander, 2014	MSN	Description of the curriculum and report on outcomes	Integrate the model into comparable program curricula and measure outcomes and compare across programs, student demographics, and geographical locations
Conceptual model for integrating scholarly writing across the curriculum	Regan & Pietrobon, 2010	Graduate	Model uses rhetoric, ethnographic, recognition, and practice principles	Apply the model and measure outcomes; compare across programs

(*continued*)

TABLE 19.1	STUDIES THAT APPLY TO CURRICULUM DEVELOPMENT (continued)			
TOPIC	AUTHOR(S)/DATES	TYPE OF PROGRAM	TYPE OF STUDY	RECOMMENDATIONS
		DOCTORAL PROGRAMS		
Curriculum content for research-focused degrees	Anderson, 2000	Doctoral	Analysis of the content of research-focused programs to include: body of nursing knowledge, research, and preparation for teaching role	Conduct a national survey and content analysis of research and practice doctoral programs and the use of frameworks to guide curricula; compare between the types
A description of the intention of the practice doctorate for postmaster's and BSN to DNP programs	Grey, 2013	DNP	Description and need for studies that compare BSN to DNP and postmaster's DNPs to compare to original intent(s) of the DNP	Conduct comparative studies of curricula, program outcomes, and graduates' practice across geographical locations, types of programs, and types of students

Curriculum and Program Evaluation

Table 19.2 summarizes studies that were found to be related to curriculum and program evaluation research and provides recommendation for further study. Few studies were found that applied directly to nursing education program evaluation, indicating the need for testing of evaluation models, especially in light of the emphasis on the measurement of program outcomes and student learning outcomes. Nursing may need to borrow from other disciplines to find and adapt evaluation models appropriate to nursing education and to compare models, theories, and concepts in evaluation as they apply to nursing.

TABLE 19.2	STUDIES THAT APPLY TO PROGRAM AND CURRICULUM EVALUATION			
TOPIC	AUTHOR(S)/DATES	TYPE OF PROGRAM	TYPE OF STUDY	RECOMMENDATIONS
		ALL TYPES		
A model of evaluation	DeSilets, 2010	All types of educational programs	Descriptive	Test model and compare
Model for strategic planning	Harmon, Fontaine, Plews-Ogan, & Williams, 2012	All types of schools of nursing	Descriptive	Test model and compare

(continued)

TABLE 19.2	STUDIES THAT APPLY TO PROGRAM AND CURRICULUM EVALUATION (*continued*)			
TOPIC	**AUTHOR(S)/DATES**	**TYPE OF PROGRAM**	**TYPE OF STUDY**	**RECOMMENDATIONS**
Three C's model of evaluation	Kalb, 2009	All types of schools of nursing	Descriptive	Test model and compare
Summative evaluation of technology outcomes	Newhouse, 2011	All types of educational programs	Comparison of digital measures to written assessment tools applied to technology	Test model and compare
Measurement of program/ student learning outcomes	Praslova, 2010	All types of educational programs	Descriptive	Test model and compare
Combined program evaluation and evaluation research	Spillane et al., 2010	Secondary schools but applicable to all	Mixed methodologies (quantitative, qualitative, and triangulation)	Check reliability and validity of tools; replicate across different types of programs
ASSOCIATE DEGREE/COMMUNITY COLLEGES				
Models of Program Evaluation	Bers, 2011	Associate Degree	Descriptive	Review for models to test, report of model, compare utilization of models across geographical areas and types and levels of educational programs
GRADUATE PROGRAMS				
Description of models of evaluation to measure outcomes in schools of nursing	Horne & Sandmann, 2012	Graduate nursing programs	Integrative review of the literature	Review for models to test, report of model, compare utilization of models across geographical areas and types and levels of educational programs
Benchmarks and trends for DNP programs	Udlis & Manusco, 2012	DNP programs	National survey of DNP programs	Replicate. Investigate identified characteristics and benchmarks

Research Topics that Apply to Curriculum Development and Evaluation

The NLN provides nursing educators with a list of priorities for research for 2012 through 2015 (NLN, 2014). The three major priorities include (a) Leading Reform in Nursing Education, (b) Advancing the Science of Nursing Education, and (c) Developing National and International Leaders in Nursing Education. For the purposes of this chapter, research and scholarship ideas are presented as they apply to curriculum development and evaluation and are based on the NLN's list of priorities for the advancement of the science of nursing education. Please note that the NLN priorities are italicized and that the suggested lists of ideas are not meant to be inclusive.

Evaluation of new curriculum models related to interprofessional education and practice.

1. Integrated review of the literature for programs/curricula that report on interprofessional education and practice.
2. Replicating and testing educational models from the list generated from the review of the literature across representative geographical areas, types of program (associate degree in nursing [ADN] through doctoral), and types of institution (private or public).

Identification of the effectiveness of clinical residency programs in facilitating transitions in practice.

1. Review of the literature for reports on clinical residency programs' effectiveness across all types of programs (ADN through doctoral, and types of institutions: private or public)
2. National survey and analysis of findings from schools of nursing that provide residencies
3. Replicating and testing residency models for comparisons of their effectiveness for graduates' practice and employers' satisfaction

Development and evaluation of partnerships for studies linking simulated learning experiences with program outcomes and graduate competencies.

1. Follow-up studies to measure graduates' and their employers' satisfaction with practice competencies and comparison to graduates not experiencing simulated learning experiences
2. Surveys of patient, student, and faculty satisfaction following simulated clinical experiences compared to nonsimulated laboratory practice experiences
3. Replication of studies to measure validity and reliability of tools to measure student learning outcomes and satisfaction with simulated experiences

Measurement of the cost-effectiveness of technologies, for example, online, simulation, videoconferencing, etc. used to expand capacity in nursing education.

1. Integrative review of the literature for reports and studies on the measurement of cost-effectiveness and models for the study of technology applications to nursing education (note: not exclusive to nursing literature).

2. Testing of models from the literature for measuring cost-effectiveness across geographical areas, types of programs, and types of institutions
3. Comparisons of the effect of technologies applied to nursing education on student enrollments and institution capacity

Identification of institutional characteristics that best contribute to the success of diverse national and international educators in academic settings.

1. National and international surveys of schools of nursing for international programs and exchange programs; analysis and classification of types of programs
2. Integrative review of the literature to identify international programs and their models of success
3. Replication, testing, and comparisons of international models for nursing education

Promote the development of multisite, multimethod research studies to determine suitable measures for the assessment of learning outcomes, particularly those relevant for a practice discipline.

1. Integrative review of the literature to identify studies that focus on the measurement of program/student learning outcomes
2. National survey of schools of nursing for measurement tools and studies related to learning/program outcomes
3. Analysis of the outcomes and measures to compare similarities and differences across geographical areas, types, and levels of programs

Identification of ways to measure the link between educational innovations and practice outcomes.

1. Comparisons of graduates' and employers' satisfaction and perceptions of clinical competencies from utilization of technologies, for example, simulations, and online education to those from traditional style programs
2. Replications of studies measuring student competencies and student, faculty, patient, and practice colleagues' satisfaction with educational innovations

Examination of innovative program evaluation models.

1. Integrative review of the literature for models of evaluation that apply to nursing education and curricula
2. Testing and replication of program evaluation models across geographical areas, types, and levels of nursing education programs

Identification and testing of valid and reliable instruments for educational research.

1. Integrative review of the literature for identification of reliable and valid instruments for measuring curriculum and program outcomes

2. Replication of studies that claim reliability and validity representative of the population and types of program under study and that can be generalized

Evaluation of effectiveness of new and existing doctoral education models that have been designed to ensure that graduates acquire competency in evidence-based pedagogy.

1. Update of national surveys of doctoral programs for content related to curriculum development and evaluation and pedagogies
2. Survey of recent graduates of doctoral programs for their experience and education in pedagogy, plans for teaching, and application of education type courses to the employment setting
3. Comparisons of types of doctoral program graduates' employment history, research and scholarship productivity, and impact on health care policy

SUMMARY

Chapter 19 reviewed the qualifications expected for nursing faculty and the types of research, translational science, and scholarship activities expected of faculty according to type of institution. Descriptions of scholarship, research, and translational science activities were discussed. Examples of research possibilities were presented using Boyer's (1990) scholarship of teaching model. Additional ideas for research, translation of research, and scholarship in nursing education were listed under the NLN's (2014) priorities for research in nursing education. Two tables reviewed articles from the literature found throughout this text that merit further investigation or replication.

DISCUSSION QUESTIONS

1. In your opinion, what is the major factor that interferes with faculty's role in scholarship and research? What strategies do you suggest to resolve the issue?
2. Differentiate between scholarship, translational science, and research as they apply to the faculty role. Give examples for each.

LEARNING ACTIVITIES

STUDENT LEARNING ACTIVITIES

Divide your class into four groups based on Boyer's (1990) concepts on the scholarship of teaching (discovery, integration, application, and teaching) and provide at least two examples for each. Describe how you would carry out each project including personnel, costs, and time commitment. Present your examples to the total group and critique them according to their rigor, practicality, and contribution to nursing education science.

NURSE EDUCATOR/FACULTY DEVELOPMENT ACTIVITIES

Identify a researchable problem in your practice as a nurse educator. Share it with a colleague and discuss the problem, refine it into a research statement and hypotheses, if indicated. Discuss an appropriate review of the literature, a conceptual or theoretical framework for the study, and possible methodologies. Discuss how it could be funded and the time commitment required. Develop a plan to carry it out.

REFERENCES

Aduddell, K. A., & Dorman, G. E. (2010). The development of the next generation of nurse leaders. *Journal of Nursing Education, 49*(3), 168–171.

American Association of Colleges of Nursing. (1999). *Defining scholarship for the discipline of nursing.* Retrieved from https://www.aacn.nche.edu/publications/position/defining-scholarship

American Psychological Association. (2014). A graduate student's guide to determining authorship credit and authorship order. Retrieved from http://www.apa.org/science/leadership/students/authorship-paper.aspx

Anderson, C. A. (2000). Current strengths and limitations of doctoral education in nursing: Are we prepared for the future? *Journal of Professional Nursing, 16,* 191–200.

Andre, K., & Barnes, L. (2010). Creating a 21st century nursing workforce: Designing a bachelor of nursing program in response to the health reform agenda. *Nurse Education Today, 30*(3), 258–263.

Association for the Study of Higher Education. (2014). ASHE Principles of ethical content. Retrieved from http://www.ashe.ws/?page=180

Bers, T. (2011). Program review and institutional effectiveness. *New Directions for Community Colleges, 152,* 63–73.

Booker, K., & Hilgenberg, C. (2010). Analysis of academic programs: Comparing nursing and other university majors in the application of a quality, potential, and cost model. *Professional Nursing, 26,* 201–206.

Boyer, E. L. (1990). *Scholarship reconsidered: Priorities of the professoriate.* Princeton, NJ: The Carnegie Foundation for the Advancement of Learning. Retrieved from http://depts.washington.edu/gs630/Spring/Boyer.pdf

Brewer, C. S., Kovner, C. T., Poornima, S., Fairchild, S., Kim, H., & Djukic, M. (2009). A comparison of second-degree baccalaureate and traditional-baccalaureate new graduate RNs: Implications for the workforce. *Journal of Professional Nursing, 25*(1), 5–14.

Comer, L., Whichcello, R., & Neubrander, J. (2013). An innovative master of science program for the development of culturally competent nursing leaders. *Journal of Cultural Diversity, 20*(2), 89–93.

Dacey, M., Murphy, J. I., Anderson, D. C., & McCloskey, W. W. (2010). An interprofessional service-learning course: Uniting students across educational levels and promoting patient-centered care. *Journal of Nursing Education, 49*(12), 696–699.

D'Antonio, P. O., Brennan, A. M. W., & Curley, M. A. Q. (2013). Judgment, inquiry, engagement, voice: Reenvisioning an undergraduate nursing curriculum using a shared decision-making model. *Journal of Professional Nursing, 29*(6), 407–413.

Davis, B. W. (2011). A conceptual model to support curriculum review, revision, and design in an associate degree nursing program. *Nursing Education Perspectives, 32*(6), 389–394.

Dearman, V., Lawson, R., & Hall, H. R. (2011). Concept mapping a baccalaureate nursing program: A method for success. *Journal of Nursing Education, 50*(11), 656–659.

DeBrew, J. K. (2010). Perceptions of liberal education of two types of nursing graduates: The essentials of baccalaureate education for professional nursing practice. *The Journal of General Education, 59,* 42–58.

De Geest, S., Sullivan Marx, E. M., Rich, V., Spichiger, E., Schwendimann, R., & Spirig, R., & Van Malderen, G. (2010). Developing a financial framework for academic service partnerships: Models of the United States and Europe. *Journal of Professional Scholarship, 42*(3), 295–304.

DeSilets, L. (2010). Another look at evaluation models. *Journal of Continuing Education in Nursing, 41*(1), 12–13.

Flood, L., Gasiewicz, N., & Delpier, T. (2010). Integrating information literacy across a BSN curriculum. *Journal of Nursing Education, 49*(2), 101–104.

Giddens, J. F., & Brady, D. P. (2007). Rescuing nursing education from content saturation: The case for a concept-based curriculum. *Journal of Nursing Education, 46*(2), 65–69.

Giddens, J. F., Wright, M., & Gray, I. (2012). Selecting concepts for a concept-based curriculum: Application of a benchmark approach. *Journal of Nursing Education, 51*(9), 511–515.

Goode, C. J., Lynn, M. R., & McElroy, D. (2013). Lessons learned from 10 years of research on a post-baccalaureate nurse residency program. *Journal of Nursing Administration, 13*(2), 73–79.

Grey, M. (2013). The doctor of nursing practice: Defining the next steps. *Journal of Nursing Education, 52*(8), 462–465.

Hagler, D., Morris, B., & White, B. (2011). Cognitive tools as a scaffold for faculty during curriculum redesign. *Journal of Nursing Education, 50*(7), 417–422.

Harmon, R. B., Fontaine, D., Plews-Ogan, M., & Williams, A. (2012). Achieving transformational change: Using appreciative inquiry for strategic planning in a school of nursing. *Professional Nursing, 28,* 119–124.

Horne, E. M., & Sandmann, L. R. (2012). Current trends in systematic program evaluation of online graduate nursing education: An integrative literature review. *Journal of Nursing Education, 51*(10), 570–576.

Kalb, K. (2009). The Three Cs Model: The context, content, and conduct of nursing education. *Nursing Education Perspectives, 30*(3), 176–180.

Klemm, P. (2012). Conducting nursing research with undergraduate students: A collaborative, participatory approach. *Nurse Educator, 17*(1), 10–11.

Klich-Heartt, E. I. (2010). Special needs of entry-level master's-prepared nurses from accelerated programs. *Nurse Leader, 8*(5), 52–54.

Martin, C., & Hodge, M. (2011). A nursing department faculty-mentored research project. *Nurse Educator, 36*(1), 35–39.

McNiesch, S. G. (2011). The lived experience of students in an accelerated nursing program: Intersecting factors that influence experiential learning. *The Journal of Nursing Education, 50*(4), 197–203.

Merrill, J. A., Yoon, S., Larson, E., Honig, J., & Reame, N. (2013). Using social network analysis to examine relationships among PhD and DNP student and faculty in a research-intensive university school of nursing. *Nursing Outlook, 61,* 109–116.

National Council of State Boards of Nursing. (2009). Report of findings from the effect of high-fidelity simulation on nursing students' knowledge and performance: A pilot study. NCSBN Research Brief, 40. Chicago, IL: Author.

National League for Nursing. (2014). NLN Research priorities in nursing education 2012-2015. Retrieved from http://www.nln.org/researchgrants/researchpriorities.pdf

Newhouse, C. P. (2011). Using IT to assess IT: Towards greater authenticity in summative performance assessment. *Computers & Education, 56,* 388–402.

Penprase, B., & Koczara, S. (2009). Understanding the experiences of accelerated second-degree nursing students and graduates: A review of the literature. *The Journal of Continuing Education in Nursing, 40*(2), 74–78.

Powell-Cope, G., Hughes, N. L., Sedlak, C., & Nelson, A. (2008). Faculty perceptions of implementing an evidence-based safe patient handling nursing curriculum module. *Online Journal of Issues in Nursing, 13* (3).

Praslova, L. (2010). Adaptation of Kirkpatrick's four level models of training criteria to assessment of learning outcomes and program evaluation in higher education. *Educational Assessment and Evaluation, 22,* 215–225.

Rafferty, M., & Lindell, D. (2011). How nurse managers rate the clinical competencies of accelerated (second-degree) nursing graduates. *Journal of Nursing Education, 50*(6), 355–357.

Regan, M., & Pietrobon, R. (2010). A conceptual framework for scientific writing in nursing. *Journal of Nursing Education, 49*(8), 437–443.

Roberts, S. J., & Glod, C. (2013). Faculty roles: Dilemmas for the future of nursing education. *Nursing Forum, 48*(2), 99–105.

Sheu, L., Lai, C. J., Coelho, A. D., Lin, L. D., Zheng, P., Hom, P., Diaz, V., & …O'Sullivan, P. S. (2010). Impact of student-run clinics on preclinical sociocultural and interprofessional attitudes: A prospective cohort analysis. *Journal of Health Care for the Poor and Underserved, 23*(3), 1058–1072.

Skiba, D. (2012). Technology and gerontology: Is this in your nursing curriculum? *Nursing Education Perspectives, 33*(3), 207–209.

Spillane, J. P., Pareja, S., Dorner, L., Barnes, C., May, H., Huff, J., & Camburn, E. (2010). Mixing methods in randomized controlled trials (RCTs): Validation, conceptualization, triangulation, and control. Education, *Assessment, Evaluation, Accountability, 22,* 5–28.

Thompson, B. W., & Skiba, D. J. (2008). Informatics in the nursing curriculum: A national survey of nursing informatics requirements in nursing curricula. *Nursing Education Perspectives, 29*(5), 312–317.

Udlis, K. A., & Manusco, J. M. (2012). Doctor of Nursing Practice programs across the United States: A benchmark of information. Part I: Program characteristics. *Journal of Professional Nursing, 28*(5), 265–273.

Weathers, S. M., & Hunt Raleigh, E. D. (2013). 1-year retention rates and performance ratings: Comparing associate degree, baccalaureate, and accelerated baccalaureate degree nurses. *Journal of Nursing Administration, 43*(9), 468–474.

Welfare, L. E., & Sackett, C. R. (2011). The authorship determination process in student–faculty collaborative research. *Journal of Counseling & Development, 89,* 479–487.

Ziehm, S. R., Uibel, I. C., Fontaine, D. K., & Scherzer, T. (2011). Success indicators for accelerated master's entry nursing program: Staff RN performance. *Journal of Nursing Education, 50*(7), 395–403.

Issues and Challenges for Nurse Educators

Sarah B. Keating

OBJECTIVES

Upon completion of Chapter 20, the reader will be able to:

1. Analyze the issues and challenges raised throughout the text that apply to curriculum development and evaluation
2. Consider some strategies for resolution of the issues raised and ways to meet the challenges with an eye to the future
3. Study the proposed parallel Unified Nursing Curriculum for its application to current and future unified nursing education programs

Chapter 20 summarizes the text and discusses trends, issues, and challenges raised throughout the text. It ends with a sample curriculum that progresses from the lower division level of higher education to the doctorate and features step out points along the way for nurses wishing to enter the workforce at various levels. It integrates some newer prerequisite courses from other disciplines to support the knowledge base for nursing in a complex and ever changing health care system. It continues the career ladder concept of nursing education so that its practitioners can enter subsequent levels of education without repeating previously learned knowledge and skills. At the same time, it promotes a nonstop, progressive curriculum for those who wish to enter at the doctorate level. It is a blueprint for an 8-year prenursing and nursing curriculum that graduates the student in 8 years with either a doctor of nursing practice (DNP) or a research and theory-building doctorate, that is, the PhD or doctor of nursing science (DNS). The author is the first to admit that it is not perfect. Its intent is to raise issues, provoke thought, and generate discussion for future planning.

CHAPTER 1: HISTORY OF NURSING EDUCATION IN THE UNITED STATES

Chapter 1 describes the history of nursing education as it moved from apprentice-type programs into higher education programs. The chapter raises many of the issues related to nursing's role in academe and its impact on the profession and entry into practice. The Institute of Medicine's (IOM) (2011) recommendation from *The Future of Nursing: Focus on Education* calls for nurses to be prepared at higher levels of education to meet the health care needs of the 21st century. In response, programs and enrollments in RN to bachelor of science in nursing (BSN) and RN to master of science in nursing (MSN) programs are expanding (American Association of Colleges of Nursing [AACN], 2014a). The explosion of DNP programs for advanced practice (AACN, 2014b), the recognition of the PhD and DNS as the discipline's research and theory-building degrees, the effect of health care legislation, and the impact of technology on the profession will be the major forces that influence continued evolvement of nursing in the 21st century.

CHAPTER 2: CURRICULUM DEVELOPMENT AND APPROVAL PROCESSES IN CHANGING EDUCATIONAL ENVIRONMENTS

Chapter 2 reviews the processes that schools of nursing undergo to bring about curriculum revision or develop new programs. Several issues related to curriculum development activities are raised including budgetary constraints and faculty shortages that result in turning away qualified applicants. As recommended by the AACN (2012), local and regional partnerships with health care facilities, foundations, and other stakeholders are possible solutions to relieving financial burdens.

The integration of technology into the curriculum challenges faculty to develop newer instructional strategies such as online classes, simulated laboratory experiences, electronic communications, and smart classrooms. The issue of content saturation must be confronted, else the temptation to crowd the curriculum beyond the point of reason will overwhelm students' learning capacity. Curriculum assessment and content analyses/maps help to identify areas of redundancies or content overload that lead to curriculum revision. Based on the assessment and evaluation, faculty can develop a curriculum that is up to date that guides and facilitates conceptual approaches to learning.

CHAPTER 3: THE ROLE OF FACULTY IN CURRICULUM DEVELOPMENT AND EVALUATION

Chapter 3 reviews the role of faculty in curriculum development and evaluation. Issues raised include the need for new, inexperienced faculty to be oriented to the curriculum and mentored by senior faculty. In the interest of expediency, many part-time and new faculty members are oriented to the particular course in which they teach but not to the total program, thus risking curriculum erosion and failure to meet planned student learning outcomes. The advantages and challenges related to orientation programs and mentorships are discussed and ideas for them are presented. The issue of the lack of pedagogical knowledge for many new master's and doctorally prepared faculty is raised. To meet this need, opportunities for faculty development through workshops, continuing education, and academic courses in education are discussed.

The importance of the role of faculty in curriculum development and evaluation is discussed. Faculty members have the responsibility to assess the curriculum and its implementation in order to identify need for revision. The necessity to include students and colleagues in practice for curriculum evaluation and development processes is discussed. Research topics and opportunities for study related to faculty role and responsibilities are considered.

CHAPTERS 4 AND 5: LEARNING THEORIES AND USING CONTEXTUAL CURRICULUM DESIGN WITH TAXONOMIES TO PROMOTE CRITICAL THINKING

Chapter 4 reviews six major categories of learning theories commonly accepted in today's education system and their application to nursing education. The rationale for analyzing learning theories and their relationship to instructional strategies for enhancing the student's ability to meet learning outcomes is explained. Combinations of learning theories depend on the faculty's philosophy of learning, the knowledge and skills to be imparted, the learning environment, and the students' and faculty's characteristics. Learning theories provide the foundation for the curriculum and its program goals. Issues that arise when considering learning theories include faculty conflicts related to individual philosophies of teaching and learning and the ability to respond to individual student learning needs when coping with heavy academic responsibilities. The challenge to faculty is to apply learning theories to curriculum designs that prepare nurses to meet the health needs of the people and the future health care delivery system.

Chapter 5 reviews the classic and newer educational taxonomies and domains of learning as they apply to nursing education. It continues with an overview of the development of critical thinking and the major role it plays in clinical decision making in nursing practice. Several models that apply the newer taxonomies to curriculum development and promote active learning are presented. Readers are challenged to use the Contextual Approach to Navigate Delivery of Outcomes (CANDO) when developing the curriculum. The model analyzes several theories including general systems, complexity, adult learning, and constructivism in light of external and internal program contexts. These analyzes result in the development of the end-of-program outcomes with the remaining components of the curriculum developed through the application of a backward design, that is, starting from the expected program outcomes to development of level and course objectives.

CHAPTERS 6 AND 7: A NEEDS ASSESSMENT MODEL FOR CURRICULUM DEVELOPMENT

Section III of this text introduces the Frame Factors model, a conceptual model that describes the major external and internal factors that influence, facilitate, or impinge upon the curriculum. Chapters 6 and 7 review the major components of a needs assessment that include analysis of these factors. While the principal activities of faculty in curriculum development and evaluation are on the curriculum plan and the need for improvement based on evaluation of its implementation and the program outcomes, the needs assessment should become part of the repertoire of the faculty. Even if faculty are not involved in the details of the needs assessment, it should be aware of all of the factors that have an influence on the curriculum.

These factors can mean the life or death of an education program; thus, faculty members sophisticated in the assessment of external and internal frame factors have an advantage in viewing the curriculum and its place in the scheme of financial security, position within the health care system and the profession, role in meeting the health care needs of the community and industry, and significance to the parent institution.

It is recommended that nurse educators in both the academic and practice settings use the Frame Factors model when evaluating education programs, considering revisions of existing programs, or initiating new programs. While administrators may take the leadership role in conducting needs assessments, faculty should participate in the decisions for what type and how much data to collect and what decisions are made that affect the curriculum based on the analysis of the needs assessment.

CHAPTER 8: FINANCIAL SUPPORT AND BUDGET PLANNING FOR CURRICULUM DEVELOPMENT OR REVISION

Chapter 8 reviews the costs, income, and resources related to the financial support of curriculum development, evaluation, and accreditation activities. Specific costs include faculty released time, administrative and staff support, and office equipment, technology support, and supplies. These are costs over and above the usual budget demands and must be planned for in advance. The challenge is to earmark funds for these activities to avoid unexpected shortfalls and an impact on other program expenditures. Knowledge of possible resources external to the program is useful for generating funds that help to initiate new programs and the chapter reviews several potential funding sources. In addition to a review of budget planning, the roles and responsibilities of administrators and faculty are described and the importance of faculty participation and contributions to budgetary planning is noted.

CHAPTER 9: COMPONENTS OF THE CURRICULUM AND ISSUES ARISING FROM TODAY'S NURSING CURRICULA

Chapter 9 organizes the components of the curriculum in the traditional way, that is, mission, philosophy, goal, organizational framework, student learning outcomes (objectives), and implementation plan. The components of the curriculum provide an organizing framework for initiating or revising an educational program. Major concepts related to the underlying philosophy and the beliefs faculty hold about nursing and education are examined in light of their contribution to and place in the curriculum. Examples include beliefs about teaching and learning processes, critical thinking and its application to nursing, liberal education and the sciences, the health care system, and so on. When revising the curriculum or developing new programs, faculty should initiate the change processes by discussing these concepts and theories and how they apply to the level of nursing education in their program. Most faculty members will agree that these concepts are fundamental to nursing education. The challenge occurs when deciding at what level of competency for each concept/essential they expect from their graduates, that is, undergraduate and/or graduate levels.

While it may seem cumbersome at times, in the long run, examining the curriculum by its major components results in a logical order for planning and evaluation. When faculty members contemplate change in response to a needs assessment of the external and internal frame factors, each component of the curriculum is examined for its congruence with the proposed changes. This may lead to a radical revamping of the curriculum, for it may be discovered that the demands for graduates or from the health care system have so dramatically changed that the mission, philosophy, and goals of the program are outdated or irrelevant.

Approaching the curriculum holistically by viewing all of its components leads to orderly revisions rather than the "Band-Aid" approach that attempts to mend one portion of the program without considering its effects on the other components. Nurse educators are frequently guilty of this maneuver in order to respond to obvious need for changes. The problems associated with this method are their possible detrimental effects on other parts of the program and adding to an already overloaded and content saturated curriculum.

CHAPTERS 10 THROUGH 15: CURRICULUM PLANNING

Chapters 10 and 11 discuss the two current, major curricula for entry into practice, that is, the associate degree in nursing (ADN) and the baccalaureate/BSN. Both of these programs have been in existence since the mid-20th century, replacing the hospital-based diploma programs that continue to exist, but are decreasing in numbers. Chapter 11 describes generic (entry-level) baccalaureate programs as well as fast-track baccalaureate programs for college graduates and RN to BSN programs. The old issue of entry into practice rears its ugly head as the ADN and baccalaureate are examined; however, with the need to produce more nurses as rapidly as possible to meet health care demands and the need for higher education in nursing, the authors of Chapters 10 and 11 describe curricula that embrace both programs and foster career ladder opportunities. Each chapter provides excellent examples of curricula for preparing nurses for the current health care system and can serve in the interim as nursing meets the challenge to educate clinicians, educators, practitioners, scientists, and researchers for the future.

Chapters 12 and 13 examine graduate education at the master's and professional doctoral degree levels including entry-level master's programs for nonnursing college graduates. The traditional place for advanced practice roles such as the nurse practitioner, nurse anesthetist, nurse midwife, and clinical specialist has been at the master's level. However, the DNP degree is replacing the master's in response to the AACN recommendation that the DNP be the terminal practice degree by 2015 (AACN, 2004). This position and the IOM's (2011) recommendation for nurses prepared at higher degree levels led to an explosive growth of DNP programs across the nation, starting first with postmaster's degrees and moving to the BSN to DNP program. Many issues arise from this situation with the profession struggling with where master's-prepared case managers, clinical nurse leaders, nurse managers, administrators, nurse educators, and community/public health nurses fall. Chapters 12 and 13 raise these issues as graduate/doctorate levels of nursing education continue to evolve.

Graduate programs are particularly hard hit by the looming shortage of doctorally prepared teachers as faculty members age and retire and the numbers of new graduates from doctoral programs do not meet the demand. This situation provides the impetus for accelerating access to graduate education for both new entrants into the discipline and practicing nurses and educators who have an interest in teaching. Additional incentives for the faculty role need to be in place to make the educator role competitive with that of practice, administration, and research. Chapter 14 discusses research-focused degree programs and their role as "Stewards of the Discipline" through their research and leadership activities and as faculty members in schools of nursing.

An issue related to doctoral-prepared faculty is the debate that continues about the doctor of nursing practice (DNP) versus the research-focused degrees, that is, the DNS and the PhD and their place in nursing education. It is posed that PhD and DNS-prepared educators are suitable for tenure-track positions in schools of nursing, while DNP graduates are meant for clinically focused teaching positions. However, a counter-argument is that the DNP prepares nurses for applied research, translational science, and evidence-based practice and they could compete in tenure-track roles. It is also argued that DNP graduates are the experts in the practice role and can be role models for the students. There are persuasive arguments on both sides but the majority of those expressing opinions agree that for either degree, nurses planning to teach in schools of nursing need additional knowledge and skills (courses) in education, for example, curriculum development, instructional strategies, educational technology/simulation, and student and program evaluation.

Chapter 15 applies the principles of curriculum development and evaluation to staff development in the practice setting. Nurse educators in academe and in the practice setting have much to offer each other. Nurse educators who focus on staff development can provide faculty with their perspectives on the knowledge and competency expectations for students and graduates. Their wisdom is valuable in helping faculty prepare new graduates for practice in the reality setting. Nursing faculty members, on the other hand, have expertise in instructional strategies and program development, which they can share with nurse educators in the practice settings. They also have clinical specialty knowledge and skills for offering in-service opportunities for nursing staff in health agencies. Faculty also provides orientation and educational services to nurse preceptors and mentors for students and new graduates.

Research partnerships between nursing service and education benefit nursing faculty members as they earn promotion and tenure and keep abreast of changes in health care, while students can carry out their graduate theses or dissertations in the practice arena in collaboration with staff. All levels of students apply the newest knowledge from research to evidence-based practice, which in turn, is shared with nursing staff members who reciprocate with their knowledge and clinical skills in the latest advances in health care.

There are increasing instances of industry and education partnerships, with industry working with schools of nursing to develop quality clinical experiences for students and to assist with the costs for additional faculty members to meet faculty shortages (Burns et al., 2011; Jeffries et al., 2013). Qualified staff members from the agencies serve as instructors, while continuing in their practice roles in the agencies. It is imperative that instructors from the service area are well oriented to the curriculum and its goals and objectives in order to protect the integrity of the curriculum. There must be opportunities for new instructors' participation in faculty and curriculum meetings as well as for their responsibilities to the curriculum. Experienced faculty members act as mentors to share the curriculum plan and the knowledge and skills necessary to the learner-centered teaching role.

CHAPTERS 16 AND 17 PROGRAM EVALUATION AND ACCREDITATION

Chapter 16 reviews common definitions, concepts, and theories in evaluation that apply to nursing curricula and programs evaluation. Nursing education evaluation is evolving from an emphasis in the past on the use of models of evaluation in education to the adaptation of business and health care models to measure productivity, outcomes, cost-effectiveness, and quality. Issues that are raised in Chapter 16 relate to the increasing emphasis on outcomes and benchmarks to measure quality and the possible loss of equal attention to the processes that lead to the outcomes. Owing to many accreditation standards, educational programs usually have master plans of evaluation in place to facilitate the process of collecting and analyzing data. These data relate to the standards expected for accreditation and the goals and objectives of the program. One flaw in many of the master plans is the lack of specific plans to follow-up on the analyzes and their recommendations. Implementing strategies to act on the recommendations closes the loop between data collection and actions for change in the curriculum, thus maintaining an up to date and vibrant program.

Chapter 17 discusses in detail accreditation agencies, their purpose, and their role in total quality management. Included in the chapter is a description of the process for undergoing accreditation. While accreditation is voluntary, it carries certain advantages for the institution and its students and graduates. For example, an accredited institution demonstrates to the public that it meets quality standards or criteria set by education and the profession, and therefore increases its marketability. For students and graduates, an accredited program signifies that they are eligible for certain financial aid programs and, in most cases, admission to an institution of higher education for the next degree level(s).

Two major issues are raised regarding accreditation. The first is the question of these agencies keeping their standards and criteria up to date. With the expansion of technology-driven distance education programs and rapid changes in the health care system, it becomes difficult to make changes in the curriculum in response to the changes and at the same time, ensure that the program continues to meet program approval standards and accreditation criteria.

Many state boards of nursing and accreditation agencies require notification of any major (or even minor) changes in the existing program. Although this ensures quality and maintenance of approval or accreditation, it can hamper creativity and a speedy response to external changes and demands on the program. The advantage of notifying program approval and accreditation agencies of pending changes is the preservation of quality, while the disadvantage is a lowered motivation for creating change. In these cases, the wise strategy is to consult with the agencies when the idea for change begins to form and to continue the consultation throughout the planning stages so that the appropriate paperwork and visits, if necessary, are ready for timely approval processes.

Educators have a responsibility to participate in accreditation processes including review of standards and criteria, becoming site visitors, and becoming members on review boards and committees of the agencies. These kinds of activities contribute to faculty's professional development and the ability of the approval and accrediting agencies to keep abreast of changes occurring in education and the profession that call for modifications of standards and criteria.

CHAPTER 18: EFFECTS OF INFORMATICS AND TECHNOLOGY ON CURRICULUM DEVELOPMENT AND EVALUATION

The growth of technology and informatics and their impact on nursing education is explored in Chapter 18. A major concern about the integration of nursing informatics and technology into the curriculum is the lack of planning in advance and the lack of using standards developed by nursing informatics experts (TIGER, 2014). Many times, classes on technology and informatics such as its application to electronic records, utilization of literature and health information databases, and experiences in simulation labs are developed without analyses for their relationship to the curriculum. It is necessary that faculty reviews the curriculum for the student learning outcomes and the organizational framework that relate to informatics and technology, utilize nursing informatics standards as guidelines, and plan for their placement into the program accordingly.

The information age and high technology require faculty to keep abreast of changes and gain the knowledge and skills required for facilitating learning, transmitting new knowledge to students, and conducting research and other scholarly activities. In some cases, faculty preparation does not keep pace with the rapid growth of the utilization of technology. Studies demonstrate the need for faculty development to not only meet the application of technology to instructional strategies but to prepare students to meet the needs of the health care system that utilizes informatics and technology for the delivery of care. Faculty and their student and clinical partners have tremendous opportunities for research that measures the effectiveness of technology and nursing informatics in education and the health care systems.

CHAPTER 19: RESEARCH AND EVIDENCE-BASED PRACTICE IN NURSING EDUCATION

Chapter 19 discusses the need for research in nursing education for evidence-based practice. It reviews Boyer's (1990) and AACN's (2014c) statements on the scholarship of teaching that serve as guiding principles for faculty to conduct research and produce scholarship that deepens our understanding of education and learning processes. The temptation for faculty is to rely on tried and true strategies for developing curricula and instructional strategies. However, with the rapid changes in the health care delivery system and the impact of technology, educators must provide curricula that are responsive to changes and prepare nurses for the future. Nurses must be able to think critically and creatively, use and generate technology for safe and quality patient care, collaborate with other health professionals and the clients they serve, provide leadership for health care policies, and participate in or conduct research that, in the end, produces high-quality health care. Each chapter of this text reviews the classic and recent literature related to curriculum development and evaluation in nursing. Chapter 19 summarizes the literature review from previous chapters, and using National League for Nursing's (NLN) *Priorities for Nursing Education* (2014), suggests topics for further study and research. It is hoped that many studies are replicated for their generalizability and usefulness to nursing educators and that new research findings lead toward evidence-based practice in education and practice.

FROM WHENCE WE CAME AND WHERE TO GO

Chapter 1 reviews the history of nursing education from the mid- to late 1800s to the 21st century. It is interesting to see the visions of nurse leader educators over the centuries that called for a unified approach to curriculum development in nursing and placement of nursing as a discipline and science into academic institutions of higher learning. It is equally interesting to see the influence that international wars and the major changes in the health care system and society had on nursing education. Nursing education programs found that with government help, they could accelerate nursing programs in institutions of higher learning and produce graduates for high demand eras. Advanced practice roles at the master's level came about as high technology and managed care systems began to change the health care delivery system and research-focused doctoral programs came about as nursing sought its professional identity and began to build the scientific body of knowledge. The explosive growth of the DNP in less than a decade's time after AACN's (2004) position paper on the DNP as the terminal degree in nursing for advanced practice is remarkable. As the graduates of these programs increase and impact the health care system at the same time that the Affordable Care Act (ACA) for reform takes place, the role of nursing becomes even more crucial (U.S. Department of Health and Human Services, 2014). Some of the major challenges facing nursing education for the future are discussed below.

THE FUTURE EDUCATIONAL PREPARATION FOR NURSING

The IOM's recommendations regarding nursing's future had an impact on nursing education along with the AACN (2004) statement on the DNP as the entry for advanced practice nurses and they might be called the "tipping points" for change in nursing education in the 21st century. Gladwell (2002) introduced the concept of tipping points as "little things that happen that result in making a big difference." Although the IOM recommendations and AACN's position are not "little things," they have influenced change. Lane and Kohlenberg (2010) review the rationale for a nursing workforce prepared at the baccalaureate or higher degree levels. They list the various professional organizations and health care systems that endorsed the need for a better prepared nursing workforce and some of the initiatives that occurred on the state legislative levels. Associate degree and baccalaureate nursing programs' collaboration for curricula that provide seamless entry into the bachelor's degree for associate degree students/graduates are increasing exponentially. As a by-product of these collaboratives, practice colleagues participate in the planning of curricula and development of the expected practice competencies of graduates (Nielsen, Noone, Voss, & Mathews, 2013; Sroczynski, Gravlin, Route, Hoffart, & Creelman, 2011). Out of these project comes a spirit of colleagueship that overcomes decades of intra-professional resentment and unhealthy competition. Nielsen et al. (2013) and Sroczynski et al. (2011) describe two recent major collaborative undertakings on the West and East Coasts of the United States and provide models for the growth of similar programs throughout the nation.

Another phenomenon is the growth of community colleges that offer baccalaureates in nursing. Daun-Barnett (2011) reviewed community colleges that offer them and found that the majority of these types of programs can be found in Florida, Texas, and Washington. The growth of these programs did not seem to affect enrollments in baccalaureate, private, and other types of nursing programs and produced more nurses for the workforce than if they not been in existence. The question as to the original purpose of community colleges remains, that is, to offer higher education opportunities at lower costs for transfer to upper division programs and to prepare graduates for technical-based careers. If these programs become more numerous, what effect will they have on these original purposes of the community colleges? And are these degrees equivalent to the baccalaureates from traditional 4-year institutions? These are the issues that will need investigation.

The growth of DNP programs and the increase in enrollments in research-focused doctorates indicate an expansion of the nursing workforce prepared at the doctorate level who will be the scientists, faculty, advanced practice heath care providers, and nurse leaders (Kirschling, 2014). It is a forecast of the role that nursing will play in leading health care policy changes for the benefit of the population and providing evidence-based practice built upon collaborative translational science and research.

A key component of professional education is the faculty members who are responsible for developing and implementing curricula that prepare nurses for the future. It is agreed that over the recent past, the focus of instruction changed from teacher-centric to participative, learner-centric modalities. As mentioned previously, nursing is in the process of producing additional doctorally prepared nurses who will serve as faculty members for the newer models of education. Some will be advanced practice nurses/leaders who focus on translational science, while others will be researchers exploring and identifying new knowledge for the science of nursing. They will encounter the same challenges facing current educators to fulfill the role of academic faculty, that is, teaching, service, and scholarship/research. The enigma to be solved is how faculty roles are defined to, first, provide high-quality instruction that prepares professionals who meet current and future health care needs and, then, to meet the other faculty expectations, that is, remain current in practice, provide service, and maintain research and scholarship. Roberts and Glod (2013) discuss these dilemmas and stress the need for nursing to find a solution that maintains quality education and research in academe and, at the same time, prepares competent professionals for the health care system.

NURSING INFORMATICS AND TECHNOLOGY

Throughout the chapters of this text, nursing informatics, clinical simulations, and technology applications are discussed as they apply to curriculum development and evaluation. Previous reviews in this chapter alluded to the need for alignment of these advances to the curriculum plan (organizational framework and student learning outcomes). Many of yesterday's technological advances such as personal digital assistants (PDAs) rapidly become outdated as smartphones and tablets with additional features provide rapid access to databases for health care information. It is hard to imagine the future and additional expansions of technology and their application to nursing and education. Thus, it becomes the responsibility of nursing educators to become or remain sophisticated in the use of informatics, clinical simulations, and other applications. While there are numerous studies on the application of these strategies in nursing education (Brewer, 2011), there remains the need for replication of studies and comparisons of programs across the country to validate their effectiveness and to provide information on best practices. Brewer, in her review of the literature, found several similarities of strategies that produced the most effective learning in simulated clinical experiences; they included student preclass assignments so they were prepared to participate in scenario/case studies, clear clinical evaluation criteria, postconferences for reflective thinking activities, cooperative team work, and linkages to didactic content.

CAREER PATHWAYS AND PROMOTING PROFESSIONAL DEVELOPMENT FOR THE FUTURE

Career Ladder Pathways in Nursing

Nursing, as a profession, prides itself on providing career ladder opportunities through experience in the workforce and progression of degree opportunities from the licensed practical nurse/licensed vocational nurse (LPN/LVN) through to the doctorate. Entry into practice as RNs remains multilayered with graduates of diploma, ADN, BSN, and entry-level master's degrees eligible for licensure. These multiple pathways continue to confuse the public and those seeking education to become RNs. However, according to the report on the nursing workforce by the Health Resources and Services Administration (HRSA) (2014), there are trends toward higher education that give credence to the IOM (2011) recommendations. From 2001 to 2011, the growth in the nursing workforce exceeded that of the general population for the first time and increased in diversity from 20% non-White to 25%. Fifty-five percent of the nursing workforce was prepared at the bachelor's or higher degree level with many of those receiving an ADN as the first degree. Both the number of bachelor's prepared nurses taking National Council Licensure Examination (NCLEX) and the number of nonbachelor's degree nurses doubled. Positive trends in higher education were demonstrated from 2007 to 2011 with an 86% increase of RNs earning a BSN. Also, there was a 60% growth of nurses earning their master's, and the number of doctoral graduates tripled (HRSA, 2014). While these trends are promising, there remains a concern about the preparation of nurses for today and tomorrow's far more complex health care demands that require providers prepared at higher levels of knowledge and skills. Although 86% of ADN nurses returned for their BSNs during 2007 to 2011, the ADN-prepared general nursing workforce remains at 60%.

Orsolini-Hain (2012) conducted a study of ADN-prepared staff nurses with years of experience to identify their reasons for not returning for the BSN. Reasons cited were the absence of a salary differential, their perceptions that their competencies were equivalent to or better than BSN-prepared nurses, and through their employer, they participated in research and projects to help improve patient care systems. They viewed master's prepared nurses as those who were not engaged in direct care but, rather, provided staff development, patient education, and management services. On the other hand, RNs who were graduates of an RN to BSN program viewed the upper division level of nursing education as adding to their communication skills with patients, a gain in cultural competence, and providing an academic background for growing professionally (DeBrew, 2010).

Baccalaureate schools of nursing have a long history of offering user-friendly programs for RNs, doing away with past practices of requiring the RNs to repeat lower division nursing courses and integrating them into classes with generic BSN students. The RN to BSN or RN to MSN programs are for the most part accelerated, usually with 1 year of full-time study to earn the baccalaureate and for the RN to MSN programs, 2 to 2.5 years of full-time study. Courses are geared toward adult learning strategies with classes scheduled 1 day a week, while others offer the program totally online, or a combination of both. The majority of programs have part time options as well.

Brown, Kuhn, and Miner (2012) describe a successful accelerated ADN to BSN program with a 10% attrition rate, a 95% rate of student/graduate satisfaction with the program, and 83% of the students reported they would pursue graduate education. Other successful programs reported in the literature include Wagner's (2013) study that described a program that introduced RN students to activities involved in professional activities such as attending legislative sessions, board of nursing meetings, and so on. Cobb (2011) discusses the influence of social presence (interactions with peers and faculty) in an online course and its positive contributions to the students' perceived learning and satisfaction with the program. Robbins and Hoke (2013) conducted a qualitative study of RN to BSN students to identify factors influencing their academic success. The study examined various ethnic groups, particularly Hispanic, as the study took place in a university with a high Hispanic population. The major positive themes identified included the faculty's belief in the potential for student success, a transparent curriculum (program of study), and a commitment to respect of the students. Student factors that had a positive influence were family support, individual resources, and employment considerations. While additional studies to replicate these findings are indicated for generalizability, they provide useful information for programs offering RN to BSN or MSN programs.

For some time, ADN and diploma graduates did not have an incentive to return to school for their baccalaureate or higher degrees owing to, among other factors, the absence of differentiation of practice in the worksite. However, some health care systems moved in that direction. For example, the VA system and hospitals seeking or having magnet status prefer the BSN for their RN staff and have tuition assistance programs for nurses to continue their education by obtaining a baccalaureate and/or higher degree.

Preparation of Interprofessional and International Providers for the Future

Although this text focuses on curriculum development and evaluation in nursing in the United States and as we contemplate the future with its promise and challenges, there is a need to envision a broader, global perspective about nursing and the education required for its professionals. Cyberspace communications give us the ability to share knowledge and expertise with colleagues in health care and discover commonalities and differences that enrich the profession and lead to improved delivery of health care. International colleagues share the same concerns of U.S. nursing educators for preparing quality health professionals to meet the needs of the world's populations from the poorest nations to the richest. Garrett (2012) likens the issues facing nursing education on an international level to the IOM's (2011) recommendations on *The Future of Nursing* in the United States. He summarizes the needs as follows:

- Inclusive, stratified and integrated regulatory frameworks for all types of health care providers (from home care aides to senior physicians), and review of specialized education to meet current needs
- Coordinated educational reform incorporating increased interdisciplinary education, teamwork and globalization of the curriculum to provide educational preparation at a wide variety of levels and specializations
- Accessible and flexible career pathways for health care professionals to support career mobility
- Expand educational programs to support specialist and advanced practice nursing
- Legislative reform to considerably expand prescribing and treatment rights to advanced practice nurses
- Better harmonization of international health care qualifications (p. 81)

These recommendations/goals serve as guidelines for nursing educators across the globe and American educators can use them to compare to their curricula and the progress toward realization of the goals.

A Proposed Unified Nursing Curriculum

For too long, nursing has been dominated by other disciplines in academe that have a major influence on the prerequisites, length, composition, and type of degree nursing will have. It is difficult to convince other disciplines in higher education of the need to educate nurses with a strong foundation in liberal arts and sciences and, at the same time, prescribing the nursing curriculum that remains within the usual number of units for associate (65–70) and bachelor's degrees (120–125). There are numerous courses that nursing values as foundations for practice such as the arts, political science, computer science, and business as they apply to health care. And yet there is little or no room for these courses in the 125-unit nursing degree program. The proposed unified curriculum in Table 20.1 is ideal but unrealistic owing to the aforementioned issues. Yet nurse educators should strive to revise or build curricula that are close to the usual credit requirements of other disciplines. At the same time, uniform curricula for entry into practice levels that allow seamless entry into the next level are necessary to provide the existing nurse workforce with career ladder opportunities and options to step out as personal situations may require.

These issues related to undergraduate education elucidate the need for nursing to move into graduate education. Following the nonstop curriculum for the doctorate in Table 20.1 and comparing it to the step-out options reveal a rigorous academic program common to professional education, and yet there is an efficiency of time and quality of courses that provides the student with opportunity to build on courses sequentially and integrate nursing knowledge and skills into the supporting arts and sciences. One needs only to interview nurses with baccalaureates in the 40+ years of age range to discover the excess number of credits in their degree work to realize the enormity of the problem and the injustices nurses suffered in gaining education beyond the diploma and associate degree with no academic recognition of their additional work. Going one step further, nurses in that age group or older who hold master's and/or doctorate's suffer the same overabundance of credits, earning far more than their colleagues in medicine, pharmacology, education, engineering, religion, and law.

Based on the curricula in Table 20.1 the argument for "entry into practice" ends with the idea that a candidate is eligible for licensure at various points of the education track commencing with the completion of the associate degree (lower division) and 3-month internship; or completion of the bachelor of science with a residency; or a master's degree with either two functional role practica or three advanced practice clinical practica with a residency prior to licensure; and finally, a doctorate that includes a clinical residency. Thus, students have a choice for entering practice through licensure at the associate, bachelor's, master's, or doctorate degree levels. At the same time, the curricula contain the same courses or content, thus allowing nurses to enter at the next step of their education to continue their career opportunities. If these generic curricula were adapted by schools of nursing

TABLE 20.1 PROPOSED UNIFIED NURSING CURRICULUM

CAREER LADDER PROGRAM (WITH STEP-OUT OPTIONS)			NONSTOP ENTRY-LEVEL DOCTORAL PROGRAM (DNP OR PhD/DNS)	
PREREQUISITES		NURSING COURSES	PREREQUISITES	
		YEAR 1		
COURSES	CREDITS	COURSES	CREDITS	COURSES	CREDITS
Verbal and Written Communications	6	Introduction to Nursing and Health Care	3	Verbal and Written Communications	6
Anatomy and Physiology	6	Basic Health Assessment and Skills	3	Anatomy and Physiology	8
Microbiology	4	Nursing Process and Skills	4	Chemistry	4
Language or General Education	3	Care of the Older Adult	3	Psychology	3
Total Credits	19		13	Sociology/ Anthropology	6
				Language or General Education	3
				Total Credits	30
		YEAR 2		
Sociology/ Anthropology	3	Parent Child Nursing	6	Human Development	3
Human Development	3	Psychiatric/Mental Health Nursing	4	Microbiology	4

(continued)

TABLE 20.1　PROPOSED UNIFIED NURSING CURRICULUM (continued)

CAREER LADDER PROGRAM (WITH STEP-OUT OPTIONS)		YEAR 2		NONSTOP ENTRY-LEVEL DOCTORAL PROGRAM (DNP OR PhD/DNS)	
General Education	3	Adult Acute Care Nursing	6	Statistics	3
Introduction to Health Care Informatics	3	12-Week Paid Internship Prior to Licensure	Work Study/no credit	Chemistry	4
Nutrition	3			U.S. Health Care System and Health Professions	3
Introduction to Pharmacology	2			Nutrition	3
				Introduction to Health Care Informatics	3
				Language or General Education	3
				Genetics	3
				Introduction to Nursing and Health Care	3
Total Credits	17		16	Total Credits	32

Step out for ADN: Total credits: 65

(continued)

TABLE 20.1 PROPOSED UNIFIED NURSING CURRICULUM (continued)

YEAR 3

| CAREER LADDER PROGRAM (WITH STEP-OUT OPTIONS) | | | | NONSTOP ENTRY-LEVEL DOCTORAL PROGRAM (DNP OR PhD/DNS) | | | |
| COGNATES | | NURSING COURSES | | COGNATES | | NURSING COURSES | |
COURSES	CREDITS	COURSES	CREDITS	COURSES	CREDITS	COURSES	CREDITS
Genetics	3	The Nursing Profession	3	Economics	3	Basic Health Assessment and Skills	3
Pharmacology	3	Critical Care Nursing	4	Pharmacology	3	Nursing Process with Skills	4
Chemistry	4	Transcultural Nursing	4			Care of the Older Adult	3
Statistics	3	Research in Nursing	3			Parent Child Nursing	6
General Education	3					Psychiatric/Mental Health Nursing	4
						The Nursing Profession	3
						Research in Nursing	3
Total Credits	16		14		6		26

(continued)

TABLE 20.1 PROPOSED UNIFIED NURSING CURRICULUM (*continued*)

YEAR 4

| CAREER LADDER PROGRAM (WITH STEP-OUT OPTIONS) | | | | NONSTOP ENTRY-LEVEL DOCTORAL PROGRAM (DNP OR PhD/DNS) | | | |
| COGNATES | | NURSING COURSES | | COGNATES | | NURSING COURSES | |
COURSES	CREDITS	COURSES	CREDITS	COURSES	CREDITS	COURSES	CREDITS
General Education Electives	6	Community Health Nursing	6	Bioethics	3	Adult Acute Care Nursing	6
Bioethics	3	Nursing Leadership and Interprofessional Collaboration	3	General Education	3	Transcultural Nursing	4
Economics	3	Health Care Delivery System	3			Community Health Nursing	6
		Nursing Informatics	3			Nursing Leadership and Interprofessional Collaboration	3
		Capstone Practicum	3			Nursing Informatics	3
		12-Week Paid Residency Prior to Licensure	Work Study/no credit			Critical Care Nursing	4
Total Credits	12		18		6		26

Step out for BSN: Total credits: 65 (lower division) + 60 (upper division) = 125

(*continued*)

TABLE 20.1 PROPOSED UNIFIED NURSING CURRICULUM (*continued*)

CAREER LADDER PROGRAM (WITH STEP-OUT OPTIONS)				NONSTOP ENTRY-LEVEL DOCTORAL PROGRAM (DNP OR PhD/DNS)			
		YEAR 5					
NURSING COGNATES	CREDITS	NURSING COURSES	CREDITS	NURSING COGNATES	CREDITS	NURSING COURSES	CREDITS
Nursing Theory	3	Functional Role Theory I, for example, Advanced Practice, Clinical Nurse Leader, Clinical Specialty, Education, Management	2	Nursing Theory	3	Capstone Practicum (upper division)	3
Analysis of Health Care Organizations	3	Functional Role Practicum I	4	Analysis of Health Care Organizations	3	Functional Role Theory I, for example, Advanced Practice, Clinical Nurse Leader, Clinical Specialty, Education, Management	2
Nursing Research Evidence-based Practice	3			Nursing Research Evidence-based Practice	3	Functional Role Practicum I	4

(*continued*)

TABLE 20.1 PROPOSED UNIFIED NURSING CURRICULUM (continued)

CAREER LADDER PROGRAM (WITH STEP-OUT OPTIONS)				NONSTOP ENTRY-LEVEL DOCTORAL PROGRAM (DNP OR PhD/DNS)			
YEAR 5							
NURSING COGNATES	CREDITS	NURSING COURSES	CREDITS	NURSING COGNATES	CREDITS	NURSING COURSES	CREDITS
Advanced Nursing Informatics	3			Advanced Nursing Informatics	3		
Advanced Pathophysiology*	3			Advanced Pathophysiology*	3		
*This course is not required for nonadvanced practice MSN roles							
Total Credits	15/12			Total Credits	15		9
YEAR 6 SEMESTER 1							
NURSING COGNATES	CREDITS	NURSING COURSES	CREDITS	NURSING COGNATES	CREDITS	NURSING COURSES	CREDITS
Advanced Health Assessment*	2	Functional Role Theory II, for example, Advanced Practice, Clinical Nurse Leader, Clinical Specialty, Education, Management, and so on.	3	Advanced Health Assessment*	3	Functional Role Theory, II for example, Advanced Practice, Clinical Nurse Leader, Clinical Specialty, Education, Management, and so on.	2
Advanced Pharmacology*	4	Functional Role Practicum II	3	Advanced Pharmacology*	3	Functional Role Practicum II	4

(continued)

TABLE 20.1 PROPOSED UNIFIED NURSING CURRICULUM *(continued)*

YEAR 6 SEMESTER 1

CAREER LADDER PROGRAM (WITH STEP-OUT OPTIONS)						NONSTOP ENTRY-LEVEL DOCTORAL PROGRAM (DNP OR PhD/DNS)	
NURSING COGNATES	CREDITS	NURSING COGNATES	CREDITS	NURSING COGNATES	CREDITS	NURSING COURSES	CREDITS
Population Health	3	Master's Project/Thesis**	3-6				
		For entry-level master's: Twelve Week Paid Residency Prior to Licensure	Work Study/no credit				
Total Credits*	9/3	Total Credits	6/9-12**	Total Credits	6		6

* These three courses are not required for non-advanced practice roles
** Required of nonadvanced practice master's degree candidates

Step out for nonadvanced practice master's degree with 30-33 credits

YEAR 7

	DNP		RESEARCH-FOCUSED DEGREE (PhD OR DNS)				
COGNATES	CREDITS	COURSES	CREDITS	COGNATES	CREDITS	NURSING COURSES	CREDITS
Health Care Economics	3	Translational Science	3	Quantitative Research	3	Nursing History and Philosophy	3
		Foundations for the DNP in Practice and Leadership	3	Qualitative Research	3	Nursing Science, Analysis of Theories	3

(continued)

TABLE 20.1 PROPOSED UNIFIED NURSING CURRICULUM (continued)

YEAR 7

CAREER LADDER PROGRAM (WITH STEP-OUT OPTIONS)				RESEARCH-FOCUSED DEGREE (PhD OR DNS)		NONSTOP ENTRY-LEVEL DOCTORAL PROGRAM (DNP OR PhD/DNS)	
		DNP					
COGNATES	CREDITS	COURSES	CREDITS	COGNATES	CREDITS	NURSING COURSES	CREDITS
	3	Advanced Communications and Interprofessional Health Care	3	Mixed Methods	3	Seminar: Dissertation I	3
	3	Advanced Nursing Informatics	3	Health Care Economics	3	Advanced Communications and Interprofessional Health Care	3
		DNP Project I, II	6				
		Quality Nursing Care and Outcomes Management	3				
Total	3		21		12		12

(continued)

TABLE 20.1 PROPOSED UNIFIED NURSING CURRICULUM (continued)

	CAREER LADDER PROGRAM (WITH STEP-OUT OPTIONS)		NONSTOP ENTRY-LEVEL DOCTORAL PROGRAM (DNP OR PhD/DNS)		
	YEAR 8 FIRST SEMESTER DNP AND PhD/DNS				
	DNP			RESEARCH-FOCUSED PhD OR DNS	
COURSES	CREDITS	COGNATES	CREDITS	NURSING COURSES	CREDITS
Role Specific Evidence-Based Practice Residency	6				
DNP Project III	3	Electives (Education courses for faculty roles or cognates to support research)	6	Nursing Science, Theory Development	3
Advanced Practice and Leadership Role Development	3			Seminar: Dissertation II	3
For entry level DNP: Twelve Week Paid Residency Prior to Licensure	Work Study/no credit				
Total	12		6		6

Postmaster's DNP: Total 36 credits
Non-stop DNP Total: 198 advanced practice credits

there would be no need for challenge examinations and repetition of knowledge and skills already assimilated.

Schools of nursing bear the responsibility for evaluating the credentials of applicants with prior education or degrees not in nursing. There is a need for flexibility in granting credit for courses equivalent to those pre- and co-requisites in nursing and nursing courses (for RNs with degrees not in nursing) to enter into the curriculum and to complete the next academic level. Examples are RNs with baccalaureates or master's in other disciplines and nonnurses with baccalaureates or higher degrees who matriculate directly into master's programs rather than repeating the baccalaureate. Of course, RNs need upper-division-level nursing courses or their equivalent and nonnurses need nursing courses equivalent to the baccalaureate but offered at the graduate level prior to entering master's or doctorate level nursing courses.

The advantages to the entry-level doctorate program are numerous. It would facilitate high school graduates' entry into a nursing program with graduation 8 years away, thus producing expert clinicians, researchers, and educators who are relatively young in age. The 8-year total curriculum plan provides the time for in-depth education and the production of quality graduates prepared for practice, teaching, and research roles. If the profession embraces this transformation of nursing education, then it must come to grips with the reality that there are roles for personnel such as the licensed practical/vocational nurses. It is logical that these programs fall into the community college genre, thus raising the specter of the "Civil War" in nursing yet again. This author leaves that debate to the nurse educators reading this text and the nursing profession over the next few decades.

SUMMARY

Chapter 20 summarized each of the previous chapters in the text and raised issues from each topic. While the world order, the national society, and the health care system change rapidly, it is difficult to predict the future. There are prevailing trends that should have an impact on the development and evaluation of nursing curricula over the next decade. If nursing chooses not to respond to these changes, the profession will continue to be splintered with less opportunity for it to help in shaping public policy toward optimal health care for the populace. Nurse educators have a responsibility to work with their colleagues in practice and research to develop curricula that prepare nurses for the future, who are competent and caring, excellent clinicians and practitioners, leaders and change agents, and scholars and researchers. A nursing education system for the future will have the following characteristics:

1. Clearly defined levels of education and differentiated practice in the health care system based on education and experience
2. Entry into practice for staff nurse positions following a 3-month residency in a selected arena of practice
3. Quality institutions of higher education that specialize in the preparation of staff nurses for entry into evidence-based practice in a timely fashion

4. Quality institutions that focus on the faculty role of excellence in teaching, community service, research, and the translation and application of knowledge from nursing science and related disciplines

5. Quality institutions of higher education that specialize in the preparation of nurses to provide evidence-based advanced practice nursing and interprofessional services for individuals, families, communities, and aggregates

6. Students, graduates, and faculty who are active participants and generators of new knowledge in nursing and related disciplines' research

7. Quality institutions of higher education that specialize in the preparation of nurse leaders who will influence health care policy and change the health care system for the benefit of the populations they serve

8. Academic and health science centers that specialize in nursing research and advancement of nursing science through translational science and evidence-based practice; testing of theories; the development of new theories, concepts, and models; and educational innovations on the national and international levels

DISCUSSION QUESTIONS

1. Given the rapid changes in the health care and education systems and the ongoing shortage of nurses, what changes in nursing education do you envision within the next 5 to 10 years?

2. What strategies for changing nursing education worked in the past and how can they apply to needed changes in nursing education today? What are the lessons from the past that prohibited nursing from moving its educational agenda forward? How can today's nurse educators use these lessons to bring about change?

LEARNING ACTIVITIES

STUDENT LEARNING ACTIVITIES

Synthesize the information in this text into a "Dream School of Nursing." Develop a curriculum that prepares nurses for practice 10 years hence, keeping in mind that practice and the setting in which it is delivered will be different. Let your imagination run wild!

NURSE EDUCATOR/FACULTY DEVELOPMENT ACTIVITIES

Hold a faculty meeting focused on brainstorming and let creative thoughts flow freely. List the characteristics of the ideal nurse prepared to practice 5 to 10 years hence. Examine these characteristics and decide how a curriculum can be developed that provides the kind of education necessary to prepare this kind of nurse. Focus on creativity and newer theories of learning. Compare these ideas to your existing curriculum. How can it be transformed into the one you envision and still meet accreditation and professional standards and criteria?

REFERENCES

American Association of Colleges of Nursing. (2004). *AACN position statement on the practice doctorate in nursing.* Retrieved from http://www.aacn.nche.edu/publications/position/DNPpositionstatement.pdf

American Association of Colleges of Nursing. (2012). *AACN-AONE Task force on academic-practice partnerships: Guiding principles.* Washington, DC: Author.

American Association of Colleges of Nursing. (2014a). *Degree completion program for registered nurses: RN to master's degree and RN to baccalaureate programs.* Retrieved from http://www.aacn.nche.edu/media-relations/fact-sheets/degree-completion-programs

American Association of Colleges of Nursing. (2014b). *DNP fact sheet.* Retrieved from http://www.aacn.nche.edu/media-relations/fact-sheets/dnp

American Association of Colleges of Nursing. (2014c). *Defining scholarship for the discipline of nursing.* Washington, DC: Author. Retrieved from American Association of Colleges of Nursing http://www.aacn.nche.edu/publications/position/defining-scholarship

Boyer, E. L. (1990). *Scholarship reconsidered: Priorities of the professoriate.* Princeton, NJ: The Carnegie Foundation for the Advancement of Learning. Retrieved from http://depts.washington.edu/gs630/Spring/Boyer.pdf

Brewer, E. P. (2011). Successful techniques for using human patient simulation in nursing education. *Journal of Nursing Scholarship, 43*(3), 311–317.

Brown, R. A., Kuhn, S., & Miner, M. (2012). Innovative accelerated RN-to-BS model: Implementation and evaluation. *The Journal of Nursing Education, 51*, 582–585.

Burns, P., Williams, S. H., Ard, N., Enright, C., Poster, E., & Ransom, S. A. (2011). Academic partnerships to increase nursing education capacity: Centralized faculty resources and clinical placement centers. *Journal of Professional Nursing, 27*(6), e14–e19.

Cobb, S. C. (2011). Social presence, satisfaction, and perceived learning of RN-to-BSN students in web-based nursing courses. *Nursing Education Perspectives, 32*,115–119.

Daun-Barnett, N. (2011). Community college baccalaureate: A fixed effects, multi-year study of the influence of state policy on nursing degree production. *Higher Education Policy, 24*, 377–398.

DeBrew, J. K. (2010). Perceptions of liberal education of two types of nursing graduates: The essentials of baccalaureate education for professional nursing practice. *The Journal of General Education, 59*, 42–58.

Garrett, B. M. (2012). Changing the game: Some thoughts on future health care demands, technology, nursing and interprofessional education. *Nurse Education in Practice, 12*, 179–181.

Gladwell, M. (2002). *The tipping point. How little things can make a big difference.* New York, NY: Little Brown & Company.

Health Resources and Services Administration. (2014). *The U.S. nursing workforce: Trends in supply and education.* Retrieved from http://bhpr.hrsa.gov/healthworkforce/reports/nursingworkforce/nursingworkforcefullreport.pdf

Institute of Medicine. (2011). *The future of nursing: Focus on education.* Retrieved from http://www.iom.edu/Reports/2010/The-Future-of-Nursing-Leading-Change-Advancing-Health/Report-Brief-Education.aspx

Jeffries, P. A., Rose, L., Belcher, A. E., Dang, D., Hochhuli, J. F., Fleischmann, D., ... Walrath, J. M. (2013). A clinical academic practice partnership: A clinical education redesign. *Journal of Professional Nursing, 29*(3), 128–136.

Kirschling, J. M. (2014). *Reflections on the future of doctoral programs in nursing.* Retrieved from http://www.aacn.nche.edu/dnp/JK-2014-DNP.pdf

Lane, S. H., & Kohlenberg, E. (2010). The future of baccalaureate degrees for nurses. *Nursing Forum, 45*(4), 218–227.

National League for Nursing. (2014). *NLN research priorities in nursing education 2012–2015*. Retrieved from http://www.nln.org/researchgrants/researchpriorities.pdf

Nielsen, A. E., Noone, J., Voss, H., & Mathews, L. R. (2013). Preparing nursing students for the future: An innovative approach to clinical education. *Nurse Education in Practice, 13*(4), 301–309.

Orsolini-Hain, L. (2012). Mixed messages: Hospital practices that serve as disincentives for associate degree-prepared nurses to return to school. *Nursing Outlook, 60*, 81–90.

Robbins, L. K., & Hoke, M. M. (2013). RN-to-BSN culture of success model: Promoting student achievement at a Hispanic-serving institution. *Journal of Professional Nursing, 29*(1), 21–29.

Roberts, S. J., & Glod, C. (2013). Faculty roles: Dilemmas for the future of nursing. *Nursing Forum, 48*(2), 99–105.

Sroczynski, M., Gravlin, G., Route, P. S., Hoffart, N., & Creelman, P. (2011). Creativity and connections: The future of nursing education and practice: The Massachusetts initiative. *Journal of Professional Nursing, 27*(6), e64–e70.

TIGER. (2014). *The TIGER initiative*. Retrieved from http://tigersummit.com/About_Us.html

U.S. Department of Health and Human Services. (2014). *About the law*. Retrieved from http://www.hhs.gov/healthcare/rights

Wagner, D. (2013). Promoting professionalism in RN–BSN education. *Journal of Nursing Education and Practice, 3*(5), 9–13.

Glossary

Accelerated programs: Programs consisting of intensive full-time study with no breaks that give students the opportunity to finish the program in a shorter time than traditional programs. They include accelerated RN to BSN and RN to MSN programs and entry-level BSN and MSN programs for graduates with bachelor's (or higher) degrees not in nursing.

Accreditation: A process that education programs and curricula undergo to receive recognition for meeting basic standards or criteria set by national, regional, or state organizations. Although it is voluntary, most programs undergo accreditation to demonstrate their quality to the consumers (students, parents, alumni, and employers).

Adult learning theory, andragogy: A model of instruction geared toward adult learning that takes into account the adult's autonomy, life experiences, personal goals, and need for relevancy and respect.

Assessment: A process that gathers information that results in a conclusion such as a nursing diagnosis or problem identification.

Asynchronous: Learning activities that occur at various times.

Behaviorism, behaviorist learning theory: A group of learning theories, often referred to as stimulus-response, that view learning as the result of the stimulus conditions and the responses (behaviors) that follow, generally ignoring what goes on inside the learner.

Benchmark: Something that serves as a standard by which others may be measured or judged (Merriam-Webster Online Dictionary, 2014).

Body politic: The people/power(s) behind the official government within a community. It is composed of the major political forces and the people who exert influence within the community.

Classical conditioning: Respondent or Pavlovian conditioning that emphasizes the stimulus and associations made with it in the learning process; these associations are often unconscious.

Cognitivism, cognitive learning theory: A group of learning theories focused on cognitive processes such as decision making, problem solving, synthesizing, and evaluating.

Constructivism, constructivist learning theory: A learning perspective arguing that individuals construct much of what they learn and understand, producing knowledge based on their beliefs and experiences.

Continuous quality improvement (CQI): The implementation of a system designed to provide for ongoing evaluation, analysis of findings, and implementation of plans for improvement within an organization.

Curriculum: The formal plan of study that provides the philosophical underpinnings, goals, and guidelines for delivery of a specific educational program.

Demographics: Data that describe the characteristics of a population, for example, age, gender, socioeconomic status, ethnicity, education levels, and so on.

Distance education: Any learning experience that takes place a distance away from the parent educational institution's home campus.

Domains of learning: Categories of learning that affect the process of learning, for example, cognitive, affective, and psychomotor behaviors.

Entry-level/generic programs: Programs that prepare students for eligibility to take the licensure examination (NCLEX) for registered nurses (RNs). The programs include diploma, associate degree, baccalaureate, and master's levels. Students entering master's entry-level programs have a baccalaureate in another field as a minimum. Students in entry-level programs do not have previous education in nursing.

Evaluation: A process by which information about an entity is gathered to determine its worth/value.

Formal curriculum: The planned program of studies for an academic degree or discipline.

Formative evaluation: The assessment that takes place during the implementation of the program or curriculum. It can also be viewed as process evaluation. In education, this type of evaluation is often linked to course or level objectives.

Frame factors: The external and internal factors that influence, impinge upon, and/or enhance educational programs and curricula. As a conceptual model, they serve to collect, organize, and analyze information that is useful for the development and evaluation of curricula. There are two major categories of frame factors, external and internal factors:

> **External frame factors**—Factors outside of the home institution in which the nursing program is housed.

> **Internal frame factors**—Factors within the institution and the nursing program that influence the curriculum.

Goal: Overall statement(s) of what the program prepares the graduates for. Statements are usually long term and stated in global terms.

Goal-based evaluation: Based on the stated goals of the entity undergoing evaluation. It is frequently used in education and tied to the stated goals, purpose, and end-of-program objectives (student learning outcomes) of the program or curriculum.

Goal-free evaluation: A method for evaluators to assess and judge some thing or entity. That person has no prior knowledge of the entity (program or curriculum) that he or she is evaluating. The person must be an expert in the field of evaluation and the type of entity that is evaluated. The value of this type of evaluation is that it is relatively bias-free.

High-fidelity mannequins: Provide students with clinical experiences in laboratory settings to practice skills on realistic mannequins programmed to specific case scenarios.

Humanism, humanistic learning theory: An approach to teaching that assumes people are inherently good and possess unlimited potential for growth; therefore, it emphasizes personal freedom, choice, self-determination, and self-actualization.

Informal curriculum: Sometimes termed as the hidden curriculum, co-curriculum, or extracurricular activities; planned and unplanned influences on students' learning.

Institutional accreditation: Provides a comprehensive review of the functioning and effectiveness of the entire college, university, or technical institution. The state mandate or institutional mission provides the lens used to guide the review.

Learning: A "change in behavior (knowledge, attitudes, and/or skills) that can be observed or measured and that occurs … as a result of exposure to environmental stimuli" (Bastable & Alt, 2014, p. 14).

Learning-centered paradigm: Power in the classroom is shared between teacher and students, content becomes less important than the reflective construction of knowledge, teachers become coaches, students assume responsibility for their learning, and authentic learning assessment is incorporated into the curriculum (Weimer, 2002).

Learning theory: A "coherent framework of integrated constructs and principles that describe, explain or predict how people learn" (Braungart, Braungart, & Gramet, 2014).

Low-fidelity models or mannequins: Provide students with laboratory experiences to practice skills on partial body parts or on full mannequins for fundamental skills.

Metacognition: Cognition about cognition, or thinking about thinking; monitoring the learning progress by checking the level of understanding, evaluating the effectiveness of efforts, planning activities, and revising as necessary.

Mission statement: The institution's beliefs about its responsibility for the delivery of programs through teaching, service, and scholarship.

National accreditation agency: Any accreditation agency that accredits colleges, universities, or technical institutes within an entire country. These include agencies that accredit faith-related or career-related institutions.

Needs assessment: The process for collecting and analyzing information that can influence the decision to initiate a new program or revise an existing one.

Nonsectarian: Not associated with a religious organization.

Objectives: The steps necessary for reaching the overall goal of the program that include the learner, a behavior that is measurable, a timeframe, at what level of competency, and the topic or behavior expected.

> **Course objectives**: Have the same properties as end-of-program and mid-level objectives but apply to specific courses and relate to and lead toward mid-level and end-of-program objectives.

> **End-of-program objectives**: Highest level of learner behaviors that demonstrate the characteristics, knowledge, and skills expected of the graduate and relate to the overall goal. They focus on the learner and must include a behavior that is measurable, a timeframe, at what level of competency, and the topic or behavior expected. These can also be defined as student learning outcomes.

> *Example:* X School of Nursing prepares competent, compassionate nurse clinicians and leaders who serve the health care needs of the people of state and the health care system.

> **Mid-level (intermediate) objectives**: Have the same properties as end-of-program objectives but occur mid-way through an educational program and are usually higher than the first-level objectives.

> **Student (individual) learning outcomes**: All of the above objectives are student or individual learning outcomes and should be learner-centered and describe what behavior (outcome) is expected.

> *Example:* At the end of the Health Assessment course, the student will present a complete health assessment of a client that includes an accurate health history, a write-up of all components of the physical examination, a list of problems and actual or potential nursing diagnoses, and a plan for follow-up of the problems and diagnoses.

Operant conditioning: Rewarding a behavior to strengthen its likelihood of repetition. These behaviors are emitted responses or operants, voluntary operations performed by the individual, in contrast to classical conditioning, in which behavior follows a stimulus

Pedagogy: Teaching methods; although it originally applied to methods used to educate children, it can be used to apply to all age groups.

PhD program or, in the case of nursing, the PhD or DNS: Degrees that emphasize nursing theory and research and educate nurses prepared to conduct research and foster the development of new knowledge in health care and nursing.

Philosophy: "The critical analysis of the rational grounds of our most fundamental beliefs and logical analysis of the basic concepts employed in the expression of such beliefs" (Merriam-Webster Online Dictionary, 2014).

Private educational institution: An institution supported through private funding.

Program approval: A process whereby regulating bodies review programs to ensure consumer safety. Nursing education programs are subject to the state regulations that are usually administered by the State Board of Nursing.

Programmatic or specialized accreditation: Focuses on the functioning and effectiveness of a particular program or unit within the larger institution (e.g., medicine, nursing).

Public institution: An institution whose main financial support comes through governmental funds.

Quality: "A high level of value or excellence" (Merriam-Webster Online Dictionary, 2014).

Quality assurance: "The systematic monitoring and evaluation of the various aspects of a program to ensure that standards of quality are being met" (Merriam-Webster Online Dictionary, 2014).

Quality control: "An aggregate of activities designed to ensure adequate quality in the product" (Merriam-Webster Online Dictionary, 2014).

Regional accreditation agency: One of seven private, voluntary accreditation agencies within six defined regions of the United States, formed for the purpose of peer evaluation and setting of standards for higher education.

Regulatory: A form of approval, recognition, or accreditation required by a federal, state, or provincial government agency.

Reinforcement: Any consequence that strengthens the behavior it follows.

Respondent conditioning (also called classical or Pavlovian conditioning): Emphasizes the stimulus and associations made with it in the learning process, depending on associations that are often unconscious.

Role modeling or observational learning: Behavioral, cognitive, and affective changes resulting from observation of others.

Scholarship in nursing: "Those activities that systematically advance the teaching, research, and practice of nursing through rigorous inquiry that (1) is significant to the profession, (2) is creative, (3) can be documented, (4) can be replicated or elaborated, and (5) can be peer-reviewed through various methods" (American Association of Colleges of Nursing [AACN], 2014).

Scholarship of teaching: Application of teaching activities to scholarship that includes four components, that is, discovery, integration, application, and teaching (Boyer, 1990).

Sectarian: Associated with or supported by a religious organization.

Self-efficacy: "People's judgments of their capabilities to organize and execute courses of action required to attain designated types of performances" (Bandura, 1986, p. 391).

Social cognitive theory: An explanation for learning that emphasizes the importance of observing and modeling behaviors, attitudes, and emotional responses of others.

State-regulatory: Those agencies that are required to recognize or approve colleges, universities, or programs for operation with the state as governed by state statutes.

Summative evaluation: Takes place at the end of the program and measures the final outcome. In education, summative evaluation is often linked to the goal(s) or purpose of the program.

Synchronous: Learning activities that take place simultaneously.

Taxonomies: Classifications of educational objectives.

Total quality management: An educational program's commitment to and strategies for collecting comprehensive information on the program's effectiveness in meeting its goals and the management of its findings to ensure the continued quality of the program.

Transformative learning: How learners construct, validate, and reformulate their understandings of their experiences.

Translational science: Research translated/applied into practice.

Vision statement: A mission that is outlook oriented and reflects the institution's plans and dreams about its direction for the future.

Voluntary: A form of accreditation not required by law or regulation. Voluntary accreditation processes are managed by private, voluntary organizations composed of peer member institutions or programs.

REFERENCES

American Association of Colleges of Nursing. (2014). *Defining scholarship for the discipline of nursing.* Retrieved from http://www.aacn.nche.edu/publications/position/defining-scholarship

Bandura, A. (1986). *Social foundations of thought and action. A social cognitive theory.* Englewood Cliff, NJ: Prentice-Hall.

Bastable, S., & Alt, M. (2014). Overview of education in health care. In S. Bastable (Ed.), *Nurse educator: Principles of teaching and learning for nursing practice* (4th ed., pp. 3–30). Burlington, MA: Jones & Bartlett.

Boyer, E. L. (1990). *Scholarship reconsidered: Priorities of the professorate.* Princeton, NJ: The Carnegie Foundation for the Advancement of Learning. Retrieved from http://depts.washington.edu/gs630/Spring/Boyer.pdf

Braungart, M., Braungart, R., & Gramet, P. (2014). Applying learning theories to health care practice. In S. Bastable (Ed.), *Nurse educator: Principles of teaching and learning for nursing practice* (4th ed., pp. 63–110). Burlington, MA: Jones & Bartlett.

Merriam-Webster's Online Dictionary. (2014). Retrieved from http://www.merriam-webster.com/word-of-the-day

Weimer, M. (2002). *Learner-centered teaching.* San Francisco, CA: Jossey-Bass.

Index